ROBOTICS
IN UROLOGIC SURGERY

ROBOTICS IN UROLOGIC SURGERY

JOSEPH A. SMITH, JR., MD
William L. Bray Professor and Chairman
Department of Urologic Surgery
Vanderbilt University School of Medicine
Nashville, Tennessee

ASHUTOSH TEWARI, MD
Cornell Institute of Robotic Surgery
Department of Urology
New York Weill Medical Center
New York, New York

SAUNDERS
ELSEVIER

SAUNDERS
ELSEVIER

1600 John F. Kennedy Blvd.
Ste 1800
Philadelphia, PA 19103-2899

ROBOTICS IN UROLOGIC SURGERY ISBN: 978-1-4160-2465-1

Notice

Knowledge and best practice in this field are constantly changing. As new research and experience broaden our knowledge, changes in practice, treatment, and drug therapy may become necessary or appropriate. Readers are advised to check the most current information provided (i) on procedures featured or (ii) by the manufacturer of each product to be administered, to verify the recommended dose or formula, the method and duration of administration, and contraindications. It is the responsibility of the practitioner, relying on their own experience and knowledge of the patient, to make diagnoses, to determine dosages and the best treatment for each individual patient, and to take all appropriate safety precautions. To the fullest extent of the law, neither the Publisher nor the Editors assume any liability for any injury and/or damage to persons or property arising out of or related to any use of the material contained in this book.

The Publisher

Library of Congress Cataloging-in-Publication Data
Robotics in urologic surgery/ [edited by] Joseph A. Smith Jr., Ashutosh Tewari.—1st ed.
p. ; cm.
Includes bibliographical references and index.
ISBN 978-1-4160-2465-1
1. Surgical robots. 2. Genitourinary organs—Surgery I. Smith, Joseph A., 1949- II. Tewari, Ashutosh.
[DNLM: 1. Urologic Surgical Procedures—methods. 2. Prostatectomy—methods. 3. Robotics—methods. WJ 168 R6665 2008]

RD571.R58 2008
617.4'610597—dc22 2007052080

Acquisitions Editor: Scott Scheidt
Developmental Editor: Elizabeth Hart
Senior Project Manager: David Saltzberg
Design Direction: Ellen Zanolle

Printed in China

Last digit is the print number: 9 8 7 6 5 4 3 2 1

This text is dedicated to the robotic surgical teams at Weill Cornell Medical College and Vanderbilt University, which have contributed to the success of the programs and to helping provide the best possible results for our patients.

CONTRIBUTORS

CLÉMENT-CLAUDE ABBOU, MD
Service d'Urologie
Centre Hospitalier Universitaire Henri Mondor
Creteil, France
8: *Extraperitoneal Laparoscopic Robotic-Assisted Radical Prostatectomy*

THOMAS E. AHLERING, MD
Professor
Department of Urology
University of California, Irvine
Professor
Department of Urology
University of California, Irvine Medical Center
Irvine, California
13: *Oncologic Outcomes of Robotic Radical Prostatectomy*

JUSTIN M. ALBANI, MD
Clinical Associate/Laparoscopy & Robotics Fellow
Division of Urology
Department of Surgery
University of Pennsylvania Health System
Penn Presbyterian Medical Center
Philadelphia, Pennsylvania
16A: *Robotic Renal Surgery: Pyeloplasty*

KETAN K. BADANI, MD
Robotic Fellow
Vattikuti Urology Institute
Henry Ford Health Systems
Vattikuti Urology Institute-Henry Ford Hospital
Detroit, Michigan
7: *Vattikuti Institute Prostatectomy (VIP) Technique and Current Analysis of Results;* 15: *Robotic Radical Cystectomy*

ERIC BARRET, MD
Department of Urology
University Rene Descartes
Department of Urology
Institut Mutaliste Montsouris
Paris, France
14: *Robotic versus Standard Laparoscopic Prostatectomy*

GLEN W. BARRISFORD, MD
Resident in Urology
Harvard Urology Program
Brigham and Women's Hospital
Boston, Massachusetts
18: *Robotically Assisted Techniques in Pediatric Urology*

GEORG BARTSCH, MD
Professor and Chairman
Department of Urology
University of Innsbruck
Innsbruck, Austria
11: *Anatomic Foundations of Nerve Sparing in Radical Prostatectomy*

JAMES F. BORIN, MD
Laparoscopy/Endourology Fellow
Clinical Instructor
Department of Urology
University of California, Irvine Medical Center
Orange, California
13: *Oncologic Outcomes of Robotic Radical Prostatectomy*

XAVIER CATHELINEAU
Clinique Hartmann
Paris, France
14: *Robotic versus Standard Laparoscopic Prostatectomy*

BEN CHALLACOMBE
Department of Urology
Guy's Hospital
London, United Kingdom
1: *Equipment and Technology in Robotics*

W. RANDOLPH CHITWOOD, JR., MD
Senior Associate Vice Chancellor for Health Sciences
Professor and Chief
Division of Cardiothoracic and Vascular Surgery
Brody School of Medicine
East Carolina University
Greenville, North Carolina
19: *Use of Robotics in Other Surgical Specialties*

RALPH V. CLAYMAN, MD
Professor and Chair
Department of Urology
University of California, Irvine Medical Center
Orange, California
16A: *Robotic Renal Surgery: Pyeloplasty*

PROKAR DASGUPTA, MSC (Urol.), MD, DL FRCS, FRCS (Urol.), FEB (Urol.)
Department of Urology
Guy's Hospital
London, United Kingdom
1: *Equipment and Technology in Robotics*

J. DEL PIZZO, MD
Assistant Professor
Director, Laparoscopic and Robotic Surgery
Director, Laparoscopic Living Kidney Donor Program
Brady Urologic Institute
Cornell University Medical Center
New York, New York
17: *Miscellaneous Adult Robotic Surgery*

MICHAEL J. FUMO, MD
Urology Resident
Vattikuti Urology Institute
Henry Ford Hospital
Detroit, Michigan
7: *Vattikuti Institute Prostatectomy (VIP) Technique and Current Analysis of Results; 15: Robotic Radical Cystectomy*

MATTHEW T. GETTMAN, MD
Department of Urology
Mayo Clinic
Rochester, Minnesota
16B: *Robotic Renal Surgery: Partial Nephrectomy and Nephropexy*

INDERBIR S. GILL, MD, MCh
Glickman Urological Institute
Cleveland Clinic Foundation
Cleveland, Ohio
4: *Laparoscopic Foundations for Robotic Surgery*

KHURSHID GURU, MD
Attending Surgeon
Department of Urologic Oncology
Director
Robotic Surgery
Roswell Park Center for Robotic Surgery
Assistant Professor of Oncology
Roswell Park Cancer Institute
Buffalo, New York
3: *Training in Robotic-Assisted Laparoscopic Radical Prostatectomy: The Vattikuti Urology Institute Program*

JUSTIN HARMON, DO
Assistant Professor
Department of Urology
Robert Wood Johnson Medical School
Assistant Professor
Department of Urology
Cooper University Hospital
Camden, New Jersey
14: *Robotic versus Standard Laparoscopic Prostatectomy*

NICHOLAS J. HEGARTY, MD
Department of General Urology
Guy's and St. Thomas' NHS
Guy's Hospital
St. Thomas' Hospital
London, United Kingdom
4: *Laparoscopic Foundations for Robotic Surgery*

ASHOK K. HEMAL, MD
Professor, Department of Urology
Director, Robotics and Minimally Invasive Surgery
Wake Forest University School of Medicine
Wake Forest University Health Sciences
Winston-Salem, North Carolina
5: *Role of Patient Side Surgeon in Robotics*

S. DUKE HERRELL III, MD
Assistant Professor
Department of Urologic Surgery
Vanderbilt University Medical Center
Nashville, Tennessee
10: *Establishment of a Robotic Prostatectomy Program; 20: Financial Considerations of Robotic-Assisted Prostatectomy*

WOLFGANG HORNINGER, MD
Department of Urology
University of Innsbruck
Innsbruck, Austria
11: *Anatomic Foundations of Nerve Sparing in Radical Prostatectomy*

ANDRÁS HOZNEK, MD
Service d'Urologie
Centre Hospitalier Universitaire Henri Mondor
Creteil, France
8: *Extraperitoneal Laparoscopic Robotic-Assisted Radical Prostatectomy*

MELISSA R. KAUFMAN, MD
Department of Urologic Surgery
Vanderbilt University Medical Center
Nashville, Tennessee
10: *Establishment of a Robotic Prostatectomy Program; 20: Financial Considerations of Robotic-Assisted Prostatectomy*

AMY E. KRAMBECK, MD
Resident
Department of Urology
Mayo Clinic
Rochester, Minnesota
16B: *Robotic Renal Surgery: Partial Nephrectomy and Nephropexy*

RAJEEV KUMAR, MCh
Assistant Professor of Urology
All India Institute of Medical Sciences
New Delhi, India
5: *Role of Patient Side Surgeon in Robotics*

ALAN P. KYPSON, MD
Assistant Professor of Surgery
Division of Cardiothoracic Surgery
Brody School of Medicine
East Carolina University
Greenville, North Carolina
19: *Use of Robotics in Other Surgical Specialties*

DAVID I. LEE, MD
Assistant Professor
Division of Urology
Department of Surgery
University of Pennsylvania Health System;
Penn Presbyterian Medical Center
Philadelphia, Pennsylvania
16A: *Robotic Renal Surgery: Pyeloplasty*

ANDREAS LUNACEK, MD
Department of Urology
University of Innsbruck
Innsbruck, Austria
11: *Anatomic Foundations of Nerve Sparing in Radical Prostatectomy*

MANI MENON, MD
Director
The Raj & Padma Vattikuti Distinguished Professor and Director
Vattikuti Urology Institute
Henry Ford Hospital
Detroit, Michigan
7: *Vattikuti Institute Prostatectomy (VIP) Technique and Current Analysis of Results; 15: Robotic Radical Cystectomy*

SIMON C. MOTEN, MB, BS, FRACS
Clinical Instructor
Division of Cardiothoracic and Vascular Surgery
Brody School of Medicine
East Carolina University
Greenville, North Carolina
19: *Use of Robotics in Other Surgical Specialties*

VIPUL R. PATEL, MD
Director of Robotic and Minimally Invasive Urologic Surgery
Associate Professor of Urology
Associate Professor of Bioinformatics
The Ohio State University
Columbus, Ohio
12: *Perioperative Outcomes of Robotic Radical Prostatectomy*

JAMES O. PEABODY, MD
Henry Ford Hospital
Detroit, Michigan
3: *Training in Robotic-Assisted Laparoscopic Radical Prostatectomy: The Vattikuti Urology Institute Program*

REINHARD PESCHEL, MD
Department of Urology
University of Innsbruck
Innsbruck, Austria
16B: *Robotic Renal Surgery: Partial Nephrectomy and Nephropexy*

CRAIG A. PETERS, MD, FACS, FAAP
John Coles Professor of Urology
Department of Urology
University of Virginia Health System
Charlottesville, Virginia
18: *Robotically Assisted Techniques in Pediatric Urology*

RAJAN RAMANATHAN
Department of Urology
New York Weill Medical Center
New York, New York
6: *Athermal Robotic Radical Prostatectomy: Technique and Results*

SANDHYA R. RAO
Department of Urology
New York Weill Medical Center
New York, New York
6: *Athermal Robotic Radical Prostatectomy: Technique and Results*

KIRSTEN ROSE, MD
Department of Urology
Thomas Guy House
Guy's Hospital
London, United Kingdom
1: *Equipment and Technology in Robotics*

FRANÇIOS ROZET, MD
Department of Urology
University Rene Descartes;
Department of Urology
Institut Mutaliste Montsouris
Paris, France
14: Robotic versus Standard Laparoscopic Prostatectomy

LAURENT SALOMON, MD
Service d'Urologie
Centre Hospitalier Universitaire Henri Mondor
Creteil, France
8: Extraperitoneal Laparoscopic Robotic-Assisted Radical Prostatectomy

RICHARD C. SARLE, MD, MS
Associate
Michigan Institute of Urology, P.C.
Dearborn, Michigan
3: Training in Robotic-Assisted Laparoscopic Radical Prostatectomy: The Vattikuti Urology Institute Program

LEE R. SCHACHTER, MD
Department of Urologic Surgery
Vanderbilt University
Nashville, Tennessee
10: Establishment of a Robotic Prostatectomy Program; 20: Financial Considerations of Robotic-Assisted Prostatectomy

CHRISTIAN SCHWENTNER, MD
Department of Urology
University of Innsbruck
Innsbruck, Austria
11: Anatomic Foundations of Nerve Sparing in Radical Prostatectomy

SAGAR R. SHAH, MD
Medical College of Georgia
Augusta, Georgia
12: Perioperative Outcomes of Robotic Radical Prostatectomy

DOUGLAS W. SKARECKY, BS
Research Associate
Department of Urology
University of California, Irvine Medical Center
Orange, California
13: Oncologic Outcomes of Robotic Radical Prostatectomy

JOSEPH A. SMITH, JR., MD
William L. Bray Professor and Chairman
Department of Urologic Surgery
Vanderbilt University School of Medicine
Nashville, Tennessee
9: Principles of Open Radical Prostatectomy: Applied to Robotic-Assisted Laparoscopic Prostatectomy

HANNES STRASSER, MD
Department of Urology
University of Innsbruck
Innsbruck, Austria
11: Anatomic Foundations of Nerve Sparing in Radical Prostatectomy

ATSUSHI TAKENAKA, MD, PhD
Assistant Professor
Department of Urology
Kobe University Graduate School of Medicine
Kobe, Hyogo, Japan
2: Anatomic Foundations

ASHUTOSH TEWARI, MD
Cornell Institute of Robotic Surgery
Department of Urology
New York Weill Medical Center
New York, New York
2: Anatomic Foundations; 6: Athermal Robotic Radical Prostatectomy: Technique and Results; 11: Anatomic Foundations of Nerve Sparing in Radical Prostatectomy

GUY VALLANCIEN, MD
Professor
Department of Urology
University Rene Descartes;
Department of Urology
Institut Mutaliste Monstsouris
Paris, France
14: Robotic versus Standard Laparoscopic Prostatectomy

CONTENTS

PREFACE

Urology has long been recognized as a speciality that embraces technologic advances. From the earliest cystoscopes and resectoscopes to flexible ureteroscopes to extracorporeal lithotripsy to laparoscopy, urologists are at the forefront in adapting and applying surgical technology. It is not surprising, then, that use of surgical robots to date has been dominated by urologists. Over the past decade, minimally invasive approaches have virtually revolutionized surgery, both within urology and in other disciplines. Robotic surgery has accelerated these changes and seems likely to have an even greater impact in the future.

Without question, robotic-assisted laparoscopic prostatectomy is the procedure that has firmly established the role of robotic-assisted surgery. Already, robotic-assisted laparoscopic prostatectomy is the dominant form of surgical treatment for carcinoma of the prostate in the United States, and its use is rapidly expanding worldwide. However, the realm of robotic-assisted surgery has expanded well beyond radical prostatectomy within the domain of urology. Robotics is impacting virtually every aspect of urologic surgery, including kidney removal and reconstruction, bladder removal, female urology, and pediatric urology. Furthermore, it is not difficult to envision changes in both the robotic instrumentation and its applications, which will permit new opportunities, some that could be anticipated and others completely unforeseen.

Introduction of robotics into a surgical practice creates challenges for both the clinician and the hospital. Training, economics, and the logistics of forming an appropriate surgical team must all be considered. Sometimes difficult decisions about whether and how to incorporate robotics into a surgeon's practice must be made. The initial enthusiasm for any new technology must be tempered by an objective analysis of comparative outcomes and patient-focused results.

Even though robotic surgery has been introduced into urology relatively recently, there is a need for a comprehensive text on the subject. In fact, it is the very newness of the topic that increases the significance of a book that dispassionately addresses the current but rapidly evolving state of the art. The goal of this text is to provide objective, comprehensive presentations of all aspects of robotic urologic surgery. There is a heavy emphasis on technical aspects of the procedure as well as patient-related outcomes and results. Establishment of an appropriate operative team is important to the success of any robotic surgery program and is presented in detail. Furthermore, in any situation, the economic consequences of expensive technology must be part of the equation and are specifically addressed in this text. The aim is not to promote robotic surgery but to help clinicians establish its appropriate role.

The editors are indebted to the many contributors who are responsible for the success of this endeavor. Many are true pioneers in the field, and all have done an outstanding job in preparing timely submissions. No attempt was made to develop a consensus of opinion, but all of the contributors provided both personal perspective and balance in their presentations.

Without doubt, robotic urologic surgery is here to stay. Equally certain is that the role of robotics in virtually all surgical disciplines, including urology, will expand. It is hoped that this text will help with the incorporation of robotics into urologic surgical practice to provide the best treatment outcomes for our patients.

Joseph A. Smith, Jr.

Ashutosh Tewari

SECTION I
FOUNDATIONS

CHAPTER 1

Prokar Dasgupta • Kirsten Rose • Ben Challacombe

Equipment and Technology in Robotics

INTRODUCTION

The word *robot* comes from the Czech *robota,*[1] meaning "forced work." It was first used by Karel Capek, a Czechoslovakian playwright and author in the 1920s. His work was often centered around his views on the potential danger of these machines, incorporating the idea of human makes robot, robot kills human. Machines performing tasks were looked at with fear at this time, with robots taking over the human race being a popular science fiction theme. Capek is now credited with the introduction of the term *robot.*

The definition of the term *robots* would state that they are "mechanical devices that sometimes resemble human beings and are capable of performing a variety of complex human tasks on command, or by being programmed in advance." Robots as we know them today were developed after World War II, resulting from the increased demand for automation in automobiles. However, the requirements of the surgical robots we use today, which are designed to be precise, accurate, and safe, have little in common with these industrial robots, which were characterized by their fast, strong, and repeatable actions.

Surgical robots were first used in the subspecialties of orthopedics and neurosurgery. In neurosurgery, stereotactic frames were developed using the fixed landmarks of the rigid cranium. These reference points were then used in conjunction with robots such as the Unimate Puma 560 (Programmable Universal Machine for Assembly, Danbury, CT) or the PUMA 200. This enabled the surgeon to maneuver the surgical arms to perform biopsies or the resection of mid-brain tumors in children using three-dimensional (3D) imaging. It was not until the 1990s that robots such as the ROBODOC (Integrated Surgical Systems, Sacramento, CA) were used in orthopedics. The combination of increased precision with the digitally stored osseous image enabled bones to be reamed with 10 times greater accuracy, allowing a reported 90% prosthesis contact.[2]

The National Aeronautics and Space Administration's (NASA's) Ames Research Center has also long been a pioneer in robotics and human/robot field testing. Starting in 1993 with the deployment of TROV, a teleoperated underwater vehicle, into the McMurdo Sound in Antarctica, through numerous remote science operations using the Russian-built Marsokhod Rover, to current tests using the Mars exploration rover prototype K9, Ames has tested human interface and autonomous technologies in many challenging environments. The Computational Sciences Division at NASA Ames Research Center has a long history and extensive experience in field robotics and human/robot field testing. Ames has been running robotic field experiments and has developed the staff and expertise to design and build robotic test platforms and embedded control systems. In 1999, in collaboration with Johnson Space Center, Ames ran ASRO, the first astronaut/rover field experiment, in which the Marsokhod rover acted as a scout, photographer, and field assistant to a suited astronaut. Field tests in 2003 and 2004 tested the Mobile Agents Architecture (MAA) for human-machine work systems.

In the early 1980s, surgical technique experienced a revolution with the introduction of minimally invasive surgery. The goal of minimally invasive surgery was to reduce patients' pain and recovery time from surgical procedures by minimizing the trauma of the larger incisions of traditional open surgery. The introduction of endoscopes and specialized tools to perform this type of surgery has also increased the technical complexity for the surgeon. The immediate difficulties facing an endoscopic surgeon were sixfold:

1. Lack of hand eye coordination
2. Lack of depth perception
3. Counterintuitive movements
4. Amplification of hand tremor
5. Limited degrees of freedom (DOF) as compared with open surgery
6. Surgical fatigue

The issues encountered by the surgeon include having to look at a screen that projects the image from the endoscope rather than looking at his or her own hands, thus interrupting hand-eye coordination. Conventional endoscopes also provide only a two-dimensional image, which means the surgeon loses depth perception. Some stereoscopic endoscopes do exist, but their performance has so far been limited by the resolution and contrast they are able to produce. Finally, the tools used are introduced into the body through ports placed in the abdominal wall. As the port acts as a fulcrum, the movement of the tip of the instrument occurs in the opposite direction to that of the surgeons' hand, making it counterintuitive and a difficult skill to master. The body wall also limits the movement of the instrument to only two directions, giving it just four DOF instead of six. All these issues make minimally invasive laparoscopic surgery a complex new skill mix for the surgeon to learn, with most procedures having longer learning curves than their open equivalents.

Although the previously mentioned difficulties can be compensated for by intensive practice, not every surgeon can become proficient in laparoscopic surgery. While pioneering laparoscopic surgeons were struggling to overcome these problems, the Defense Advanced Research Project Administration (DARPA) was funding telesurgical projects in the United States with the chief aim of enabling surgeons at remote hospitals to operate on soldiers injured in battle.[3]

EARLY ROBOTIC SYSTEMS: THE WICKHAM ERA

The limitations of laparoscopic surgery encouraged the introduction of robotic systems that can carry out precise tasks quickly and repeatedly without tiring. There is now mounting evidence for the use of these robotic systems within the field of urology. The first clinical use of a robot in urology was the PROBOT in 1989, which was used to assist in transurethral resection of the prostate (TURP).[4] The TURP robotic frame was developed in the late 1980s as a joint project between Guy's Hospital and the Mechanical Engineering Department at Imperial College, London, United Kingdom (Figure 1–1). The frame was constructed

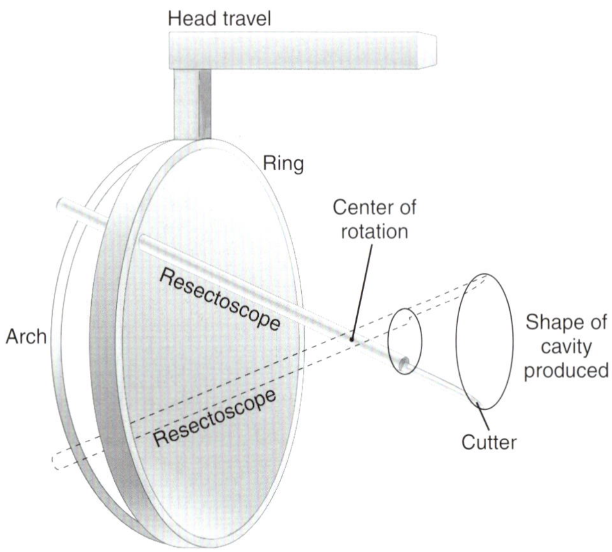

FIGURE 1–1 The Wickham TUR frame. *(Courtesy J. Wickham and S. Nathan.)*

to support a six-axis Unimate Puma robot with a Wickham Endoscope Liquidiser and Aspirator.[5] Initially this device was tested on prostate-shaped potatoes, which confirmed that this robotic system was feasible and rapid. This was followed by a series of clinical trials, initially just on five patients, where it was shown to be safe and provided good hemostasis. Further studies also included the patients' postoperative flow rate, which was found to have significantly improved.[6]

SCARA

Because the prostate is a relatively fixed structure, it continued to be an ideal organ to further develop robotic-assisted procedures. The SR8438 Sankyo Scara robot was developed to perform transrectal ultrasound-guided prostate biopsies. The system allowed the surgeon to choose the biopsy site from the ultrasound images provided by the rectal probe before taking robotic-assisted biopsies of the prostate. Initial trials on animal models showed this method of obtaining prostate biopsies to be quicker and more accurate than the traditional method.[7] It also has good reliability because of the system's lack of drift. The robot can be remotely controlled and has been used with Integrated Services Digital Network (ISDN) lines as an early demonstration of telesurgery.

ENDOUROLOGIC SYSTEMS

As interest in robotics in urology grew, so did its clinical applications. Yet again, Wickham's group developed the first percutaneous nephrolithotomy (PCNL) robot in collaboration with Imperial College. The PCNL robot was a passive five DOF manipulator with an access needle that was mounted onto the operating table and guided by a C-arm. Positional sensors were used to record the position of the device, which was matched to the C-arm's coordinates. A personal computer displayed the access needle's trajectory on each fluoroscopic image, and the surgeon could manipulate its position. Initial experiments showed a targeting accuracy of less than 1.5 mm.[8]

The state-of-the-art robot for PCNL, the PAKY-RCM, has been developed to accurately position and insert a standard 18-gauge needle percutaneously into the kidney. This acronym stands for the **P**ercutaneous **A**ccess of the **K**idne**Y** robot-**R**emote **C**enter of **M**otion and was designed, engineered, and patented by the team at the Urobotics Laboratory, Johns Hopkins, Baltimore.[9] The PAKY-RCM robot consists of a seven DOF lockable manipulator, or passive arm,[10] connected to a three DOF active arm with a radiolucent needle driver (Figures 1–2 through 1–4). This is used to guide and actively drive a trocar needle in percutaneous access procedures. The RCM is a compact robot for surgical applications that can implement a fulcrum point located distal to the mechanism (usually the skin entry point). The robot can therefore

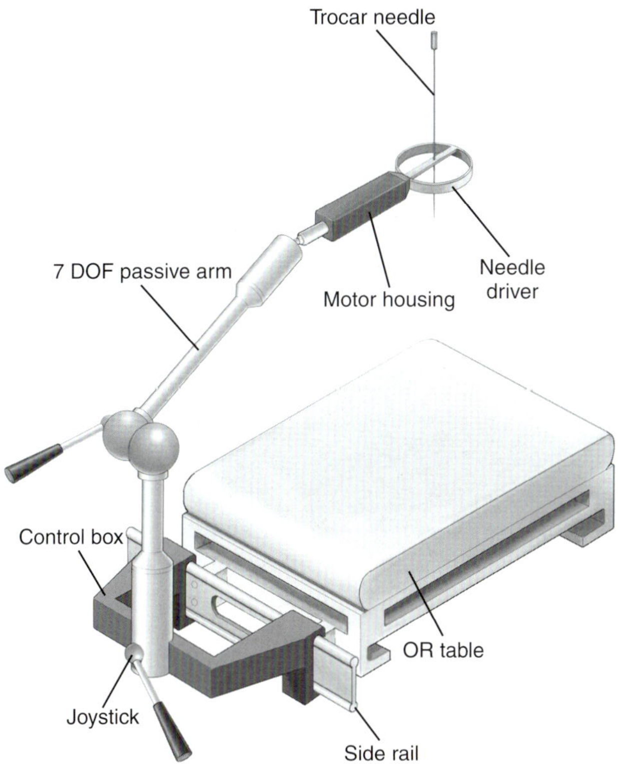

FIGURE 1–2 PAKY-RCM. *(Courtesy of the Urobotics Laboratory, Johns Hopkins, Baltimore, MD.)*

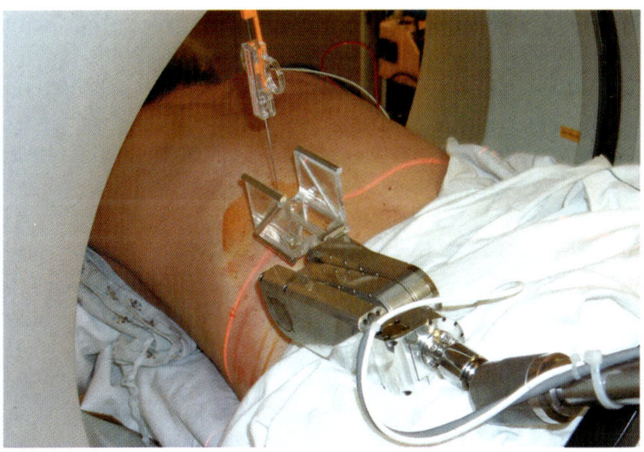

FIGURE 1–3 The z-PAKY being tested under computed tomography (CT) guidance. *(Courtesy of the Urobotics Laboratory, Johns Hopkins, Baltimore, MD.)*

precisely orientate a surgical instrument in space while maintaining the location of one of its points. The system was first evaluated using a porcine kidney model before initial clinical trials.[11] Comparison of robotic percutaneous access to the kidney to conventional methods on 23 patients proved robotic PCNL to be a feasible and safe method of obtaining renal access for nephrolithotomy. The number of attempts and time to access were comparable to those of standard manual techniques.[12] A Smart Needle has also been developed to be used in conjunction with the PAKY-RCM system. The needle detects the change in resistance upon successful entry to the renal collecting system and thus can confirm percutaneous access. The PAKY-RCM robot has been adapted for use in computed tomography (CT)-guided biopsies[13] and radiofrequency ablation procedures on the kidney.

HERMES AND AESOP

The Hermes Operating Room Control Center operates on voice and handheld touch-screen commands and lays the foundation for expanding the use of voice control technology in the operating room. It consists of a computer-control unit that is networked with multiple Hermes-ready devices and is controlled by a surgeon using simple verbal commands or an interactive handheld, touch-screen pendant. The system recognizes the surgeon's voice through a prerecorded voice card that the surgeon inserts into the system before the start of surgery. The surgeon controls devices such as an endoscopic camera, an endoscopic light source, a video cassette recorder, a video printer, and a laparoscopic insufflator. The system also provides visual and digitized voice feedback to the surgical team. Hermes can accommodate the integration of additional medical devices, including diathermy and various imaging systems.

AESOP, or Automated Endoscopic System for Optimal Positioning,[14] is one of the devices potentially under Hermes voice control, although it can operate independently. It positions an endoscope in response to the surgeon's commands, using either voice, foot, or hand control.[15] By imitating the form and function of a human arm, AESOP eliminates the need for a member of the surgical team to manually reposition the medical video camera (Figure 1–5). With precise and consistent movements, AESOP gives the surgeon direct control over a steadier operative field of view. AESOP responds to a vocabulary of 23 commands. Through simple commands such as "AESOP, move up," the surgeon can reposition the endoscope exactly where it is required. AESOP was the world's first U.S. Food and Drug Administration (FDA)-cleared surgical robot capable of assisting in minimally invasive procedures. Since its introduction, AESOP has assisted in more than 45,000 minimally invasive surgical procedures in more than 350 hospitals around the world. It is now regarded as a standard tool in performing laparoscopic radical prostatectomy and enables independent operating. Laparoscopic images with the AESOP are steadier with less camera changes and inadvertent instrument collisions compared with an inexperienced human assistant.[16]

MASTER-SLAVE SYSTEMS

The most advanced surgical robots currently are the "master-slave systems." The Zeus Robotic Surgical System and the da Vinci robotic surgical system (Intutitive Surgical, Sunnyvale, CA), which help surgeons eliminate hand tremor

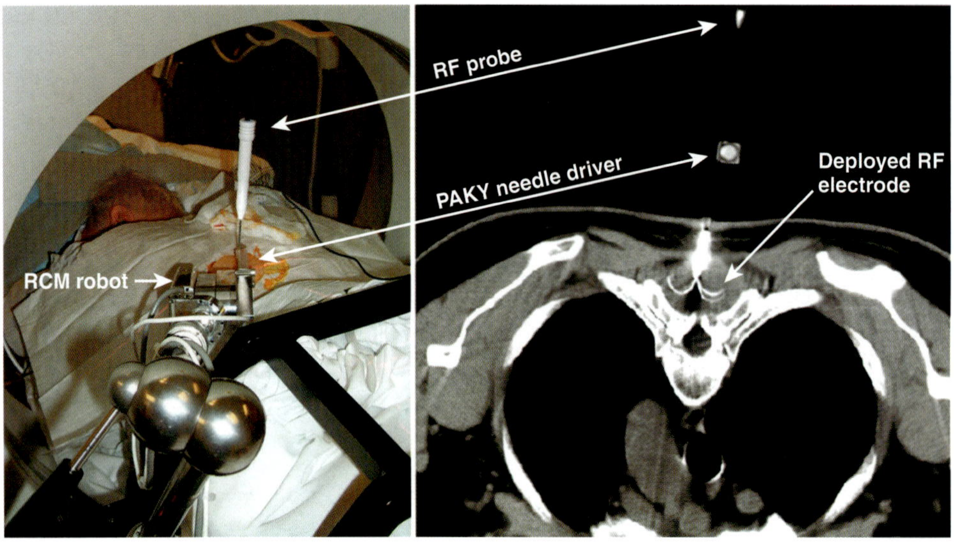

FIGURE 1–4 Computed tomography (CT)-guided remote center of motion (RCM) radiofrequency. *(Courtesy of the Urobotics Laboratory, Johns Hopkins, Baltimore, MD.)*

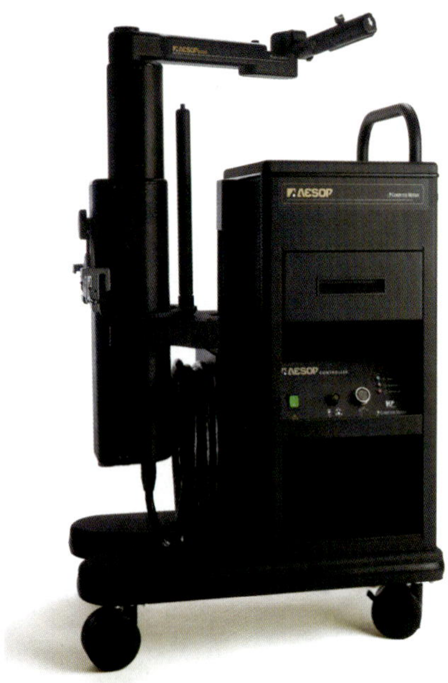

FIGURE 1–5 AESOP 3000. *(Courtesy of Intuitive Surgical.)*

and overcome dexterity and precision limitations, enable a new class of microsurgical procedures. Some who have argued that these are not true robots because they lack automation prefer the term *computer-assisted surgery* for operations performed with these machines.[17] This type of system was initially described by Bowersox in 1998, when the prototype Green Telepresence Surgical System (SRI, International, Menlo Park, CA) was used to perform nephrectomies, ureteral anastomosis, and cystotomy closure on anesthetized swine.[18]

Intuitive Surgical was founded in 1995 and licensed technology from Stanford Research Institute, Massachusetts Institute of Technology, and IBM's Watson Laboratory. The first prototype built in 1996 and tested in animals had two arms with wristed instruments and a third camera arm providing stereoscopic vision. The second version was tested on humans in Belgium in 1997. The alpha prototype of the da Vinci system was used for cardiac surgery in Paris and Leipzig. FDA trials followed in Mexico City in 1998, and the system was given approval for laparoscopic use in 2000 and thoracoscopic use in 2001.[19]

The master-slave systems comprise two major subsystems. One is the surgeon's console housing the CPU and display system, from which the surgeon handles the user interface and the electronic controller. The surgeon has a control panel, a clutch, and a camera control. The second subsystem is the patient side cart consisting of the robotic arms, of which there can be three or four including the camera arm. Both systems use 3D imaging to engulf the surgeon in a 3D video operating field. Zeus uses 3D glasses to achieve this, whereas the da Vinci uses binocular endoscopic vision. Until recently, da Vinci was in direct competition with the Zeus robot, but a corporate merger in 2003 resulted in Intuitive Surgical acquiring the rights to both machines. The Zeus has been phased out, making the da Vinci, with its superior performance, the unchallenged master-slave system. The da Vinci System (Figure 1–6) creates an immersive operating environment for the surgeon by providing both high-quality stereo visualization and restoring hand-eye coordination by projecting the image of the operative field on top of the surgeon's hand. The surgeon is made to feel like his or her hands are inside the patient's body and each of his or her movements is intuitive, unlike laparoscopic surgery. The da Vinci also restores the DOF lost in conventional

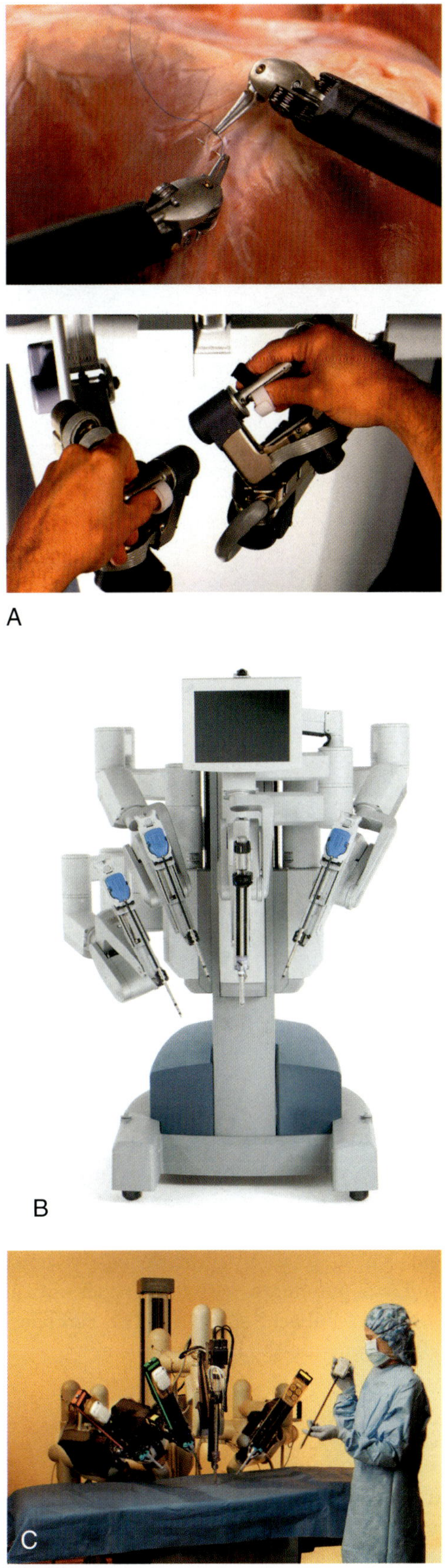

FIGURE 1–6 *A–C*, The da Vinci robot. *(Courtesy of Intuitive Surgical.)*

laparoscopic surgery by placing a three DOF wrist inside the patient. This brings a total of seven DOF to the control of the tool tip—three orientation, three translational, and one for grip. The system also uses its control system to filter out surgeon tremor, making the tool tips steadier than an unassisted hand. It allows for variable motion scaling from the master to the slave, for example, a 3:1 scale factor allows 3 cm of movement on the masters to be translated into 1 cm of movement at the slaves. In combination with the 6× to 10× magnification, motion scaling makes delicate motions easier to perform. The da Vinci comes with its entire set of articulating instruments except a harmonic scalpel, which is nonarticulating. These include scissors, a hook, graspers of different designs, bipolar forceps, Maryland forceps, and needle holders. The instrument tips are usually 7 mm in size, but finer needle drivers for microanastomosis and 5-mm instruments for pediatric use are also available. However, one must not forget the patient-side surgeons who assist the console surgeon using standard laparoscopic instruments. They are the so-called unsung heroes of robotics without whom the console surgeon would find it impossible to function.

The authors attempted to gather details about the science behind the da Vinci robot, in particular the exact hardware and software specifications, but this is proprietary information and currently a closely guarded secret. Suffice to say that although there is considerable debate about it being called a "robot," this computer, like most others in the public domain, has elements of "automation" that we cannot see. The debate is therefore merely one of terminology. The main competition to the da Vinci system can be expected from "mechanical manipulators," which can be used as traditional laparoscopic instruments and are cheaper. Most of these are in developmental stages.[20]

TRANS-OCEANIC TELEROBOTICS

Telementoring in urology has been pioneered by the Baltimore group who have telementored several procedures in Austria, Singapore, Italy, and Germany, including laparoscopic adrenalectomy, radical nephrectomy, varicocelectomy, renal cyst ablation, and PCNL.[21] Telerobotic control is achieved via ISDN lines. Internet connections can also be used and are cheaper. The fastest but most expensive telelinks use satellite connections. The concept of having a surgeon in one country performing an operation in another via a computer-assisted link became reality in 2001, when a laparoscopic cholecystectomy was performed on a patient in Strasbourg by a surgeon in New York using the Zeus telerobotic system (Lindbergh Operation).[22] French telecom provided high-speed asynchronous transfer mode (ATM) lines for this landmark procedure. Time delay can significantly affect surgical performance; however, if the lag time is less than 700 ms, the surgeon is able to learn to compensate.

RANDOMIZED, CONTROLLED TRIAL OF TELEROBOTICS

To our knowledge, the only randomized, controlled trial of telerobotics in urology was the trans-Atlantic study between Guy's and Johns Hopkins. Statistical analysis with adequate power required a total of 304 telerobotic PCNLs, which could not be ethically supported in humans and was legally unacceptable in animals in the United Kingdom. A specially designed and validated kidney model was used (Limbs and Things, Bristol, UK), and either a robotic arm (152 procedures) or a urologist (152 procedures) inserted a percutaneous needle. Thirty remote procedures were performed from Baltimore via four ISDN lines. The trial showed the robot to be slower but more accurate than humans. All urologists made fewer needle passes while using the robotic arm. A cross-over trial has subsequently demonstrated that the robot can be controlled equally well from the United Kingdom to the United States as it is in the opposite direction.[23]

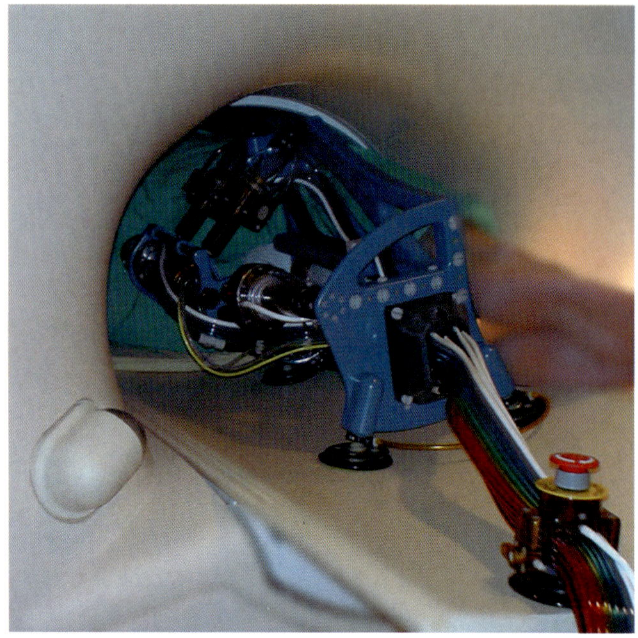

FIGURE 1–7 MrBot. *(Courtesy of D. Stoianovici, Urobotics.)*

VIRTUAL REALITY AND PREOPERATIVE PLANNING WITH KINEMATICS AND HAPTICS

Preoperative planning and simulation of robotic setup is actively being explored. This can allow accurate placement of ports and prior surgical planning based on the patient's CT or magnetic resonance imaging (MRI) images. The ultimate aim is for surgeons to be able to perform virtual surgery on the individual patient the day before the actual procedure.[24,25]

A group from Japan has gone some way toward achieving this goal. This involves geometric modeling of the da Vinci system using 3D computer-aided design (CAD) software followed by calibration of the camera. A whole-body typical patient model is then created from 400 MRI slices at 4-mm intervals. A geometric model of a CO_2 insufflated abdomen is developed from this using a PHANTOM haptic interface (www.sensable.com). Simulation of a da Vinci robotic procedure can then be achieved.[26]

MULTI-IMAGER COMPATIBLE ACTUATION PRINCIPLES IN SURGICAL ROBOTICS

It is believed that today's master-slave systems have not achieved their full potential. One way forward is to integrate them with real-time image guidance, which is a concept we are currently developing. However, imager compatibility raises significant engineering challenges for robotic systems. Although the majority of robotic components may be redesigned with MRI-compatible materials, the electromagnetic motors most commonly used in robotic actuation are incompatible. Stoianovici[27] has described two new types of pneumatic/hydraulic motors that may enable the development of better performance image-guided robots.

MrBot is the first robot for fully automated image-guided access of the prostate gland (Figure 1–7). The robot is customized for transperineal needle insertion and designed to be compatible with all known types of medical imaging equipment. This includes uncompromised compatibility with MRI of the highest field strength, size accessibility within closed-bore tunnel-shaped scanners, and clinical intervention safety. The robot is designed to accommodate various end-effectors for different percutaneous interventions such as biopsy, serum injections, or brachytherapy. For MRI compatibility, the robot is exclusively constructed from nonmagnetic and dielectric materials such as plastics, ceramics, and rubbers and is electricity free. The system uses a new type of motor specifically designed for this application, the pneumatic stepper motor (PneuStep). These uniquely provide easily controllable, precise, and safe pneumatic actuation. Fiber optical encoding is used for feedback, so all electric components are distally located outside the imager's room.[28]

ADVANTAGES OF ROBOTIC TECHNOLOGY: PERCEIVED AND REAL

Perceived advantages of robot-assisted surgery include precise movement of robotic arms, endowrist technology, and 3D stereoscopic vision. For the novice, robotics seems to make intracorporeal suturing easier compared with pure laparoscopic surgery. The "fulcrum effect" in conventional laparoscopic surgery whereby the instrument tips move in the opposite direction to the surgeon's hand around the port site (fulcrum) is counterintuitive. Conversely, robotic movements are intuitive where the instrument tips move in the same direction as the surgeon's hands. Experienced laparoscopic urologists, however, believe that these are not true advantages of robotic surgery and can easily be overcome by rigorous practice of conventional laparoscopy. Most laparoscopic surgeons, although seeing objects in two dimensions on a flat screen, think in three dimensions. They are also able to suture effectively and precisely intracorporeally without any need for a robot.[17] To justify its expense and establish its position firmly in urology, robotics has to be better than open surgery and conventional laparoscopy, not just equal.[29] Evidence as to whether an experienced laparoscopic urologist can improve his or her operative skills and outcomes using robotics is not available. Robotics does provide some real advantages, though. The surgeon's seated position at the console is thought to be more ergonomic. Motion scaling can be a helpful computational adjunct. These machines make remote surgery possible, in principle allowing a patient at a remote location to receive care from an experienced surgeon. Finally, robotic technology is sure to improve even further in the future.

DISADVANTAGES OF ROBOTIC TECHNOLOGY

The costs of installing a robotic system, its subsequent maintenance, and the price of disposable instruments are prohibitive. Pressures on health care funding differ greatly between countries, and this is reflected in the distribution of surgical robots. It is anticipated that the price of these robots will decrease and that savings for patients and hospitals, because of the advantages offered by robotics, will ultimately balance the initial expenditure. Current robotic systems lack tangible force feedback. The da Vinci is a large machine that may possibly become smaller in the future. Instrument size and design must improve, and the tools themselves need to last longer. Finally, although some robots such as the AESOP can facilitate solo surgery, this has negative implications for the training of juniors who need to learn camera and instrument manipulation as part of their laparoscopic skills.

EVALUATION OF ROBOTIC TECHNOLOGY: INTUITION IS NOT SCIENCE

Owning a robot because your neighbor has one is almost fashionable but a rather expensive prospect. Marketing savvy should not be the driving force for this technology—instead the drive to acquire these machines should stem from a true desire for robust scientific evaluation. This should involve not just urologists but health economists and social scientists. The Jet Propulsion Laboratory at the California Institute of Technology has formulated a new technique of evaluating human-robot system performance, which involves complex mathematical methodology[30]; a similar method could be used to evaluate the true performance and safety of surgical robots.[31]

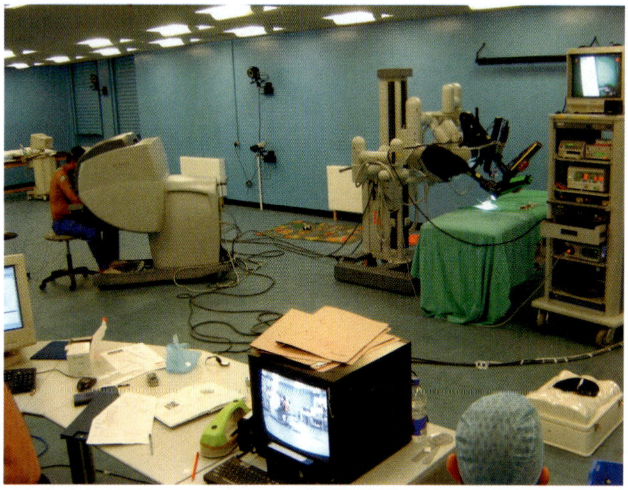

FIGURE 1–8 Studying robotic ergonomics in a motion lab. Note sensors attached to the surgeon. *(Courtesy of A. Shortland.)*

The performance (p) of system m for **primitive** k is characterized by the following:

$$p(k,m)$$

This quantifies how well the system does each primitive function.

For each system, there is also a set of parameters that reflects the resources the system needs. A performance to resource ratio and finally a composite score is derived as follows:

$$S = (½) \log S\ p2\ (k,m)$$

The ergonomics of the da Vinci system is currently being tested in our motion laboratory by attaching and recording from motion sensors on the surgeon's head, arms, and torso (Figure 1–8). This novel technique will compare the robot to traditional laparoscopy and open surgery and may lead to finer adjustments and improvements in design of the robotic console.

THE FUTURE

We appear to be heading toward a digital surgical future. Despite advances in surgical robotics, it is important to keep things in context. The robotics technology branch at the NASA Johnson Space Center has developed a humanoid robot called Robonaut (Figure 1–9) with dexterity approaching that of a suited astronaut. This robot can serve

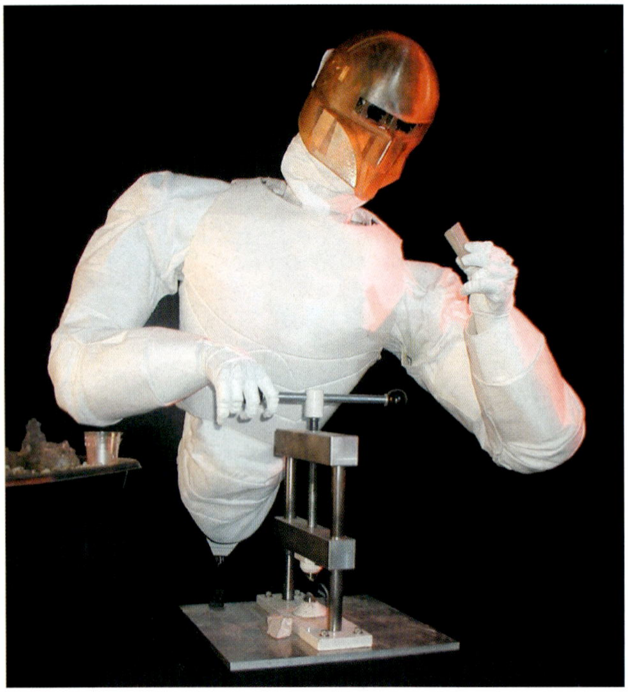

FIGURE 1–9 The Robonaut. *(Courtesy of the NASA Robonaut website.)*

with human astronauts in a rapid response capacity.[32] Compared with such technologic advances, robotic urologic surgery is still in early phases of development.

Surgical robotics does have a bright future; however, rigorous scientific evaluation is necessary. Biomedical, ethical, and moral issues need to be addressed at this time to avoid an uncontrolled and unprepared future.[33] Legal and licensing barriers will need to be overcome before telesurgery becomes clinically viable. Shared responsibility for robotic failures must be in place for telerobotic procedures. As surgeons, we may get too engrossed with new technology and forget our patient's desires and satisfaction, which need assessment by validated patient satisfaction surveys.

We have come a long way since the initial enthusiasm for urologic robotics, and this should be seen not as a revolution but as a well-grounded evolution.[34] The operating room of the future is probably going to be an operating room without people. The question is when and how? Even now, most new advances in robotic technology are being developed in defense and space research. The translation of these to surgical robotics will need adaptation of these machines to suit clinical needs. Let us not forget that humans made these machines, and however clever they become, they will never get ahead of us.

Acknowledgments

We would like to thank the Guy's and St. Thomas' Charity, British Urological Foundation, and Friends of Guy's for their project grants to support robotic and telerobotic urology at Guy's and the Robotic Steering Group for its evaluation.

REFERENCES

1. Shah J, Mackay S, Rockall T, et al: 'Urobotics': robots in urology. BJU Int 88:313–320, 2001.
2. Paul HA, Bargar WL, Mittlestadt B, et al: Development of a surgical robot for cementless total hip arthroplasty. Clin Orthop Relat Res 285:57–66, 1992.
3. Schneeberger WE, Michler RE: An overview of the intuitive system: the surgeon's perspective. Op Tech Thorac Cardiovasc Surg 6:170–176, 2001.
4. Davies BL, Hibberd RD, Coptcoat MJ, Wickham JE: A surgeon robot prostatectomy—a laboratory evaluation. J Med Eng Technol 13:273–277, 1989.
5. Harris SJ, Arambula-Cosio F, Mei Q, et al: The Probot—an active robot for prostate resection. Proc Inst Mech Eng [H] 211:317–325, 1997.
6. Nathan MS, Harris SJ, Davies B, et al: Robotic transurethral electrovaporisation of the prostate. Br J Urol 77 S1:32A, 1996.
7. Rovetta A, Sala R: Execution of robot-assisted biopsies within the clinical context. J Image Guid Surg 1:280–287, 1995.
8. Dasgupta P, Rose K, Wickham JEA: Percutaneous renal surgery: a pioneering perspective. J Endourol 20:167–169, 2006.
9. Stoianovici D, Witcomb LL, Anderson JH, et al: Lecture Notes in Computer Science 1496: Medical Imaging and Computer-Assisted Intervention—MICCAI'98, volume 1496, pp. 404–410, Springer Verlag, Berlin, Germany, October 1998.
10. Lerner G, Stoianovici D, Whitcomb L, Kavoussi L: A Passive Positioning and Supporting Device for Surgical Robots and Instrumentation. Medical Image Computing and Computer-Assisted Intervention, September 1999, Cambridge, England: Lecture Notes in Computer Science, Springer-Verlag, Vol. 1679, pp. 1052–1061.
11. Cadeddu JA, Stoianovici D, Chen RN, et al: Stereotactic mechanical percutaneous renal access. J Endourol 12(2):121–125, 1998.
12. Su LM, Stoianovici D, Jarrett TW, et al: Robotic percutaneous access to the kidney: comparison with standard manual access. J Endourol 16:471–475, 2002.
13. Masamune K, Fichtinger G, Patriciu A, et al: System for robotically assisted percutaneous procedures with computed tomography guidance. Computer Aided Surg 6:370–383, 2001.
14. Unger SW, Unger HM, Bass RT: AESOP robotic arm. Surg Endosc 8:1131, 1994.
15. Allaf ME, Jackman SV, Schulam PG, et al: Laparoscopic visual field. Voice vs foot pedal interfaces for the control of the AESOP robot. Surg Endosc 12:1415–1418, 1998.
16. Kavoussi LR, Moore RG, Adams JB, et al: Comparison of robotic versus laparoscopic camera control. J Urol 154:2134–2136, 1995.
17. Guillonneau B: What robotics in urology? A current point of view. Eur Urol 43:103–105, 2003.
18. Bowersox JC, Cornum RL: Remote operative urology using a surgical telemanipulator system: preliminary observations. Urology 52:17–22, 1998.
19. Shrivastava A, Menon M: Surgical robots: the "genie" is out. In Hemal AK (ed): Contemporary Trends in Laparoscopic Urologic Surgery. New Delhi, BI Churchill Livingstone, 2002, pp 289–296.
20. Dasgupta P, Challacombe B: Robotics in urology. BJU Int 93:247–248, 2004.

21. Link RE, Schulam PG, Kavoussi LR: Telesurgery. Remote monitoring and assistance during laparoscopy. Urol Clin North Am 28:177–188, 2001.
22. Marescaux J, Leroy J, Gagner M, et al: Transatlantic robot-assisted telesurgery. Nature 413:379–380, 2001.
23. Challacombe BJ, Kavoussi LR, Dasgupta P: Trans-oceanic telerobotic surgery. BJU Int 92:678–680, 2003.
24. Nedas T, Challacombe B, Dasgupta P: Virtual reality in urology. BJU Int 94:255–257, 2004.
25. Nedas T, Challacombe B, Dasgupta P: Robotics in urology—an update. Int J Med Robotics Comput Assisted Surg 1(2):13–18, 2005.
26. Hayashibe M, Suzuki N, Hashizume M, et al: Preoperative planning system for surgical robotics setup with kinematics and haptics. Int J Med Robotics Comput Assisted Surg 1(2):76–85, 2005.
27. Stoianovici D: Multi-imager compatible actuation principles in surgical robotics. Int J Med Robotics Comput Assisted Surg 1(2):86–100, 2005.
28. Stoianovici D, Song D, Petrisor D, et al: "MRI Stealth" Robot for Prostate Interventions. Minim Invasive Ther Allied Technol 16:241–248, 2007.
29. Dasgupta P, Jones A, Gill IS: Robotic urological surgery: a perspective. BJU Int 95:20–23, 2005.
30. Rodriguez G, Weisbin CR: A new method to evaluate human-robot system performance. Auton Robots 14:165–178, 2003.
31. Dasgupta P, Rodriguez G: A new method to evaluate human-robot performance and its application to urological robotics. J Endourol MP2.12, 2004.
32. Bluethmann W, Ambose R, Diftler M, et al: Robonaut: a robot designed to work with humans in space. Auton Robots 14:179–197, 2003.
33. Satava RM: Biomedical, ethical and moral issues being forced by advanced medical technologies. Proc Am Philos Soc 147:246–258, 2003.
34. Gallagher AG, Smith CD: From the operating room of the present to the operating room of the future. Human-factors lessons learned from the minimally invasive surgery revolution. Semin Laparosc Surg 10:127 139, 2003.

CHAPTER 2

Atsushi Takenaka • Ashutosh Tewari

Anatomic Foundations

INTRODUCTION

Robotic prostatectomy is increasing rapidly and is growing to be an important option for the management of localized prostate cancer.[1] It is possible to view almost all of the pelvic anatomic structures during robotic prostatectomy using the three-dimensional (3D) magnified laparoscope.[2,3] This enables the surgeon, in theory, to perform the operation with respect to the anatomic findings using multijointed instruments. We therefore felt the need to revisit the anatomic foundations to understand the macroscopic and microscopic findings with respect to this new instrumentation. In addition, because the surgical steps are reversed, visual angles are different from open retropubic prostatectomy, and these anatomic principles need to be retailored in the context of robotic surgery.

The goal of this chapter is to introduce some new anatomic concepts with the hope that it will benefit surgeons attempting robotic pelvic surgery. We especially focus on the anatomy concerned with erectile functioning and urinary continence.

ANATOMY OF AUTONOMIC NERVE STRUCTURE

Trizonal Concept for Nerve-Sparing Robotic Prostatectomy

In the classical concept, the neuroanatomy for nerve-sparing pelvic surgery has been described in a limited area, that is, only the posterolateral aspect of the prostate and the seminal vesicle.[4] Many urologists have imagined the preserved neural component to be a bundle-like structure. Recent studies, however, report that the origin of the cavernous nerve is a distal branch of the pelvic splanchnic nerve (PSN). Also, these nerve fibers join the hypogastric nerve (HGN) with a spray-like arrangement along the lateral wall of the rectum.[5] We should understand the pelvic neuroanatomy to be located in a wider area to perform nerve-sparing surgery. Because we approach the prostate in an antegrade fashion during robotic prostatectomy, we need to understand the anatomy around the proximal and posterior aspect of the prostate. From a practical standpoint, the relevant neural tissue that we encounter during robotic prostatectomy can be grouped into three broad zones (Figure 2–1): the proximal neurovascular plate (PNP), the predominant neurovascular bundles (PNB), and the accessory distal neural pathways (ANP).[6]

Proximal Neurovascular Plate

The PNP is an integrating center for the processing and relay of neural signals. This plate is located lateral to the bladder neck, the seminal vesicles, and the branches of the inferior vesical vessels. It is thick in the center near the seminal vesicles. Specifically, depending on variations in anatomy and prostate size, the PNP is located 5 to 10 mm (average, 5 mm) lateral to the seminal vesicles, 2 to 7 mm (average, 3 mm) thick, 5 to 25 mm (average, 7 mm) wide, and 4 to 30 mm (average, 9 mm) in length. It is located within 4 to 15 mm (average, 6 mm) of the bladder neck and within 2 to 7 mm (average, 5 mm) of the endopelvic fascia, and it overlaps 0 to 7 mm (average, 5 mm) of the proximal prostate.

The PNP extends posterolaterally to the base of the prostate, and the cavernous nerve candidates course in the most distal part. Distally, the plate continues as the classical neurovascular bundle, while a few branches travel through the fascial and capsular tissue of the prostate as accessory pathways. During robotic prostatectomy, the PNP intermingles with the vessel pedicle of the prostate. It is impossible to separate them clearly (Figure 2–2).

Predominant Neurovascular Bundles

The predominant neurovascular bundle corresponds to the classical bundle; however, it carries the neural impulses not only to the cavernous tissue but also to the urethral sphincter and to the end of the levator ani muscle, that is, the puboperinealis muscle (Figure 2–3).[7] The PNB is enclosed within the layers of levator fascia and/or lateral pelvic fascia and is located at the posterolateral aspect of the prostate. The course varies from base to the prostatic apex. We could not distinguish the PNB from the ANP histologically; that is, no clear sheath encircles the PNB.

The PNB occupies the groove between the prostate and the rectum. It is thickest at the base and has the most variable course and architecture near the apex. Our anatomic studies showed that the cavernous nerve candidate continued to the PNB through the distal part of the PNP. The fibers from the HGN are more ventral and from the PSN are more dorsal at the base of the prostate.[5]

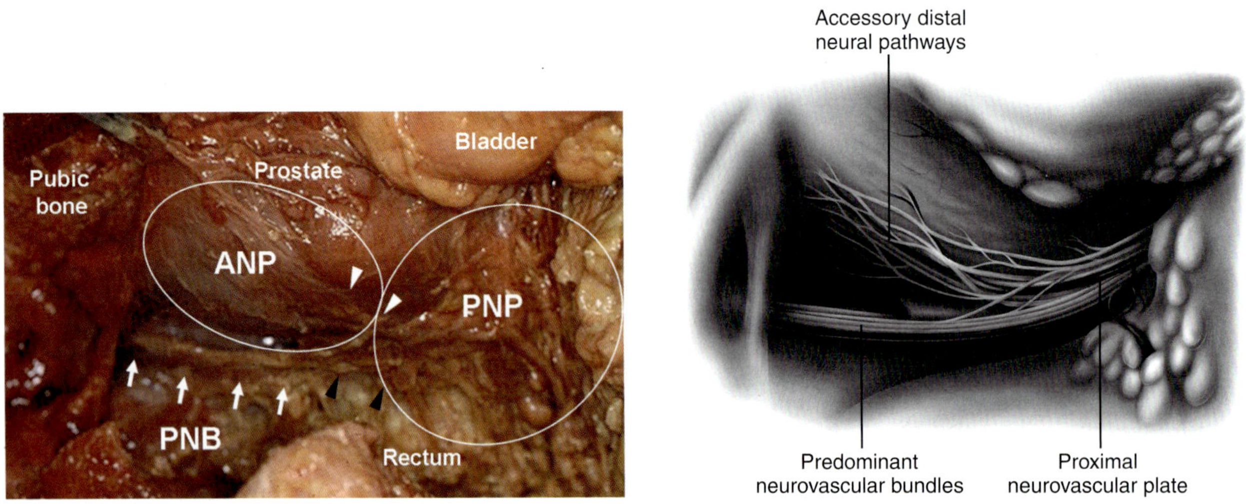

FIGURE 2–1 The trizonal concept of proximal neurovascular plate (PNP), predominant neurovascular bundles (PNB, *white arrows*), and accessory distal neural pathways (ANP). White arrowheads indicate the continuity of PNP and ANP, and black arrowheads are PNP and PNB. Fresh cadaver.

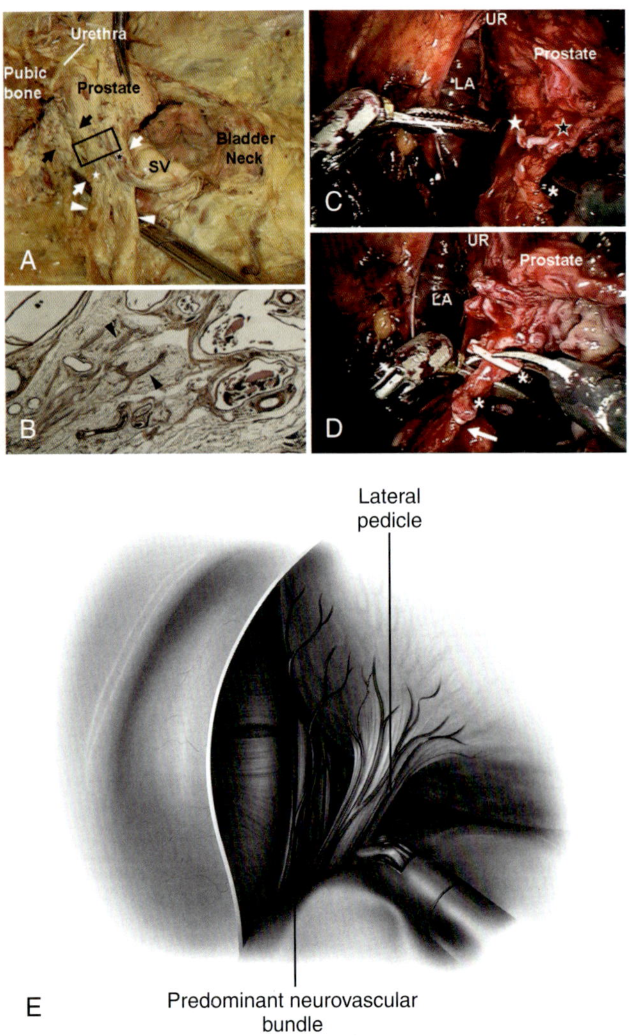

FIGURE 2–2 Control of vascular pedicle. *A,* Cadaveric dissection showing the relationship between seminal vesicle (SV) and proximal neurovascular plate (PNP, *white arrowhead*) according to the procedure of robotic prostatectomy. Bladder neck transaction is performed, and the prostate is lifted up by the forceps. PNP is intermingled with the vascular pedicle *(black star)* of the prostate. *B,* Histologic study stained by hematoxylin and eosin in small square in *A. Black arrowhead,* ganglion cell cluster; *black arrow,* PNB; *white arrow,* intermingled structure of vascular and neural *(white star)* component. *C* and *D,* Robotic procedure. Viewing these structures laterally *(C),* we should estimate the location of the approximate border between the PNP and the vessel component, although they are actually intermingled. We have already cut a part of the vessels using a clip *(asterisk). D,* We thread the left-hand instrument through the border, ligate the residual vessels using a clip, and cut sharply. *E,* The schema of the robotic procedure. LA, levator ani; UR, urethra.

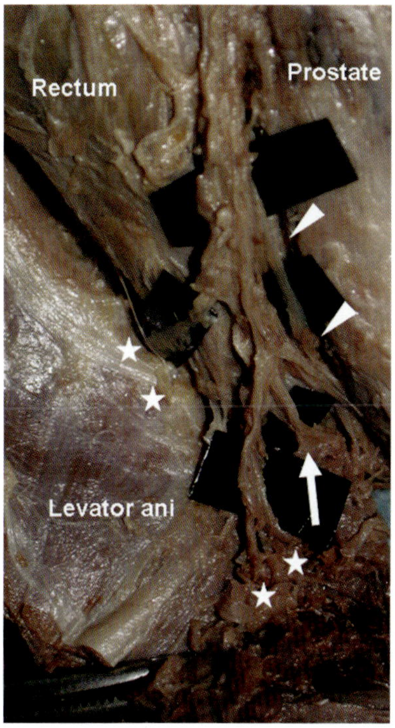

FIGURE 2–3 The distal part of the right predominant neurovascular bundles (PNB). The PNB contains many nerve fibers to the cavernous tissue *(arrow)*, urethral sphincter *(arrowheads)*, and the bottom of the levator ani muscle *(stars)*.

Accessory Distal Neural Pathways

There have been discussions about putative accessories in addition to the PNB around the prostate. They were usually described within the layers of the levator fascia and/or lateral pelvic fascia, on the anterolateral and posterior aspect of the prostate, which may serve as additional conduits for neural impulses. Many cadavers (75%) had the proximal third of the prostate covered by the PNP where these nerve fibers were most prominent.

Additional pathways were noted posteriorly. In 25% of specimens, a posterior pathway arose from the medial aspect of the PNP near the base of the seminal vesicles. Other accessory branches occasionally formed an apical plexus on the posterolateral aspect of the prostatic apex and urethra incorporating fibers from both of the PNB. This distal plexus was observed in 35% of cases, penetrating the rectourethral muscle (Figure 2–4). This could potentially act as a neural pathway for not only cavernous tissue but also the urethral sphincter. It could also serve as a safety mechanism for providing backup neural crosstalk between the two sides. In 10% of cases the fibers were circumferential at the apex.

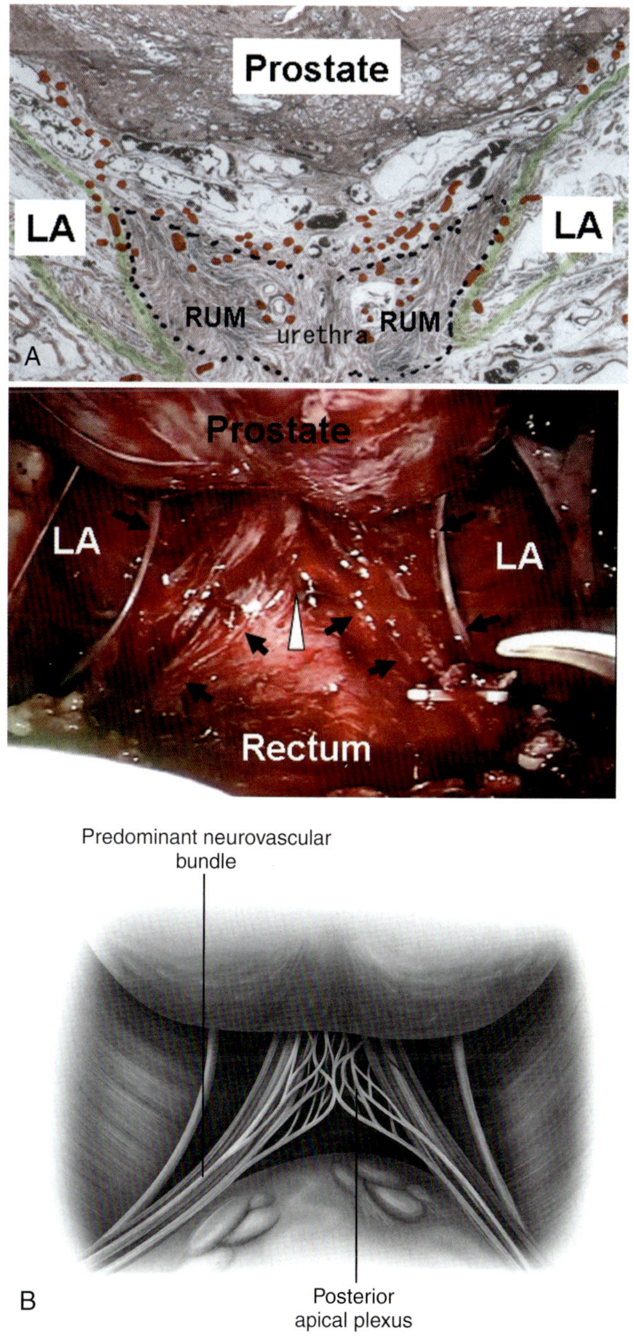

FIGURE 2–4 Apical transaction. *A*, A frontal section through the membranous urethra. Many nerve fibers *(red dots)* exist behind the apex of the prostate between bilateral levator ani (LA). Some of them penetrate the rectourethral muscle (RUM) encircled by dots. Hematoxylin and eosin staining. *B*, The surgical procedure. We can see the many nerve fibers behind the apex of the prostate during robotic prostatectomy. Bilateral predominant neurovascular bundles (PNB) *(black arrows)* overlapped behind the apex and formed the posterior plexus *(white arrowhead)*.

The Distribution and Functional Classification of the Autonomic Ganglion Cells

Distribution

In nerve-sparing prostatectomy, the major components intended for preservation include nerve bundles. However, ganglion cells (GCs) have received little consideration in this strategy. Surgical damage to GCs can result in a much worse outcome than injury to nerve fibers because GCs cannot repair themselves.[8] To our knowledge, we were the first to report the distribution of the autonomic GCs in the male pelvis.[9]

Of course, autonomic GCs existed in the macroanatomic nerve components. There were many GCs in and along the PSN, especially distally near the PNP. The HGN, previously believed to contain many sympathetic postganglionic nerve fibers, also contained GCs along its distal course near the distal ureter. GCs in the PNP were not attached to the seminal vesicle but were separated from it by just 1.0 mm. Great intersubject differences in cell number were evident in all three nerve components. Although the PNB contained more peripheral nerve fibers than the previously mentioned nerve components, GCs were evenly distributed along the prostate from base to apex.

Autonomic GCs also existed viscerally, not in the macroanatomic nerve components. At 1-mm interval sections, we examined the distribution of GCs in detail, according to the robotic procedure.[10] We detected many GCs in the PNP (250 to 1113 cells) and in the PNB (66 to 908 cells). After the bladder neck transaction, we recognized the intermingled structure of the PNP and the vascular component. GCs were distributed widely throughout the PNB, especially laterally or posteriorly (Figure 2–5). In particular, these GCs were attached to the prostatic capsule or even embedded within the capsule. In the ANP, some GCs existed in the bladder/prostate junction, dorsal aspect of seminal vesicle, and the dorsal aspect and near apex of the prostate. Almost all nerve fibers and GCs converged to the apex. There were almost no GCs in the ventral aspect of the prostate and levator ani muscle.

As shown in the macroanatomic nerve components, intersubject differences were evident in all sites. Significant variations are noted in the dorsal aspect and near the apex of the prostate. This might lead to varying postoperative outcomes with respect to patient quality of life (QOL).

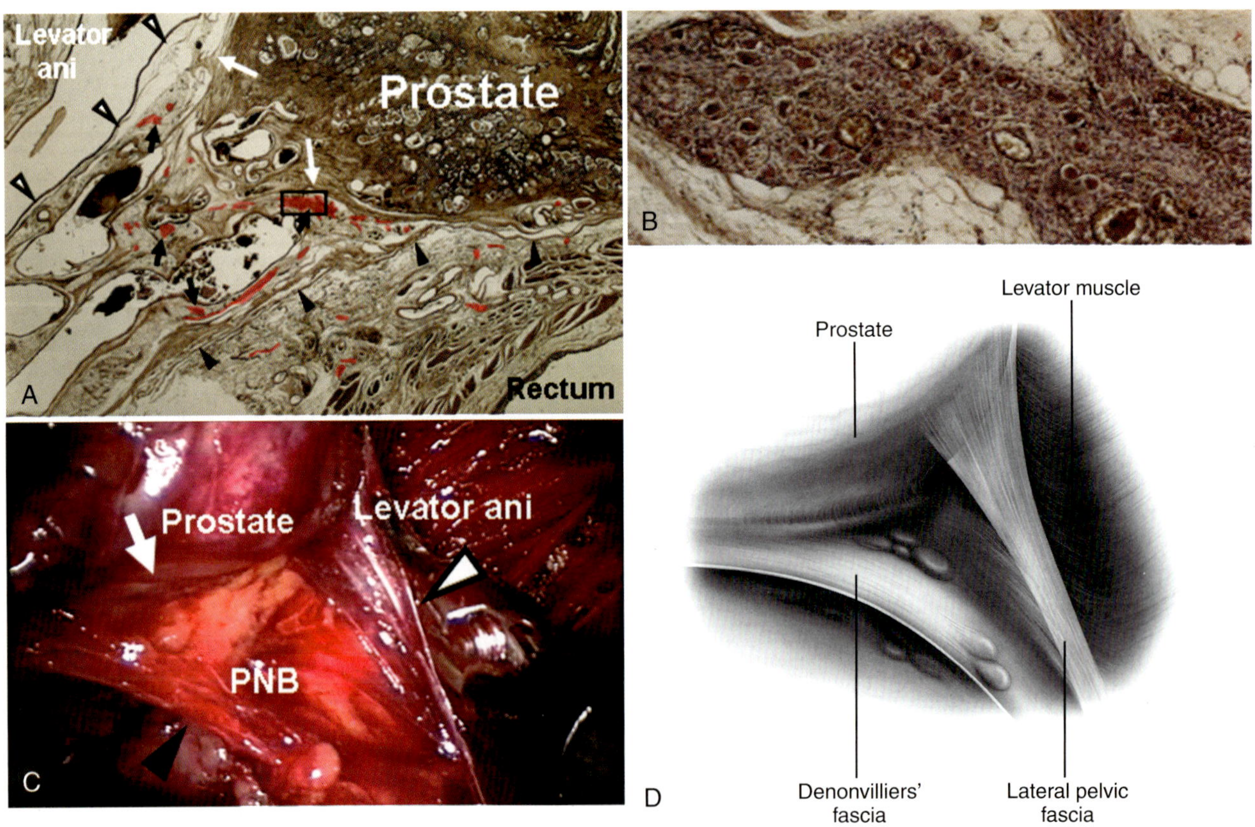

FIGURE 2–5 Release of predominant neurovascular bundles (PNB). *A,* Horizontal section of the posterolateral prostate. Ganglion cells *(black arrow)* in PNB are along or attached to the posterolateral aspect of the prostate capsule *(white arrow).* Ganglion cells exist in the triangle of the prostate capsule, lateral pelvic fascia *(white arrowhead),* and Denonvilliers' fascia *(black arrowhead).* Red, neural component. *B,* Magnification of small square in *A.* Hematoxylin and eosin stain. *C,* The robotic procedure. We should imagine the PNB as a triangle, which is seen in *A. D,* The schema of the robotic procedure.

The control of the pedicle, the release of the PNB, and the apical transaction are extremely important steps in the preservation of the GCs. This is because several GCs exist along the plane of dissection.

The Functional Classification

The functional classification of autonomic nerves was actually not very simple. Butler-Manuel et al.[11] reported that the uterosacral ligament containing the HGN showed positive immunostaining of both tyrosine hydroxylase (TH) as a sympathetic nerve marker and vasoactive intestinal polypeptide (VIP) as a parasympathetic nerve marker. We demonstrated that TH-positive and peptide histidine isoleucine (PHI, as a parasympathetic marker)-positive GCs were intermingled in one ganglion attaching to the posterolateral surface of the prostate. TH-positive cells were also seen in all GC clusters in the male pelvis, for example, the mean TH-positive cell ratio in a GC cluster was 62% in HGN and 36% in PSN.[9] Simple classification of macroanatomic pelvic autonomic nerve components as sympathetic or parasympathetic would seem misleading.

ANATOMY OF THE URETHRAL SUPPORTING SYSTEM

Fascial Anatomy

Almost all conventional textbooks on urologic surgery describe the incision of the endopelvic fascia to reach the paraprostatic space; however, few mention the existence of the levator ani fascia.

Sectional macroscopic observation depicted the levator ani fascia as a definite structure adherent to but not fused with the lateral pelvic fascia (Figure 2–6). The thin fascia overlying the levator ani fascia and lateral pelvic fascia represented the true endopelvic fascia. During surgery the true endopelvic fascia and the levator ani fascia are often fused. When surgeons cut this fusion fascia, the levator ani fascia is attached to the lateral pelvic fascia.[12]

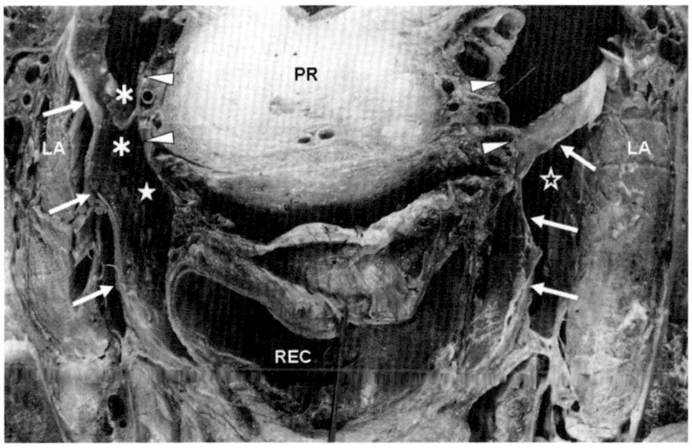

FIGURE 2–6 Macroscopic findings of the fascia around the prostate. The levator fascia *(arrow)* on the right side is not attached to the lateral pelvic fascia *(arrowhead)*. The thin fascia *(asterisk)*, which connects the levator fascia and the lateral pelvic fascia, is the endopelvic fascia. The levator fascia on the left side is attached to the lateral pelvic fascia, and there is a space between the levator fascia and the levator muscle (LA). PR, prostate; REC, rectum. Axial section of formalin-fixed specimen.

The levator fascia folds back at the anterior or lateral aspect of the prostate behind the endopelvic fascia. The overlap of the endopelvic fascia and the foldback resembles a condensed white line, that is, the fascial tendinous arch of the pelvis. In other words, the fascial tendinous arch of the pelvis is not the anatomic ligament structure. Its lowest part connects to the puboprostatic ligament.

Puboprostatic Collar: Puboprostatic Ligament and Endopelvic Fascia

When the prostate is small, the fascial tendinous arch connects to the anterior aspect of the prostate, and the puboprostatic ligament is clearly seen to connect to the bladder. When this is the case, it is called the pubovesical ligament (Figure 2–7*A*). In patients with large prostates, the location of the fascial tendinous arch is sometimes lateral and the pubovesical ligament is not easily visible (Figure 2–7*B*). When the thin endopelvic fascia is incised within the fascial tendinous arch of the pelvis, the collar and the levator ani can be separated laterally and distally (Figure 2–7*C*). The levator fascia connects the puboprostatic ligaments. Then the endopelvic fascia, levator fascia, and puboprostatic ligaments form a sheet covering the pelvic floor. The shape of the collar varies, depending on the prostate shape, volume, and the shape of the pelvis itself.

Puboperinealis Muscle

The puboperinealis muscle attaches behind the insertion of the puboprostatic ligament.[13] It is the anteromedial part of the levator ani. It is a thicker muscle than the rhabdosphincter and embraces the urethra and the rhabdosphincter. In fact, the rhabdosphincter itself is very thin muscular tissue. It terminates at the perineal body between the urethra and the anterior aspect of the rectum and forms a "hammock" around the urethra. In the case shown in Figure 2–8, the rhabdosphincter was Ω-shaped, and the dorsal fibers coursed to the puboperinealis muscle and the apex of the prostate.

Furthermore, the puboprostatic ligament and the fascial tendinous arch form together the puboprostatic collar on the pelvic floor, and the puboperinealis muscle, which forms the inner layer of levator ani muscle and connects to the urethral sphincter, attaches to the back of the puboprostatic ligament.[14] These three structures surround and support the periurethral area, horizontally, sagittally, and frontally, as a complex (Figure 2–9).

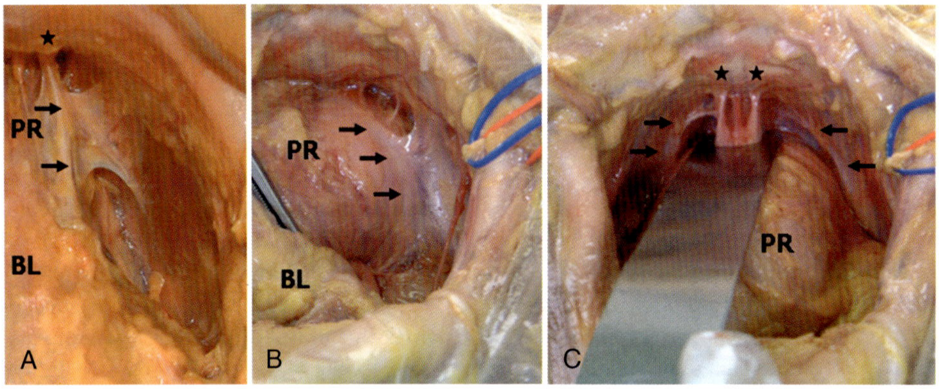

FIGURE 2–7 The various shapes of the endopelvic fascia and puboprostatic ligaments *(star)* in the fresh cadavers. *A,* The prostate is very small. We can easily understand that the fascial tendinous arch of the pelvis *(arrow)* connects to the pubic symphysis to form the puboprostatic (pubovesical, in this case) ligament. *B,* Case with large prostate. The endopelvic fascia is incised along the arrows, the condensed collar; that is, the fascial tendinous arch of the pelvis *(arrow)* and the levator ani could be separated laterally *(C)*. BL, bladder; PR, prostate.

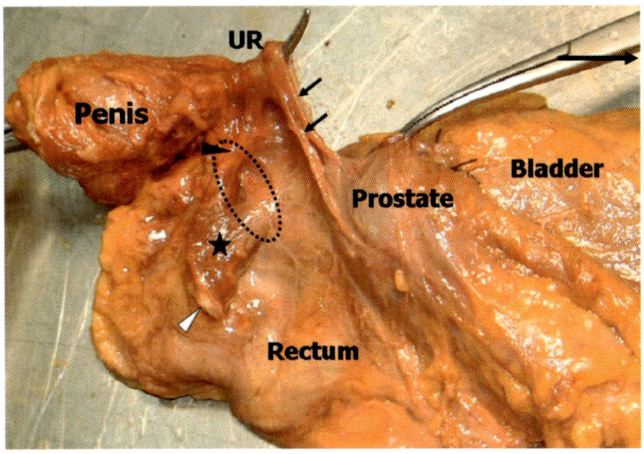

FIGURE 2-8 The rhabdosphincter, the urethra, and the puboperinealis muscle in the fresh cadaver. The urethra is cut at the apex of the prostate, and the forceps is inserted into the urethra retrogradely. The puboperinealis muscle *(star)* and puboprostatic ligaments *(white arrowhead)* are separated from the pubic symphysis and drop over the rectum. The rhabdosphincter is Ω-shaped, and the dorsal fibers coursed to the puboperinealis muscle and the apex of the prostate (*black arrowhead* and *black arrow,* respectively). The puboperinealis muscle terminated at the perineal body (encircled by dots). UR, urethra.

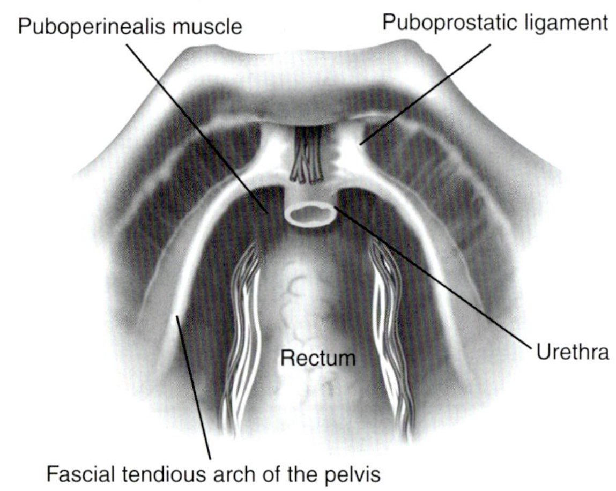

FIGURE 2-9 The schema of urethral supporting structures.

CONCLUSIONS

This manuscript summarizes some new anatomic concepts of the male pelvis. These findings were obtained from the fusion of the 3D magnified surgical view, macroanatomic studies using fresh and fixed cadavers, and histologic studies. We hope these concepts will help many urologists understand anatomic robotic surgery in the male pelvis.

Acknowledgments

We thank Professor Masato Fujisawa in the Division of Urology of Kobe University Graduate School of Medicine for the intellectual interaction about the clinical neural anatomy and Dr. Robert A. Leung in the Department of Urology of Weill Medical College of Cornell University for his assistance in preparing this manuscript. We are also grateful to Professor Gen Murakami in the Department of Anatomy of Sapporo Medical University for supplying the fresh and fixed cadavers and helpful technical comments in the anatomic study.

REFERENCES

1. Menon M, Tewari A, Peabody JO, et al: Vattikuti Institute prostatectomy, a technique of robotic radical prostatectomy for management of localized carcinoma of the prostate: experience of over 1100 cases. Urol Clin North Am 31:701-7-17, 2004.
2. Tewari A, El-Hakim A, Horninger W, et al: Nerve-sparing during robotic radical prostatectomy: use of computer modeling and anatomic data to establish critical steps and maneuvers. Curr Urol Rep 6:126–128, 2005.
3. Badani KK, Bhandari A, Tewari A, Menon M: Comparison of two-dimensional and three-dimensional suturing: is there a difference in a robotic surgery setting? J Endourol 19:1212–1215, 2005.
4. Lepor H, Gregerman M, Crosby R, et al: Precise localization of the autonomic nerves from the pelvic plexus to the corpora cavernosa: a detailed anatomical study of the adult male pelvis. J Urol 133:207–212, 1985.
5. Takenaka A, Murakami G, Soga H, et al: Anatomical analysis of the neurovascular bundle supplying penile cavernous tissue to ensure a reliable nerve graft after radical prostatectomy. J Urol 172:1032–1035, 2004.
6. Tewari A, Takenaka A, Mtui E, et al: The proximal neurovascular plate (PNP) and the tri-zonal neural architecture around the prostate gland—importance in athermal robotic technique (ART) of nerve sparing prostatectomy. BJU Int 98:314–324, 2006.
7. Takenaka A, Murakami G, Matsubara A, et al: Variation in course of cavernous nerve with special reference to details of topographic relationships near prostatic apex: histologic study using male cadavers. Urology 65:136–142, 2005.
8. Kato R, Kiryu-Seo S, Sato Y, et al: Cavernous nerve injury elicits GAP-43 mRNA expression but not regeneration of injured pelvic ganglion neurons. Brain Res 986:166–173, 2003.
9. Takenaka A, Kawada M, Murakami G, et al: Interindividual variation in distribution of extramural ganglion cells in the male pelvis: a semi-quantitative and immunohistochemical study concerning nerve-sparing pelvic surgery. Eur Urol 48:46–52, 2005.
10. Takenaka A, Leung RA, Fujisawa M, et al: Anatomy of autonomic nerve component in the male pelvis—the new concept from a perspective for robotic nerve sparing radical prostatectomy. World J Urol 24:136–143, 2006.
11. Butler-Manuel SA, Buttery LDK, A'Hern RP, et al: Pelvic nerve plexus trauma at radical and simple hysterectomy: a quantitative study of nerve types in the uterine supporting ligaments. J Soc Gynecol Investig 9:47–56, 2002.
12. Takenaka A, Hara R, Soga H, et al: A novel technique for approaching the endopelvic fascia in retropubic radical prostatectomy, based on an anatomical study of fixed and fresh cadavers. BJU Int 95:766–771, 2005.
13. Myers RP, Cahill DR, Kay PA, et al: Puboperineales: muscular boundaries of the male urogenital hiatus in 3D from magnetic resonance imaging. J Urol 164:1412–1415, 2000.
14. Takenaka A, Tewari A, Leung RA, et al: Preservation of the pubo-prostatic collar and pubo-perineoplasty for early recovery of urinary continence after robotic prostatectomy: anatomic basis and preliminary outcomes. Eur Urol 51:433–440, 2007.

CHAPTER 3

Richard C. Sarle • Khurshid Guru • James O. Peabody

Training in Robotic-Assisted Laparoscopic Radical Prostatectomy: The Vattikuti Urology Institute Program

"Robotic prostatectomy is hard to learn but easy to do."

Good judgment comes from experience, and experience comes from bad judgment. Many surgeons have heard this aphorism and understand its truth. It is self-evident that adequate training can and should take the place of the bad judgment that comes from inexperience. What constitutes an adequate training experience will depend on many factors and is likely to vary from institution to institution. In this chapter we discuss our philosophy of and experience with training in robotic surgery at the Vattikuti Urology Institute (VUI). This has developed and evolved over the almost 2400 robotic-assisted procedures, including radical prostatectomy (RP), radical cystectomy, and radical and partial nephrectomy performed by our surgical teams.

Our robotic prostatectomy program began soon after the da Vinci Surgical System was approved by the U.S. Food and Drug Administration (FDA) in October of 2001. It was one of the first to be developed and was quickly the highest-volume program in the world. A brief description of the program's development and underlying philosophy may prove instructive.

Based on review of historical data from our institution, we felt that RP achieved a better result in terms of cancer control for most prostate cancer patients. We also felt that some patients chose nonsurgical treatments for their prostate cancer because of concern about potential morbidity associated with the surgery. We were impressed with the development of the laparoscopic radical prostatectomy (LRP) program of Guillonneau and Vallancien at the Institute Mutualiste Montsouris (IMM) in Paris[1] and its potential to achieve a less morbid, safer, and better outcome. Our institute had rudimentary laparoscopic skills at that time and we felt that to safely embark on a program of laparoscopic prostatectomy an intensive mentoring by experts like those at IMM would be necessary.

Led by Dr. Mani Menon, several staff members began intensive training in laparoscopic prostatectomy. This included several visits to IMM by our team to observe cases, as well as twelve 1-week visits to the Henry Ford Health System by Vallencien and Guillonneau to proctor LRP cases. The initial cases were performed safely and effectively with the mentors' help.

After several visits by the IMM team, we leased the da Vinci robot because we believed it might facilitate our performance of the LRP procedure. The initial experience with the robotic system confirmed this impression. We believed that the robotic system had specific application to LRP. Although our first several cases were challenging, with the help of our mentors during 20 to 30 cases, we were able to establish a technique of robotic-assisted laparoscopic prostatectomy known, at our institution, as the Vattikuti Institute prostatectomy (VIP) procedure.[2]

We believe that the robotic system significantly reduces the difficult learning curve of LRP. That is not the say that the robotic system eliminates this curve by any means, but, because of the three-dimensional (3D) visualization and "wristed" instruments, it does dramatically decrease the difficulty of complex laparoscopic dissection and suturing. As such, although the LRP learning curve may be in excess of 50 cases, we believe that with proper planning, training, and mentoring, the robotic learning curve may be 20 to 30 cases in many situations.[3]

Box 3–1

The Vattikuti Urology Institute Training Program

Work with nurses and assistants to learn robotic setup and function.

- Review recordings of the procedures to gain knowledge of procedure.
- Participate as second patient side assistant (left side) on 30 Vattikuti Institute prostatectomy (VIP) cases.
- Participate as primary patient side assistant (right side) on 30 VIP cases.
- Graduate mentored experience on console from more basic to more complex portions of the procedure over 50 cases.
- Continue mentored performance of entire procedures until mastery achieved over 50 cases.

THE CURRENT STANDARD

Since the spring of 2001 we have performed more than 2000 VIP procedures. Currently we perform the procedure in an average of 2.5 hours of total operative time, with 30% of cases being completed in less than 2 hours. Our patients are discharged on postoperative day 1 approximately 95% of the time, and our transfusion rate continues to be less than 2%. Recovery of continence and potency has been excellent, and cancer control rates have improved over those we achieved with open RP.[4,5] Currently three staff members at the VUI routinely perform the VIP. Each of these surgeons has undergone an extended period of training as described later in this chapter. In addition, residents and fellows at the VUI have extensive exposure to the VIP and are proficient at both assisting and performing all aspects of the procedure (Box 3–1).

THE DECISION TO START A ROBOTIC PROSTATECTOMY PROGRAM

Our institute performed 120 to 150 RP procedures per year when we began our robotics program in March 2001. An adequate surgical volume that allows for regular performance of the procedure will facilitate a program's ability to reduce its learning curve. Frequent repetition of the procedure will allow for the entire team to ingrain the fundamentals of robotic setup, anesthesia, patient positioning, port placement, and operative technique. The largest improvements in our operative time occurred when we performed cases on consecutive days. A program without significant volume that performs the procedure irregularly will progress along the learning curve more slowly because the team is more likely to forget certain aspects of the setup and procedure during periods of inactivity, and this may impact the eventual success of a program. Although a specific number of cases is not easy to define, an institution performing less than four to five prostatectomy cases per month may be challenged to develop a successful program. With this in mind, performance of cases several days in a row at the beginning of the program can help inculcate the principles necessary in all the team members. Without significant volume, the time between cases only further delays the program's achievement of competence.

THE ROBOTIC TEAM

We organized our team around a primary surgeon and two assistant surgeons. The team was augmented by an anesthesiologist and two operating room (OR) nurses. The primary surgeon was the console surgeon for the first 30 to 40 cases performed by the team, and the assistant surgeons were consistent through the initial 50 to 60 cases. During this time, the team developed a consistent technique. The team members became familiar with the steps of the procedure by being present for all the cases and by reviewing the video recordings of the procedures as well as the pathologic results. This allowed for transition of additional team members to the console surgeon position. As the team worked together and became more familiar with the robotic system, dramatic reductions in time to system setup, port placement, and operative steps occurred and helped decrease the total OR time.

Although the robotic system can allow a nonlaparoscopic surgeon to perform complex laparoscopic maneuvers at the console, we believe that at least one of the assistants should have significant previous laparoscopic training and be comfortable with basic laparoscopic techniques, including establishment of pneumoperitoneum through various techniques, safe port placement, exposure and manipulation of tissues, suctioning passage of suture and retrieval of needles, bagging of specimens, and port closure. The fine points of these techniques are challenging and are not easily mastered by the novice laparoscopic surgeon. Assistants can benefit from mentoring and careful study of recorded cases to learn proper techniques. We believe that careful mentoring of the patient side assistants can greatly reduce the learning curve for the assistant and the team.

Although the surgeons play a crucial role, an anesthesiologist familiar with laparoscopic anesthesia is critical to patient safety, especially in the early stages of the program when cases are likely to be of longer duration. The head-down position used by many teams coupled with the intraperitoneal approach can create difficulties with high ventilatory pressures and carbon dioxide retention. Anesthetic techniques to deal with these problems should be familiar to the team.

Finally, the scrub and circulating nurses play important roles in facilitation of cases. A team that can efficiently prepare the robotic system, including the draping and

Box 3–2

Attributes of a Successful Robotic Team

- Familiarity with basic laparoscopic techniques
- Excellent laparoscopic support
- Familiarity with steps of robotic prostatectomy
- Console surgeon experienced in open anatomic radical prostatectomy
- Familiarity with laparoscopically viewed anatomy
- Understanding of patient positioning
- Familiarity with port placement for robot and setup of robot
- Facility with changing and cleaning lenses and trouble-shooting robot
- Initial cases mentored
- Review of case recordings and results

calibration of lenses, will make possible earlier start times and more rapid case turnover. The nursing staff should rehearse with the rest of the surgical team so that all parties know what equipment is regularly needed and also have available suture instruments and catheters that are needed less frequently. The steps of the operation should be known so that each item will be available as it is needed. Initial cases are also often supported by Intuitive Surgical and their representatives can provide important troubleshooting tips during the initial phases of a program (Box 3–2).

PREPARATION BEFORE THE FIRST CASE

We recommend that the surgical team spend time reviewing both DVD and live case demonstrations before performance of the initial procedure. Familiarity with the steps of the procedure and their appearance in a laparoscopic view can help an "open" surgeon appreciate subtleties of the procedure more rapidly. Even surgeons with substantial open RP experience can find the anatomy of the pelvis in the laparoscopic view somewhat disorienting. Tissue planes are approached from a different direction, and the lack of tactile feedback can initially make the dissections more challenging. Once familiar with the steps of the procedure and important anatomic landmarks, surgeons often develop an even greater appreciation of the view afforded to them of the deep pelvis by the robotic system and can perform the operations more precisely.

Surgeons and teams interested in starting a program are required to complete the Intuitive Surgical online course, which teaches them about the various components of the robotic system and instrumentation. After completing online training, surgeons usually are exposed to the robotic system in the dry lab setting. This initial exposure to the robotic system is a crucial part of training because it allows the team to begin to learn how to manipulate the system. The more quickly a team becomes familiar with the setup and manipulation of the device, the more rapidly they will proceed to successful completion of the procedures. The next step involves dry lab drills with manipulation of beads, rings, and wires and performance of suturing and knot tying. The 3D vision and "wristed" instrumentation make these initial tasks much easier than would be the case with traditional laparoscopy. These techniques are still difficult in the beginning of one's experience, and the mechanics can be practiced using a pelvic trainer. We have found that intracorporeal suturing techniques such as understanding and ingraining the fundamentals such as direction of needle passage and learning to hold proper tension on the suture are best refined at this stage. It is important for console surgeons to master these before embarking on live cases.

While the basics of these manipulations are accomplished, it is critical that the surgeon become familiar with the camera and instrument clutching mechanisms. These allow the surgeon to work in a comfortable and more ergonomic position. We have observed several novice robotic surgeons working with the camera system too far away or off center from the point of dissection, or with their hands on the masters in a nonoptimal position, compromising their ability to perform the procedure with maximum accuracy. In this way the clutching is very much like driving a car with a manual transmission. In the beginning much thought is put into meshing the clutch and gear manipulations, but over time it becomes second nature.

After completing the dry lab experience, the team should proceed to an animal lab and perform various urologic procedures, including prostatectomy. This gives the console surgeon and assistants hands-on experience with living tissues and the opportunity to manipulate these tissues, for suturing and gaining hemostasis. The opportunity to work in an environment without haptic feedback is usually a new one, and it allows the surgeon to become accustomed to the visual cues that are important in assessing tissue characteristics and strength. Performance of several procedures on each animal is recommended to maximize the opportunity for tissue dissection and reconstruction.

A cadaver lab experience is also recommended by some and will be of particular use to those teams without substantial experience with laparoscopic prostatectomy to allow increased familiarity with the surgical approach.

PATIENT SELECTION

Optimal patient selection can also help reduce OR time and complication rates in a surgeon's initial experience (Box 3–3). We recommend beginning with patients who have a low cancer burden. Patients should have a prostate-specific antigen (PSA) of less than 10 ng/mL and a lower volume of Gleason 6

Box 3–3

Criteria for Selection of Ideal Initial Patients

- Prostate size: 30–40 g
- Body mass index: 23–28
- No previous prostatic or abdominal surgery
- Erectile dysfunction
- Low-risk disease, prostate-specific antigen <10 ng/mL and Gleason score <7
- Minimal lower urinary tract symptoms
- Healthy—no chronic obstructive pulmonary disease
- No androgen ablation therapy

cancer. This will decrease the likelihood of positive surgical margins in the initial cases. In addition, to diminish the impact of suboptimal nerve sparing, patients with low sexual health inventory in men (SHIM) scores or those in whom preservation of sexual function is not important should be in the initial group of patients.

Patient height and weight are also important considerations in the initial phases of a program. Although experienced teams can routinely perform cases on patients with a body mass index (BMI) of more than 32, we recommend that initial patients have a BMI in the range 23 to 28. Thinner patients have more easily identified anatomic landmarks and less abdominal fat, making the task of newly trained assistants less difficult in regard to port placement and retraction.

Previous abdominal surgery should also be an important consideration. It is helpful in the early stages of this program to begin with patients who have not had previous abdominal surgery or inflammatory conditions in the bowel. This will decrease the possibility of bowel adhesions, which increase the OR time and the risk of bowel injury during the takedown. Although a mature program can eventually attempt the procedure on patient with extensive previous abdominal surgery, we advise an unoperated abdomen in the initial cases. We believe that most bowel injuries occur during the takedown of these adhesions prior to docking the robotic system. Previous prostatic surgery with resection and thermal therapy of laser can alter the shape of the prostate and cause periprostatic fibrosis, making the bladder neck and posterior dissections more difficult. These patients should be offered other treatment until a program has achieved a plateau on its learning curve. A large median lobe can also cause problems with dissection for a less experienced team. Preoperative ultrasound, computed tomography (CT), or cystoscopic assessment may be considered in patients with severe lower urinary tract symptoms (LUTS) to rule this out.

THE FIRST CASE AND THE MENTOR/PROCTOR

The mentor/proctor and surgeon relationship is very important. We use these terms interchangeably, but some feel that mentorship implies a longer-term relationship with more give-and-take and sharing of surgical responsibility, whereas the role of proctor is less involved and more observational. We feel strongly that most institutions starting a program will benefit from and require a mentorship relationship at the beginning of their experience. Mentors should have extensive experience performing the procedure, as well as teaching the procedure—in our view, at least 100 cases. It is important for the surgeon and the mentor to have a thorough discussion about the steps of the procedure before the operation. Ideally, the surgeon should visit the mentor's institution and observe cases being performed by the mentor and team prior to the first cases. Considerations regarding exact technique, sequence of steps, approach, and method of vascular control should be agreed on beforehand. Ideally, arrangements should be made for the mentor to assist at the patient side or console during the operation to demonstrate proper techniques.

We believe that it is advisable to perform initial cases using the intraperitoneal approach. The reduced working space using the extraperitoneal approach may negatively affect the initial cases of a new robotic team.

REVIEW OF REPORTED RESULTS

Several groups have reported their initial experience with robotic-assisted laparoscopic prostatectomy. These reports come from groups with differing initial experiences in laparoscopy and robotics. A review of these reports demonstrates how different approaches to training and different institutional resources have resulted in successful programs.

The initial reports of a structured training program were by Menon and the group from the VUI[2–5] describing their experience with development of the program at the VUI. As described previously, this program grew out of an initial mentoring collaboration with Guillonneau and Vallancien. The team transitioned to the use of the da Vinci system during this mentoring and then refined the technique to take fuller advantage of certain aspects of the robotic technology. The initial cases were closely supervised, and the VUI team gradually performed more of the procedures as they gained expertise. As the team's experience grew, surgeons from many other centers came to watch cases to learn the setup and surgical techniques.

The next report was by Aherling et al.[6] from the group at University of California at Irvine describing the transfer of open surgical skills to a laparoscopic environment using the da Vinci system. This team, from a laparoscopically enriched environment, was able to achieve operative times of less than 4 hours after 12 cases. They accomplished this by developing a skilled laparoscopic team headed by a very experienced open prostatectomy surgeon and an expert laparoscopic surgeon who had been involved in the world's first laparoscopic prostatectomies.[7] The team members trained on the robot in a dry lab and in a porcine model and viewed live and recorded cases before embarking on their first cases.

Patel et al.[8] reported on the first experience with da Vinci prostatectomy in a community setting. Their group described the excellent results of their first 200 cases performed by a two-surgeon team. Their training consisted of previous laparoscopic experience and case observations at the VUI and during the International Robotic Urology Symposiums (IRUS) in Detroit. They were careful in their initial case selection following the criteria in Box 3–1. They report that operative times were regularly less than 4 hours by 20 cases.

Costello et al.[9] reported their experience with telerobotic RP at the Royal Melbourne Hospital. They described the results of their initial 122 patients. Their training consisted of a 1-week dry and animal lab followed by a cadaver lab. Their first six cases were mentored by an expert robotic surgeon. Excellent results were obtained.

Kaul et al.[10] report the results of their initial experience at the Addenbrooke's Hospital with robotic prostatectomy following an intense mentoring experience. The team was composed of a chief surgeon with extensive open prostatectomy experience who had observed 10 to 15 live robotic prostatectomy cases. Other team members included surgeons with extensive laparoscopic prostatectomy experience and anesthesiologists and nurses well trained in laparoscopy and laparoscopic anesthesia. They were mentored by an experienced robotic surgery team consisting of a console mentor and a patient side mentor. The console proctor performed 60% of the first case; the trainee-surgeon's involvement was approximately 70% in case 2, and he completed the entire operation by case 3. Cases 4 and 5 were used for increasing speed and refining surgical technique. Additional cases were completed by the team after the mentors left with good functional results and operative times of less than 4 hours.

Herell and Smith[11] reported on their initial experience as they began their robotic prostatectomy program. Their training consisted of case observation and dry and wet lab experience. Their team consisted of a very experienced open prostatectomy surgeon and a skilled laparoscopic surgeon. The group has been comparing their results between their open and robotic procedures. The group has reported on their perceived learning curve, stating that it took several hundred robotic cases to achieve results comparable to those of their open cases.

Wicklund[12] reported on the experience from the Karolinska Institute in Stockholm, Sweden. A team of experienced open prostate surgeons trained on the robot in a dry and animal lab setting and observed live cases. He reported that operative times were consistent at 2 to 3 hours after about 20 cases but continued with a downward trend at 80 cases.

Reports from other institutions have detailed aspects of their results in comparing their initial experience with laparoscopic prostatectomy with a more recent experience with robotic-assisted laparoscopic prostatectomy.[13,14] Although the details of their training are not reported, it is clear that each group was skilled in performance of the laparoscopic procedure and was able to make a relatively easy transition to the robotic procedure by virtue of their understanding of the fundamentals of laparoscopic surgery, their familiarity with the steps of the procedure, and the relevant pelvic anatomy. For these groups, addition of the robot was the addition of a sophisticated laparoscopic tool to a procedure they were already very familiar with. Groups with this level of previous experience are likely to have a shorter learning curve.

OTHER THOUGHTS

This raises the question of deciding when a team is "trained." Typically, groups will feel accomplished when a certain time parameter is reached, usually 4 hours. Although this is an important milestone, it is clearly not the most important clinical outcome. The most important parameters are cancer control, continence, urinary control, preservation of potency, return to normal activities, and freedom from complications. These outcomes take a longer time to realize and are therefore not focused at the time of the initial surgeries. It is critical that these outcomes be monitored so that teams can evolve their techniques over time to achieve optimal results. Video recording of cases should be performed to allow teams to review cases and outcomes that are optimal and suboptimal. Modifications and improvements should result from these reviews.

The point at which a team achieves adequacy, comfort, and mastery of the technique will vary with the team's skills and with the team's previous level of accomplishment with open prostatectomy. Teams with superior skills and results may take several hundred cases to reliably exceed results obtained with open surgery, whereas less proficient open surgical teams may achieve better results with far fewer cases.[11]

The issue of credentialing is raised with any new procedure. Ultimately this is an issue for local hospitals and, at times, medical societies to decide. However, these groups have an interest in protecting the public and their patients by giving them the highest standard of care possible. With this in mind, we believe that teams should make patients aware of their level of experience, their training, and their results. It must be realized that medicine is not an exact science and results cannot be guaranteed, even in the most experienced hands. Hospitals should set a standard that assures their patients that they will be well taken care of by physicians who have adequate experience—or are mentored by physicians who have adequate experience—to perform the operation safely and effectively.

Finally, the opportunity for remote proctoring and mentoring is an exciting prospect made possible by the possibility of interface between da Vinci systems. Live video feed can be observed by a remote surgeon-mentor who can direct a team during performance of a case. Ultimately, the possibility exists for a teaching console to be placed adjacent to the primary operating console or at a site far distant from the operating console. This would allow the mentor to temporarily take over portions of the case to demonstrate particular portions of the procedure.

REFERENCES

1. Guillonneau B, Vallencien G: Laparoscopic radical prostatectomy: the Montsouris technique. J Urology 163:1643, 2000.
2. Menon M, Tewari A, Peabody JO, Members of the VIP Team: Vattikuti Institute prostatectomy: technique. J Urol 169:2289–2292, 2003.
3. Menon M, Shrivastava A, Tewari A, et al: laparoscopic and robot assisted radical prostatectomy: establishment of a structured program and preliminary analysis of outcomes. J Urol 168:945, 2002.
4. Tewari AT, Srivastava A, Menon M, VIP Team: A prospective comparison of radical retropubic and robot-assisted prostatectomy: experience in one institution. BJU Int 92:205, 2003.
5. Menon M, Tewari A, VIP Team: Robotic radical prostatectomy and the Vattikuti Urology Institute technique: an interim analysis of results and technical points. Urology 61:15, 2003.
6. Aherling TE, Skarecky D, Lee D, et al: Successful transfer of open surgical skills to a laparoscopic environment using a robotic interface: initial experience with laparoscopic radical prostatectomy. J Urol 170:1738–1741, 2003.
7. Schuessler WW, Schulam PG, Clayman RV, Kavoussi LR. Laparoscopic radical prostatectomy: initial short-term experience. Urology 50:854, 1997.
8. Patel VR, Tully AS, Holmes R, et al: Robotic radical prostatectomy in the community setting—the learning curve and beyond: initial 200 cases. J Urol 174:269–272, 2005.
9. Costello AJ, Haxhimolla H, Crowe H, et al: Installation of telerobotic surgery and initial experience with telerobotic radical prostatectomy. BJU Int 96:34–38, 2005.
10. Kaul SA, Peabody JO, Shah N, et al: Establishing a robotic prostatectomy programme: the impact of mentoring using a structured approach. BJU Int 97:1143–1144, 2006.
11. Herrell SD, Smith JA Jr: Robotic-assisted laparoscopic prostatectomy: what is the learning curve? Urology 66:105–107, 2005.
12. Wicklund NP: Technology insight: surgical robots—expensive toys or the future of urologic surgery? Nat Clin Pract Urol 1:97–101, 2004.
13. Hu J, Nelson R, Wilson T, et al: Perioperative complications of laparoscopic and robotic assisted laparoscopic prostatectomy. J Urol 175:541–546, 2006.
14. Joseph J, Vicente I, Madeb R, et al: Robot-assisted vs pure laparoscopic radical prostatectomy: are there any differences? BJU Int 96:39–42, 2005.

CHAPTER 4

Nicholas J. Hegarty • Inderbir S. Gill

Laparoscopic Foundations for Robotic Surgery

INTRODUCTION

The use of robotics in urology owes much to experience in the field of laparoscopy. True, a number of operations, notably vasovasostomy and vasoepididymostomy, have been performed with robotic assistance,[1] exploiting the robot's ability to filter out tremor and perform scaled movements, along with its tremendous magnification and three-dimensional (3D) image; however, it is hard to think of a facet of robot-assisted laparoscopic surgery that has not been influenced by laparoscopy. A variety of robots have been used and continue to be used in different urologic settings, but by far the most widely used system is the da Vinci robotic system (Intuitive Surgical, Sunnyvale, CA). This is not a robot in the true sense of the word, in that it does not execute autonomous movements but rather performs computer-assisted surgery, translating movements of the operating surgeon at the surgical console into movements of the surgical arms. This reliance on operative skill, knowledge, and judgment in the operating surgeon has added to the appeal of robotics in those already familiar with open or laparoscopic techniques, and to date, developments in the compass of procedures that can be performed robotically has been interdependent with the training and aptitude of the operating surgeon. It has also opened up the field of minimally invasive surgery (MIS) to a greater number of surgeons.

FOUNDATIONS IN LAPAROSCOPY

MIS provides advantages over traditional open surgery in many settings. In reconstructive surgery the ability to perform surgeries equivalent to open techniques with considerably less surgical trauma has resulted in shortened hospital stay and reduced costs. Patients have a swifter recovery and return to full activity and long-term have less troublesome and more cosmetically acceptable wounds. Similar benefits are present in extirpative surgeries, particularly when small surgical specimen size allows removal through one of the access ports. Other advantages such as the view that can be obtained with magnification and the ability of the laparoscope to transmit images from the furthest reaches of the abdomen and pelvis certainly facilitate the surgeon's ability to perform dissection and reconstruction in areas difficult to access at open surgery. Laparoscopic procedures frequently have lower blood loss than their open equivalents. Robotic-assisted laparoscopy has embraced the benefits of MIS. It is generally agreed that the ability to perform more complex maneuvers such as intracorporeal suturing and knot tying is more easily acquired with robotic rather than pure laparoscopy. Thus, more surgeons are embracing this form of MIS, and consequently more patients are being given access to the benefits of MIS. Two areas of technologic progress that have facilitated this transition are advances in optics and instrumentation.

Optics

The earliest viewing systems in routine clinical use relied on analog tube cameras. These were superseded by charged coupled device (CCD) chip cameras, which afforded considerably greater clarity of image. Further advances in this technology allowed the development of three-chip cameras, providing improved images while not adding significantly to the camera bulk. The resultant digital images are less susceptible to degradation than those from analog systems, providing increased sharpness, color, and depth of perception. Both continuous and still images can readily be captured from digital systems and edited for teaching or display purposes. The emergence of liquid crystal display (LCD) and more recently plasma screens has greatly reduced the bulk of viewing screens. This permits them to be suspended in closer proximity to the surgical team, and large flat screens afford a clear view of proceedings from almost any position in the operating room. This provides a tremendous view for ancillary operating room personnel and for teaching and demonstration purposes.

3D Vision

Although the flat screen systems used in laparoscopy allow perception of depth, the camera system in the robot provides a true 3D image based on overlapping images (Figure 4–1). The strength of the robotic arms and the counterbalancing system of the camera arm mean that cameras of considerable weight can be used. This has

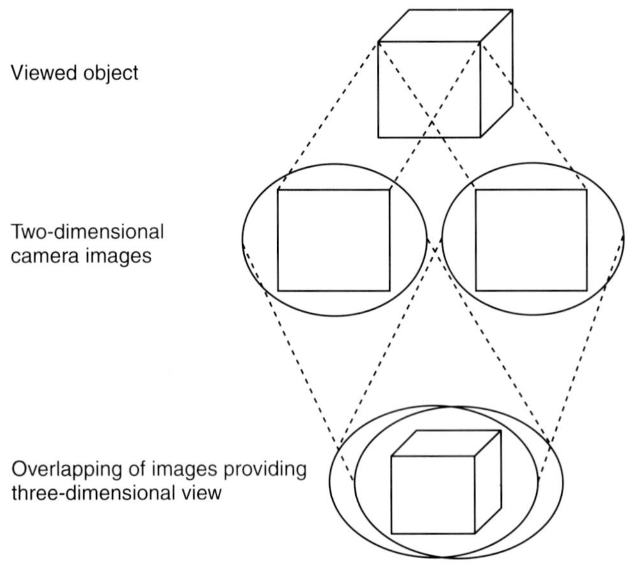

FIGURE 4–1 Three-dimensional camera image.

allowed the use of cameras incorporating two camera heads to generate the 3D image. Fixity of the surgeon's head in the operating console minimizes distortion of the 3D image from movement or viewing screens at an angle and allows enhanced perception of depth during dissection and suturing.

Scope Position

Maintaining optimal scope position during laparoscopy mandates a level of cooperation between the assistant and principal surgeon. Fundamental to this is a good understanding of the surgery being undertaken. Frequently, the camera assistant must assume an uncomfortable position to provide the best image possible, while simultaneously trying to permit the operating surgeon as much room as possible to manipulate the laparoscopic instruments. There is also the question of fatigue that may develop not only with longer surgeries but also from maintaining alterations in posture. The Automated Endoscopic System for Optimal Positioning (AESOP, Computer Motion, Goleta, CA) is a hands-free system comprising a table-mounted, computer arm that holds the camera. In its current form it is voice-controlled, allowing the operating surgeon to directly instruct on camera position and thus providing a stable image from which the surgeon can work. It reduces personnel requirements, without having any effect on operative duration or morbidity.[2]

A similar concept is used in the da Vinci system, whereby the operating surgeon controls camera position from the surgical console. This provides the surgeon with a steady image that is not subject to fatigue and can be positioned according to his or her liking. It does, however, mean that the operating surgeon may need to interrupt the flow of surgery to reposition the camera or compromise by operating outside the center of the optical field to avoid repositioning during a particular surgical maneuver.

Viewing Angle

The direction of view is also a potential advantage for robotics over laparoscopy where typically a 90-degree separation exists in the angle between screen, surgeon, and direction of operation. In robotics, the hand controls are inline with the viewed image, although foot-pedal controls remain outside this axis.

INSTRUMENTATION

The range of instruments available for laparoscopy has continued to expand rapidly. Numerous instruments are now available for grasping, dissection, cutting, retracting, and suturing, and more involved devices are available for intraoperative imaging, stapling, and application of various thermal energy forms. Nevertheless, laparoscopists will still complain that instrument design has not kept up with the demand for performing more complex surgeries. Many laparoscopic instruments have been adopted to function in robotic surgery. A significant difference in the design of most robotic instruments has been the incorporation of distal articulation, likened to the human wrist. This shifts much of the manipulation that is predominantly extracorporeal in laparoscopy close to the site of surgery. Design of such instruments has required considerable ingenuity to create instruments that are sufficiently delicate yet suitably robust to perform both delicate and coarse intracorporeal maneuvers. Moving the focus of surgery provides particular advantages for those not adept at performing advanced laparoscopic moves. A further increase in the range of instruments available will mean the operator will become less dependent on the tableside assistant for clip application and introduction of sutures as well as laparoscopic retraction, use of suction, and irrigation. Improvements in instrument longevity (current robotic instruments typically have a life span of 10–20 cases) will likely significantly reduce per case expense. The lack of tactile feedback with robotic instrumentation has presented new challenges to the surgeon. Increasingly, visual cues are used to determine appropriate suture tension. Subtle variations in grasp strength are used to avoid traumatizing tissues and to hold needles off center when required because there is a tendency for them to assume a right-angled position within the jaws of the needle driver.

Instrument Port Placement

Much has been learned from laparoscopy with regard to the confines of the anatomic cavity and the external space required to perform the requisite movements within it. Robotic camera and port positions at least initially mirror those of laparoscopic surgery. Subsequent variations have been made

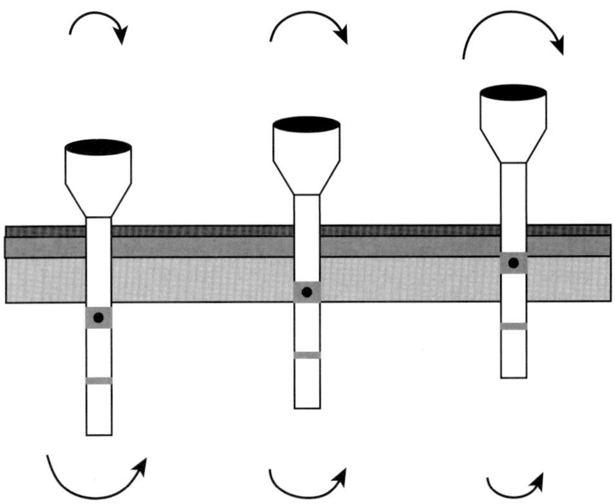

FIGURE 4–2 Fulcrum on anterior abdominal wall. *a,* Port placed too deep into abdomen provides excessive movement of distal port and increased torque on abdominal wall. *b,* Fulcrum of port located at level of fascia, providing least torque on abdominal wall. *c,* Superficial port placement resulting in increased abdominal wall torque.

based on the number of assistants required, minimizing collisions between arms and auxiliary port placement away from the robot arms and allowing access for the assistant to reach the port (without fear of injury). Ports also need to be placed at a particular depth as in laparoscopy to minimize trauma to the abdominal wall and reduce strain on instruments and robotic arms (Figure 4–2).

Patient Positioning

Careful patient positioning in robotics is also vital to surgical planning and is firmly based in laparoscopy. Protection of pressure points in the immobilized patient takes on even more importance in robotics as access to the patient can be limited during surgery. Gravity is used to aid exposure and the traction-countertraction required for laparoscopic surgery; thus, pelvic procedures are performed in steep Trendelenburg, whereas kidney procedures are done in a flank position. Strict planning takes on even greater importance with robotics because once the robot is in position any necessary change in position requires undocking of the robot. Sufficient space around the operating table is also required for positioning of the robot arms and instrument exchanges.

OTHER CONSIDERATIONS

Filter of Tremor

The software incorporated in robotic surgery provides the ability to filter tremor in the hands of the operating surgeon. This is of particular use during fine dissection or other delicate maneuvers. This does not in itself represent a particular advance for intra-abdominal surgery because the experienced laparoscopist can apply pressure on the operating instrument through the abdominal wall fulcrum to achieve a similar steadying effect.

Motion Scaling

Current robots allow a range of motion from 1:2 to 1:5 scaling. Coupled with this, the tremendous magnification and 3D vision of the robotic camera system allow the performance of very fine movements. Although most surgeries are performed without the need for scaled motion that require greater movement on the part of the surgeon, it certainly is useful for very delicate maneuvers such as anastomosis of vas[1] or nerve grafting.[3]

Mentoring

The projection of the surgical image on multiple viewing screens allows all in the operating room to have a good view of surgery. The facility with which the digital camera allows each surgery to be recorded also helps the preparation of teaching material and analysis of specific aspects of surgery. Robot design lends itself to development where dual-operating consoles may be created. This would facilitate teaching by allowing the principle surgeon and trainee to participate in combined surgeries. Telementoring and telepresence surgery have become a reality with advances in video and broadband technology. Whereas in most instances telepresence surgery has been performed to demonstrate the feasibility of such practices, individual programs have been developed to provide expert surgical technique to remote areas[4] and such an application may become more widespread in the future.

GENERAL CONSIDERATIONS

Laparoscopy has taught us that considerable thought and effort is required to replicate open techniques in a new surgical environment. Gradually with experience and improved instrument design, it has been able to replicate even complex open surgeries laparoscopically.[5] Subtle differences in technique are continuously being proposed to more faithfully replicate open surgery and thus provide improved patient outcomes. One example is the avoidance of cautery in the dissection of the neurovascular bundles to lessen nerve injury and preserve potency during prostatectomy. This modification of dissection of the prostatic pedicles first described in laparoscopy[6] has subsequently been described for robot-assisted laparoscopic radical prostatectomy.[7]

Laparoscopy has laid another important foundation for robotics as a model for the introduction of a new surgical approach. As a complementary and in many instances competitive surgical practice to the established open techniques, there have been a number of important lessons learned.

Where comparisons have been made, they have usually been to the highest standards of established open surgery particular in terms of patient outcomes, be they oncologic or functional, expense, and comorbidity. Catastrophic outcomes, when they have occurred, have received considerable publicity, and exaggerated claims have met with swift response. This is entirely laudable because it has meant that for the most part laparoscopy has been introduced with due diligence. Honesty in reporting has been extremely important, and the demonstration of benefit for any new procedure has been paramount to published studies, rather than simply proving a new technique can be performed. These principals have guided the establishment of laparoscopy as a very real clinical entity. This is important because technologic advances are generally greeted with a blend of skepticism and excitement. The enthusiasm that greets a new technology must be grounded in a treatment of substance. Phraseology such as "keyhole surgery" and lasers in surgery have in the past generated high levels of interest in the lay and frequently the medical press, and some patients may have developed unfounded expectations based on preconceptions aroused by such impressive terminology. The term *robotics* is an equally dazzling term, arousing sentiments of control beyond human capabilities. Critics have alluded to the hype and marketing that surrounds such a term. As a group, we must not pretend it is something it is not, and in our dealings with patients, we must make sure that their perceptions are in touch with reality. At the same time, we should strive to maximize the advantages that robotics do provide such that precision of dissection, delicate handling of tissues, and suturing with very fine suture materials are brought to a new level.

As in laparoscopy, we must strive to determine areas of benefit and identify shortcomings and address them to provide the maximum benefit to patients that can be accrued with this very impressive technology. There is no doubt that robotics will continue to play an increasing role in the future. Improvements with miniaturization, improved instrument design, reduced cost, and incorporation of existing and newer technologies can only enhance what is rapidly gaining broad acceptance in the urologic and wider surgical community. Robotics owes much to the foundations provided by laparoscopy and will extend the ability to perform MIS to more surgeons and thus afford more patients the benefits of MIS. Upon these foundations, robotics will continue to mimic what is already humanly possible and rise to the challenge of providing treatment strategies beyond the human compass.

REFERENCES

1. Kuang W, Shin PR, Matin S, et al: Initial evaluation of robotic technology for microsurgical vasovasostomy. J Urol 171:300–303, 2004.
2. Proske JM, Dagher I, Franco D: Comparative study of human and robotic camera control in laparoscopic biliary and colon surgery. J Laparoendosc Adv Surg Tech A 14:345–348, 2004.
3. Kaouk JH, Desai MM, Abreu SC, et al: Robot assisted laparoscopic sural nerve grafting during radical prostatectomy: initial experience. J Urol 170:909–912, 2003.
4. Anvari M, McKinley C, Stein H: Establishment of the world's first remote surgical service: for provision of advanced laparoscopic surgery in a rural community. Ann Surg 241:460–464, 2005.
5. Gill IS, Desai MM, Kaouk JH, et al: Laparoscopic partial nephrectomy for renal tumor: duplicating open surgical techniques. J Urol 167:469–476, 2002.
6. Gill IS, Ukimura O, Rubinstein M, et al: Lateral pedicle control during laparoscopic radical prostatectomy: refined technique. Urology 65:23–27, 2005.
7. Ahlering TE, Eichel L, Chou D, et al: Feasibility study for robotic prostatectomy cautery-free neurovascular bundle preservation. Urology 65:994–997, 2005.

CHAPTER 5

Ashok K. Hemal • Rajeev Kumar

Role of Patient Side Surgeon in Robotics

INTRODUCTION

Robotic surgical systems have developed significantly in the past 10 years. One of the most significant developments has been that of telesurgical systems such as the da Vinci device that allows control of operating instruments using two or three robotic arms through a remote location. The term *patient side surgeon* (PSS) has come into being as a consequence of these systems wherein the principal surgeon, called the "console surgeon," is located at the robotic controls, unscrubbed, and away from the patient. In a way, the PSS has become the primary human interface among the console surgeon, robot, and the patient and may actually have become more important for the safe conduct of surgery than a traditional first assistant would have. We review the role of this surgeon in current robotic urologic surgery.

The initial development of the robotic program in urology began with intensive mentoring and hands-on training of laparoscopy naïve surgeons with expert laparoscopists. Menon et al.[1,2] reported the development of this structured program at the Henry Ford Hospital in Detroit. The trainee surgeons, both the console surgeon and the PSS, were exposed to a very limited amount of laparoscopic surgery and learned basic laparoscopy skills by working on trainers, animals, and human cadavers at an expert center. This was followed by on-site mentoring by visiting experts at the surgeons' institution. The console surgeon began assisting the experts during laparoscopic radical prostatectomy as the first assistant before moving on to the robot. This sequential learning, similar to that in any surgical procedure, highlights the importance of primary hands-on training as a PSS before moving on to the console.

Even after the development of a program, maintenance of high surgical standards and efficiency requires constant coordination among the console surgeon, the PSS, and other members of the team. One of the main roles of the PSS, as discussed further in this text, is to change the instruments in the robotic arms. This requires a good deal of anticipation and in-depth knowledge of the procedure and the console surgeon's preferred instrument for each surgical step so that time is not wasted in these changes. Like Menon et al.,[1,2] Ahlering et al.[3] also stress the need for a single dedicated team and believe it is of importance in achieving a decreased operative time and good results.

Before we begin looking at the specific role of the PSS, it is important to realize that robotic surgery has allowed laparoscopy naïve surgeons to progress to minimally invasive surgery without extensive laparoscopy training. The console surgeon performs the procedure similar to an open surgery albeit without direct contact with the patient. For the console surgeon, good open surgical skills may be sufficient for progressing to the robotic-assisted surgery. However, this is significantly dependent on a laparoscopy trained PSS who performs all the laparoscopic steps directly on the patient.[3]

THE ROLE OF A PSS

Among the various urologic surgeries that have been performed using a robot, radical prostatectomy for cancer of the prostate is the most common, with nearly 20% of all radical prostatectomies being performed using the device.[4] Robotic radical prostatectomy (RRP) is thus the benchmark surgery that will be used to define the role of a PSS.

Patient Positioning

Patient positioning is critical to the success of most surgeries and RRP in particular. RRP can be performed by both the transperitoneal and extraperitoneal approaches. For the former approach, it requires a steep Trendelenburg position for most of the procedure, and adequate padding and support are mandatory. It is primarily the responsibility of the PSS to ensure correct patient positioning and padding. This is particularly true at the beginning of a robotic program because, although the console surgeon and the PSS may have received training for the procedure, attendant staff and anesthetists are unlikely to have done so. The steep Trendelenburg position is rarely used in open surgery and would be familiar only to a team regularly exposed to laparoscopic radical prostatectomy or cystectomy.

Port Placement

Port placement depends on the surgical technique and the number of assistants used in the surgery. Proper positioning of the ports is one of the most important steps in any laparoscopic surgery because this determines the ability to manipulate the instruments to the best possible use.[5] The decision on the site of ports lies with the PSS. This decision cannot be premeditated for all patients. Port positioning has to be consciously decided for each individual patient because even for the same surgery, it will differ with body habitus and previous surgical scars. Ports placed too close to each other will hamper movement and cause clash of instruments, whereas ports placed too far from the site of surgery may not allow the instruments to reach the operative site. The PSS must be aware of these factors in deciding the site of placement.

Insertion of Trocars

For any laparoscopic procedure, a working space has to be created. In transperitoneal procedures, this involves the creation of a pneumoperitoneum, whereas for extraperitoneal procedures, creation of the extraperitoneal space itself requires an assistant skilled in laparoscopy to avoid inadequate room or peritoneal rent. This space is usually created by the PSS. Subsequently, the PSS is responsible for insertion of the primary and secondary trocars. Trocar insertion requires reasonable training because it can result in injuries if not properly performed. The PSS must be aware of the various types of trocars available and their use. The PSS must also ensure that robotic ports are inserted to the correct depth to avoid inadvertent port site tears and injuries resulting from movements of the robotic arms.

Adhesiolysis

Although it is always preferable to operate on patients with no previous abdominal surgeries, adhesions between the omentum, bowel, and the abdominal wall may often be present even in "virgin" abdomens. In such cases, the PSS has to divide the adhesions using the available ports and conventional laparoscopy instruments. This step requires at least basic laparoscopy skills. It is important to present a clear operative field to the console surgeon, who may then divide additional adhesions as they appear.

Robot Installation

The steps described previously are common to all laparoscopy procedures. Once the trocars have been inserted, the robot is installed and the robotic arms are attached to their respective ports. This is an important step in robotic surgery and may take significant time in the initial part of a program. The camera arm is docked to the central port while the lateral two or three arms are attached to the respective robotic trocars. While installing the robot, the PSS must ensure a proper fit and proper port position and confirm that the patient is safe and not being compressed at any point, particularly the lower limbs, by the robot. Installing the robot requires coordination between the unscrubbed personnel moving the robot and the scrubbed PSS guiding the placement. Increased experience has significantly reduced the time used for docking the robot. This step would often take up to an hour during the initial few cases but can now be achieved in less than 10 minutes. This has resulted primarily from the increased experience of the PSS.

Change of Robotic Instruments

Another specific role of the PSS in robotic surgery is change of instruments in the robotic arms. Each instrument is specifically designed for a function, and these need to be changed at various points in the procedure. The PSS should be aware of the surgical steps and the console surgeon's preference for instruments at each step so as to quickly place those instruments into the robotic arms. These expensive and fine instruments need careful handling to avoid malfunctioning and breakage. The PSS must be well versed with the articulation mechanisms.

Surgical Assistance

Active surgical assistance follows the same principles as in open surgery. However, in robotic surgery, the PSS must be laparoscopically trained. The main responsibilities of the PSS are retraction, suction, irrigation, insertion of sutures, entrapment and removal of the dissected organ, port removal, and closure. Some of the important steps during RRP that require active assistance are dissection of the bladder neck, seminal vesical identification and dissection, mobilization of the prostate from the rectum, identification and preservation of the neurovascular bundles, and, finally, the urethrovesical anastomosis. These steps require active retraction, suction, and irrigation to clear the operative field and insertion and removal of sutures. The PSS must be fully conversant with his or her expected role at each step to minimize loss of time and inadvertent movements.

Managing Complications

One of the most important, and least highlighted, aspects of the PSS's role is in managing intraoperative complications. It has already been accepted that the console surgeon may not have advanced laparoscopy skills. Although some complications may be managed entirely by the console surgeon with robotic assistance, advanced laparoscopy skills may be required for tasks such as additional mobilization, retraction, suction, compression, or freehand intracorporeal suturing. The laparoscopy skills of the PSS may be the deciding factor in whether the procedure continues laparoscopically or needs conversion to open surgery. This is particularly true for vascular complications, which not only can be prevented but also managed by PSS—or at least the bleeding structure can be held by him or her to allow further management.

Learning the Procedure

The importance of hands-on training under mentored programs is paramount in developing both laparoscopic and robotic skills. Patient side assistance is the principal means of acquiring these skills. The PSS is thus responsible not only for a safe and efficacious conduct of the surgery but also for acquiring necessary skills to graduate to the console surgeon's position. Although there are no data yet to suggest that surgeons who have worked as a PSS in robotic programs acquire console skills quicker or of a higher level, it seems reasonable that repeated assistance in the same procedure will allow the surgeon better appreciation of the anatomy and difficulties of the surgery and enable him or her to adapt to the console surgeon's role easily.

ROLE IN SPECIFIC SURGERIES

RRP is one of the few robotic urologic procedures in which the techniques of surgery have become reasonably standardized. The role of the PSS varies according to the technique being used to perform the surgery. Depending on the availability and need to train additional surgeons, the Vattikuti Institute prostatectomy (VIP),[2,6] which has become an exemplary program across the globe to develop robotic programs, allows the use of either one or two PSSs. The group at the University of California at Irvine[7] uses one PSS with a three-arm robot. One PSS is also required for prostatectomy with a four-arm robot.[8,9]

Vip Technique[2,6]

The VIP team has the largest published experience in RRP.[10] They were also the first to describe a structured program in training for RRP.[1] The VIP technique allows for the use of two PSSs, one on either side of the patient. The right-side assistant plays a more dominant role than the left-side assistant. The left-side assistant is scrubbed primarily to enhance training rather than as an essential component of the surgical team. In the VIP program, the console surgeon may or may not have advanced laparoscopy skills. However, the PSS who presents the operative field to the console surgeon and assists during the procedure should be facile in laparoscopic surgery.[6] This technique highlights the use of two PSSs for the purpose of training residents and fellows and uses six ports with a three-arm robot. Three ports are available for use by the PSS. Two of these, one 10 mm and one 5 mm, are on the right side, and one 5-mm port is on the left side. The right-side assistant is solely responsible for all the suction, irrigation, insertion and removal of sutures, application of vascular clips if needed, and removal of the specimen. Both assistants help with traction and retraction at various steps (Table 5-1).

Single Assistant, Three-Arm Robot

Similar to the VIP program, the RRP program at the University of California at Irvine,[7] which has a large experience, also depends on a laparoscopically trained PSS because the console surgeon has extensive open surgical experience but limited laparoscopy skills. These surgeons use a five-port technique with a three-arm robot. Two ports are used by the assistant, and the positioning of these ports depends on the dominant hand of the assistant. The PSS sits on the right side of the patient with both ports to the right of the midline camera port if he or she is left handed and vice versa for a right-handed PSS. The nondominant hand is used primarily for retraction, whereas the more dexterous dominant hand is required mainly for suction. The dominant hand controls the suction through a 5-mm port, whereas the 12-mm nondominant hand port is used to insert a locking grasper for retraction, a needle driver to insert and remove a suture, and a vascular stapling device for the dorsal venous complex.

Some critical steps requiring active assistance have been described. The PSS grasps the adipose tissue on the anterior bladder wall and retracts it cranially to help identify the junction between the prostate and the bladder anteriorly. Once the anterior bladder wall has been divided, the balloon of the Foley catheter is deflated and the catheter is grasped through its eye by the PSS and used to retract the prostate with an upward traction. Subsequent to division of the posterior bladder neck, the grasper is used to hold the tips of the vas deferens and retract upward, exposing the seminal vesicles for dissection. The suction instrument is used in the dominant hand to provide a clean field of vision and also countertraction for seminal vesicle dissection. During dissection of the apex of the prostate, the suction instrument is used to maintain a clear field of vision. Subsequently, during the vesicourethral anastomosis, the PSS helps maintain traction on the running suture and also provides continuous suction to remove the urine and blood from the field. Finally, the PSS removes the specimen through the 12-mm port.

Single Assistant, Four-Arm Robot[8,9,11]

Based on their earlier experience with extraperitoneal laparoscopic prostatectomy, Gettman et al.[11] described an extraperitoneal approach to RRP. This approach uses one PSS, seated on the right side of the patient. However, unlike the one-assistant transperitoneal approach described previously, six ports are used, three being available for use by the PSS.

Table 5-1 Vattikuti Institute Prostatectomy (VIP) Technique: Role of the Patient Side Surgeon (PSS)

Surgical Step	Role of PSS
Peritoneoscopy	Adhesiolysis using conventional laparoscopy instruments
Entry into space of Retzius	Retraction of medial umbilical ligaments to facilitate incision
	Countertraction on the peritoneum during bladder exposure
Control of dorsal vein complex	Introduction and removal of suture for ligation
	Retraction of the prostate for visibility
Bladder neck division	Traction on the proximal stay suture of prostate (done by left side PSS)
	Traction on the bladder to help identify the prostate vesical junction
	Retraction of the Foley catheter cranially after division of anterior bladder neck
Dissection of vas deferens, seminal vesicles, vascular bundles	Retraction of ends of the divided vas deferens and tips of seminal vesicles
	Application of hemostatic clips if required
Nerve sparing	Retraction of prostate away from the side of dissection
Apex division	Retraction of prostate
	Removal of tissue for frozen section biopsies
Pelvic lymphadenectomy	Retraction and removal of specimen
Vesicourethral anastomosis	Introduction and removal of suture
	Suture "following" if required
Completion	Introduction of specimen retrieval bag, entrapment of specimen and its removal
	Undocking of robot and closure of ports

Suction and irrigation are probably the two most important roles of the PSS. These need to be performed judiciously and carefully at all stages of the procedure to provide a clear operative view to the console surgeon while not allowing the pneumoperitoneum to decrease significantly. A specially designed long suction device may be needed in case the port used is placed cranial to the robotic camera port because the traditional devices may not reach the pelvis.

These include two on the right side of the midline camera port and one in the midline above the symphysis pubis. Similar to the open anatomic retropubic prostatectomy, the procedure is begun with dissection of the prostatic apex. The PSS is required to help visualize the apex by rotating the prostate in either direction during placement of the suture on the dorsal venous complex. Subsequently, the apex is divided and the dissection proceeds retrograde toward the bladder neck. Esposito et al.[9] modified this procedure using a four-arm robot. The fourth arm of the robot is articulated to the central column and is capable of holding an additional instrument. However, as in the three-arm procedure, one PSS is still required. This procedure uses five ports, four for the robot and one for the PSS. The fourth arm of the robot is docked to the right side port, and the PSS uses the left side 10-mm port. The fourth arm helps reduce the dependence on the PSS for retraction and dissection. The PSS is required only for suction, irrigation, insertion and removal of sutures, and the specimen retrieval. The authors believe that the addition of the fourth arm helps eliminate the need for a laparoscopically skilled PSS but agree that this approach is not suitable in teaching institutions where one of the roles of the PSS is to actively learn the procedure.

Sundaram et al.[8] describe another variation of the four-arm robot wherein the fourth arm of the robot is docked to the left side port and the PSS uses the right side port for assistance. The authors believe that the PSS is often better than the fourth arm, particularly for the dissection of the seminal vesicles because of his or her basic laparoscopy knowledge.

AESOP-Assisted Radial Prostatectomy

Although the term *RRP* has almost become synonymous with the use of the da Vinci device, other robotic devices such as the AESOP (Automated Endoscopic System for Optimal Positioning) are being widely used, and for a longer time, in urologic laparoscopic surgery. The first commercially used robotic assistant, the Aesop 1000, was developed in 1993 by Computer Motion. This device worked on the shared-control principle and was used for holding an endoscopic camera in minimal invasive laparoscopic surgery. The device was controlled by foot pedals, which were often a problem for new users because they had to look down at the pedals before they could adjust them. The device was modified in 1996, and the Aesop 2000 used voice control. The Aesop 3000 added another degree of freedom in the arm. A number of publications with series extending to more than 1000 cases describe the use of voice-controlled robot assistance for laparoscopic radical prostatectomy.[12,13]

Kavoussi et al.[14] described the use of an AESOP arm on one side and a human assistant on another side in patients requiring similar laparoscopic surgeries bilaterally and concluded that the robot was useful in holding the camera because of its untiring precision. Antiphon et al.[15] went on to describe completely solo AESOP-assisted radical prostatectomies in 16 patients and compared them with another 16 patients undergoing a standard laparoscopic radical prostatectomy. Five trocars were used in both sets of patients. In the human assistant group, the assistant held the camera through one port and an instrument through another port, leaving three ports open to the primary surgeon. In the solo group, an AESOP 3000 robotic arm was used to hold the camera while another mechanized arm (Lina Medical, Denmark) was used to hold an assisting instrument. They concluded that the AESOP-assisted group of patients had lower inadvertent and erratic movements of the camera. This report may be applicable to such mechanized arms that are used during laparoscopic surgery but cannot be relevant for telerobotic surgeries such as the da Vinci procedures in which the primary surgeon is not scrubbed.

Pyeloplasty

Laparoscopic pyeloplasty has become an accepted treatment modality for ureteropelvic junction obstructions, and robotic assistance has been used in this surgery, primarily to overcome the problem of precise intracorporeal suturing that requires deft laparoscopy skills. Existing literature describes only a transperitoneal approach using four trocars with a three-arm robot. The fourth trocar for use by the PSS may be located subcostally in the anterior axillary line,[16] below the xiphoid in the midline,[17] or in the paramedian location, contralateral to the operative side.[18] The choice of port placement depends on the preference of the operative team and the body habitus of the patient. The aim is to allow the PSS maximal access to the operative site without interference from the three robotic arms that come from the ipsilateral side of surgery, over the flank of the patient. The role of the PSS is similar to that in prostatectomy, with a lesser degree of retraction. The PSS is critical during the anastomosis of spatulated ureter with the pelvis, particularly in case of a good functioning kidney in which the urine drainage may need continuous suctioning. Another specific role of the PSS in these cases is during the placement of ureteral stent. Because a number of these procedures are performed in children, adolescents, and young adults, meticulous closure of all laparoscopy ports is also essential, and the PSS must take care that this is done properly to avoid port site hernia.

Robotic Radical Cystectomy[19]

Radical cystectomy with urinary diversion is a standard treatment option for muscle-invasive bladder cancer. Open surgery requires a relatively large incision with consequent morbidity and long recovery, and laparoscopic radical cystectomy is a technically difficult procedure. The use of robotic assistance for this surgery is still limited to a few reports but is promising because of the similarity in technique to RRP.

A five- or six-port technique is commonly used, with port placement that differs little from that for RRP as described by Hemal et al.[5] The PSS is usually seated on the right side of the patient. At the beginning of the procedure, the PSS helps identify and dissect the ureters by retraction on the divided posterior peritoneum above the rectum. The PSS applies clips to the ureter before their division and also helps control the vesical pedicles by applying hemostatic clips. During the remainder of the procedure, the role of the PSS is similar to that in radical prostatectomy, primarily being retraction, suction, and insertion and removal of sutures. The PSS, if skilled, may also be responsible for creation of the neobladder and the ureteroileal anastomosis that is performed extracorporeally through the small midline incision from which the specimen has been delivered. Once the neobladder has been constructed, it is replaced into the peritoneal cavity and the PSS closes the abdominal wound and redocks the robot to enable the urethra-neobladder anastomosis.[19] The anastomosis proceeds in a manner similar to radical prostatectomy, with the PSS being responsible for suction, irrigation, traction, and insertion and removal of sutures.

Female Urology

To date, robotics have been used in female urology or urogynecology for the limited indications, such as colposuspension, repair of vesicovaginal fistula, and sacrocolpopexy.[20] However, in these procedures, the role of PSS remains invaluable as described for other surgeries.

ADVANTAGES OF A TRAINED PSS

The use of robotic assistance may help decrease the number of assistants required during surgery. This has become evident based on the reports that currently use only one PSS. Unlike a robot, the human assistant is able to perform intuitive tasks and respond to changing situations. A trained PSS acts as a source of support and guidance to the console surgeon, often offering constructive advice during the procedure. He or she also helps overcome the need for laparoscopy training of the console surgeon and allows the console surgeon to transfer open surgical skills directly to the laparoscopy environment. The use of a human assistant is also important from the training perspective. Hands-on training is the best form of learning in surgery, and assisting on the patient side helps the trainee understand the procedure better than through any other modality.

PROGRAM DEVELOPMENT

One of the biggest advantages of a properly trained PSS is the potential development of new robotic surgery programs. Systematic training in a manner similar to the VIP program may help achieve this objective because it ensures the sequential development of all skills necessary for it. A trainee begins by observing the procedure and assisting on the left side of the patient where his or her role is minimal but gives a hands-on feel of the instruments and the device. It also helps learn the basics of robotic assistance such as port placement, docking, and instrument change. For assisting on the right side, the PSS must acquire reasonable laparoscopy skills, and active involvement in the procedure helps increase confidence for moving to the console as the primary surgeon. Thorough knowledge of the device and its use gained through this experience can be of immense help is devising and establishing a robotic program in which all other personnel may be new to the procedure and the device. Experience gained through the VIP program of training as a PSS has been widely used to establish new RRP programs all over the world.

THE PSS AS A TEACHER

Despite rapid acceptance of the robot as a tool for robot-assisted radical prostatectomy, very few centers in the world perform this surgery routinely or in enough numbers to be able to help disseminate training to other surgeons. Properly trained PSSs will be crucial to the spread of robotic skills to newer surgeons. A console surgeon who has learned all areas of robotic surgery, including maintenance and patient side assistance, will be ideally suited to help train more individuals, initially as a PSS and then as a console surgeon. This would not be possible if all console surgeons were to directly migrate from open surgery to robotic surgery without the PSS interface.

COMPLETE SOLO RRP

A natural corollary of a fully trained and competent PSS who becomes a console surgeon is the attempt to perform complete solo da Vinci–assisted prostatectomy. Because the PSS has the capability of performing all tasks, including maintenance, port placement, docking, and surgery, he or she may be able to perform a complete solo surgery with the help of only a physician or nurse assistance. The surgeon may be able to initially scrub to place the ports and install the robot before moving to the console for the actual surgery. Intraoperative assistance may be provided by an adequately trained nonsurgeon PSS.

Although this seems technically feasible, it raises certain ethical and legal issues apart from negating the basic tenets of teaching and training additional surgeons. In case of an emergency, it may take the console surgeon some time to scrub and be available patient side, and this may lead to catastrophic results in case of major vessel injuries that cannot be managed through robotic instruments or by the nurse.

AIIMS EXPERIENCE

The first RRP in India was performed at the All India Institute of Medical Sciences (AIIMS), New Delhi, in 2005. The performance of these surgeries vouches for the role of the PSS in not only performing the surgery but also establishing new programs from scratch. The console surgeon (AKH) was a part of the VIP team since its beginning and trained in all aspects of the surgery as a PSS before migrating to the console. This training allowed the development of the AIIMS team wherein only one additional member had observed RRP during a short-term fellowship with the VIP program.[21,22] This team was able to perform surgeries without complication and within an operative time of under 2.5 hours primarily because the comprehensive training as a PSS allowed the console surgeon to manage all tasks necessary for the surgery, including instrument handling, port placement, robot installation, and completion of surgery. This department acquired a four-arm da Vinci-S surgical system in July 2006 and in just over a year has performed more than 200 robotic procedures, including RRP, radical cystectomy, pyeloplasty, anterior exenteration, ureteric reimplantation, and vesicovaginal fistula repair.[23–25]

CONCLUSIONS

Telerobotic surgery has helped laparoscopy naïve surgeons offer minimal access surgery to their patients without undergoing extensive laparoscopy training. However, this has depended on the availability of laparoscopically trained assistants. Even a laparoscopically trained console surgeon cannot obviate the need for a trained PSS because the PSS has to assist throughout the procedure and it is not possible for the unscrubbed, remotely located console surgeon to use his or her laparoscopy skills during the surgery. It has thus become important for trainees who wish to participate in robotic surgery to learn at least basic laparoscopy. This training has to be in addition to the training in open surgery that guides all steps during the robotic procedure. Finally, to assist in robot docking and interchange of instruments and to further progress to the role of a console surgeon, the trainees will have to acquire robotic skills along with their basic and laparoscopy skills. It is thus likely that, unlike a number of robotic surgeons today, robotic surgeons in the future will be adept at all three forms of surgery because they may not be at liberty to directly become console surgeons from open surgeons.

REFERENCES

1. Menon M, Shrivastava A, Tewari A, et al: Laparoscopic and robot assisted radical prostatectomy: establishment of a structured program and preliminary analysis of outcomes. J Urol 168:945-949, 2002.
2. Menon M, Hemal AK, VIP Team: Vattikuti Institute prostatectomy: a technique of robotic radical prostatectomy: experience in more than 1000 cases. J Endourol 18:611-619, 2004; discussion 619.
3. Ahlering TE, Skarecky D, Lee D, et al: Successful transfer of open surgical skills to a laparoscopic environment using a robotic interface: initial experience with laparoscopic radical prostatectomy. J Urol 170:1738-1741, 2003.
4. http://www.davinciprostatectomy.com/cuttingedge.htm; Accessed January 4, 2006.
5. Hemal AK, Eun D, Tewari A, et al: Nuances in the optimum placement of ports in pelvic and upper urinary tract surgery using the da Vinci robot. Urol Clin North Am 31:683-692, 2004.
6. Menon M, Tewari A, Peabody J, Members of the VIP team: Vattikuti Institute Prostatectomy: technique. J Urol 169:2289-2292, 2003.
7. Lee DI, Eichel L, Skarecky DW, et al: Robotic laparoscopic radical prostatectomy with a single assistant. Urology 63:1172-1175, 2004.
8. Sundaram CP, Koch MO, Gardner T, et al: Utility of the fourth arm to facilitate robot-assisted laparoscopic radical prostatectomy. BJU Int 95:183-186, 2005.
9. Esposito MP, Ilbeigi P, Ahmed M, et al: Use of fourth arm in da Vinci robot assisted extraperitoneal laparoscopic prostatectomy: novel technique. Urology 66:649-652, 2005.
10. Menon M, Tewari A, Peabody JO, et al: Vattikuti Institute prostatectomy, a technique of robotic radical prostatectomy for management of localized carcinoma of the prostate: experience of over 1100 cases. Urol Clin North Am 31:701-717, 2004.
11. Gettman MT, Hoznek AS, Salomon L, et al: Laparoscopic radical prostatectomy: description of the extraperitoneal approach using the da Vinci robotic system. J Urol 170:416-419, 2003.
12. Rassweiler J, Marrero R, Hammady A, et al: Transperitoneal laparoscopic radical prostatectomy: ascending technique. J Endourol 18:593-599, 2004.
13. Guillonneau B, el-Fettouh H, Baumert H, et al: Laparoscopic radical prostatectomy: oncological evaluation after 1,000 cases at Montsouris Institute. J Urol 169:1261-1266, 2003.
14. Kavoussi LR, Moore RG, Adams JB, et al: Comparison of robotic versus human laparoscopic camera control. J Urol 154:2134-2136, 1995.
15. Antiphon P, Hoznek A, Benyoussef A, et al: Complete solo laparoscopic radical prostatectomy: initial experience. Urology 61:724-729, 2003.
16. Gettman MT, Neururer R, Artsch G, et al: Anderson-Hynes dismembered pyeloplasty performed using the da Vinci robotic system. Urology 60:509-513, 2002.
17. Atug F, Woods M, Burgess SV, et al: Robotic assisted laparoscopic pyeloplasty in children. J Urol 174:1440-1442, 2005.
18. Patel V: Robotic-assisted laparoscopic dismembered pyeloplasty. Urology 66:45-49, 2005.
19. Hemal AK, Abol-Enein H, Tewari A, et al: Robotic radical cystectomy and urinary diversion in the management of bladder cancer. Urol Clin North Am 31:719-729, 2004.
20. Sundaram BM, Kalidasan G, Hemal AK: Robotic repair of vesicovaginal fistula: a case-series of 5 patients. Urology 67:970–973, 2006.
21. Menon M, Hemal AK: Robotic urologic surgery: is this the way of the future? World J Urol 24:119, 2006.
22. Kumar R, Hemal AK, Menon M: Robotic renal and adrenal surgery: present and future. BJU Int 96:244–249, 2005.
23. Rao R, Nayyar R, Panda S, et al: Surgical techniques: robotic bladder diverticulectomy with the da Vinci-S surgical system. J Robotic Surg 1:217–220, 2007.
24. Nayyar R, Wadhwa P, Hemal AK: Pure robotic extended pyelolithotomy: cosmetic replica of open surgery. J Robotic Surg 1:207–211, 2007.
25. Kumar R, Yadav R, Kolla SB: Case report: simultaneous bilateral robot-assisted dismembered pyeloplasties for bilateral ureteropelvic junction obstruction: technique and literature review. J Endourol 21:750–753, 2007.

SECTION 2
PROCEDURES

CHAPTER 6

Ashutosh Tewari • Sandhya R. Rao • Rajan Ramanathan

Athermal Robotic Radical Prostatectomy: Technique and Results

INTRODUCTION

It is estimated that in 2007, approximately 218,890 new cases of prostate cancer will be diagnosed and 27,050 men will die of the disease.[1] Radical retropubic prostatectomy remains the gold standard of treatment for localized prostate cancer[2,3] but is associated with significant postoperative morbidity.[4] Both laparoscopy and robotics are minimally invasive modalities, but laparoscopic radical prostatectomy has a steep learning curve. Robotic-assisted laparoscopic prostatectomy, which provides three-dimensional (3D) visualization, wristed instrumentation, and intuitive finger controlled movements and an ergonomic position for the surgeon, may soon become the standard of care for localized prostate cancer.

Prostate cancer surgery is a challenging procedure with the competing goals of cancer control and maintenance of erection. The surgeon's ability to develop a precise plane between the nerves and the prostatic capsule is hampered by the difficulty in recognizing microscopic invasion of neurovascular tissue by the cancer, and this issue becomes even more relevant in robotic surgery in which there is no tactile feedback. The concerns with robotic surgery are deviation from the principles of open radical surgery, the use of thermal energy, and the inability to examine the specimen before completion of the surgery.

We present here the athermal trizonal nerve-sparing technique of robotic prostatectomy,[5] which addresses these concerns. This technique maximizes cancer control, preserves neurovascular tissue (in appropriate candidates), and is based on the anatomic principles laid down by Walsh[6,7] and the Vattikuti Institute prostatectomy (VIP) procedure developed by Menon.[8,9] The modifications we have introduced include absolute avoidance of all thermal energy and coagulative necrosis in posterior dissection, avoidance of bulldog clamps on neurovascular tissue, a simplified maneuver to identify the bladder neck, use of a scissors instead of hook for the entire procedure, an anatomic technique for restoration of the continence mechanism, and integration of specimen examination prior to the completion of surgery. In line with the principles of anatomic radical prostatectomy, our technique includes obturator lymph node dissection in all patients and more extensive dissection in high-risk patients.

ANATOMIC CONSIDERATIONS

Our technique is based on anatomic and clinical studies conducted by the Cornell Institute of Robotic Surgery, New York, in close collaboration with the Institute of Urology at the University of Innsbruck in Austria. The anatomic studies were primarily aimed at providing an intraoperative neural map for robotic prostatectomy by depicting the location of neurovascular tissue in relation to the various steps of robotic prostatectomy.

Based on these studies, we found that relevant neurovascular plate around the prostate could be grouped into three zones called the trizonal neural architecture, which has been described at length in Chapter 2.[5] These zones are the proximal neurovascular plate (PNP), the predominant neurovascular bundle (PNB), and the accessory neural pathways (ANP).

Proximal Neurovascular Plate (PNP)

The PNP, located lateral to the bladder neck and seminal vesicle, is an integrating center for the processing and relay of erectogenic neural signals. This plate can get damaged during incision of the posterolateral aspect of the bladder neck, lateral dissection of the seminal vesicle, and/or mass clipping or cautery of prostatic pedicles.

Predominant Neurovascular Bundle (PNB)

The PNB lies in the depth of the prostatorectal groove and carries neuronal impulses to cavernous tissue. In 65% of cases, there is a medial extension behind the prostate, which converges medially at the apex in 30% of cases.

Accessory Neural Pathways (ANPs)

The ANPs lie within the layers of levator fascia and/or lateral pelvic fascia on the anterolateral or posterior aspect of the prostate and form a plexus near the apex in 35% of cases. This plexus acts as a neural pathway for both cavernous tissue and the urethral sphincter.

Fascial Layers

The prostatic capsule is surrounded by prostatic fascia, lateral pelvic fascia, levator fascia, and finally levator muscles. Interposed between the prostatic fascia and lateral pelvic fascia are the neurovascular tissue and the periprostatic venous plexus. This venous plexus and neurovascular tissue travel distally to innervate distal structures, including the sphincter, urethra, and cavernous tissue. Proper nerve sparing should leave an intact capsule covered preferably by a safety layer of prostatic fascia (and some veins) on the specimen. During aggressive nerve sparing, a plane can develop deep to the prostatic fascia and veins that, although it provides maximum chances for potency, increases the risk of capsular incision.

INDICATIONS FOR SURGERY

The indications for robotic prostatectomy are the same as those for radical prostatectomy. Appropriately counseled and consenting patients with clinically localized prostatic cancer and a life expectancy of more than 10 years are candidates for the procedure. Although no absolute contraindications exist, certain conditions may pose challenges to the novice robotic surgeon. These include obese patients (body mass index [BMI] > 35), multiple previous abdominal or pelvic surgeries with likelihood of adhesions, previous hernia repair, large-volume prostate (>100 g), neoadjuvant hormone therapy, and previous radiotherapy.

DECISION MAKING FOR NERVE SPARING

Based on previously recommended criteria,[10] patients were grouped into low-risk, intermediate-risk, and high-risk categories. Special emphasis was placed on intraoperative digital rectal examination (DRE) to evaluate palpability, location, and size of the tumor. To understand the utility of intraoperative DRE, an immediate reexamination was performed soon after the specimen was retrieved. This technique used detailed examination of the specimen for adequacy of surrounding tissue, area of nerve preservation, indurations, capsular breech, apical contour, shape and completeness, seminal vesicles, vas, and lymph nodes. Intraoperative frozen sections were taken to supplement visual clues while making decisions regarding wide excision of neurovascular bundles.

PREPARING THE PATIENT FOR SURGERY

The chief preoperative measures that we advocated were the strict implementation of a walking regimen, weight loss, and stopping blood thinners. The abdomen was examined for scars of previous surgery to aid in planning the port placement.

POSITIONING OF THE PATIENT

Before induction of anesthesia, the supine patient's buttocks are positioned a little beyond the leg break of the table so as to compensate for an expected cephalad slide of patient in extreme Trendelenburg. This avoids repositioning once the patient is anesthetized. The patient's legs are also supported in stirrups and kept in lithotomy position. After applying lower extremity sequential compression device cuffs, the arms of the patient are secured to the patient's side. Both hands are also protected using egg crate foam resting on the arm sleds. The sleds are positioned to give enough space for the assistants and to avoid inadvertent pressure on the hands by robotic arms. Similarly, foam and adhesive tape are used to support both shoulders in a crisscross manner over the chest, counteracting the gravity effects on the patient in the extreme Trendelenburg position. Custom-made foam, or a Shea headrest, is kept over the face to protect the intubation tube and to avoid inadvertent injury to the face.

In patients with restricted movement of abduction and flexion at the hip joint, preoperative positioning simulation is advisable. For these special patients, instead of using stirrups in the conventional manner, spreader bars or leg support at the table edge should be used, depending on the height of the patient.

PORT PLACEMENT

Port placement is an integral part of the surgery, and success of the procedure depends on this intricate task.

Camera Port

We create a pneumoperitoneum using a Veress needle introduced through a periumbilical puncture. The camera port position is usually 2.5 cm below the level of the umbilicus. However, this cannot be applied as a universal rule. The umbilical position varies depending on the height and weight of the patient, and the port position must be appropriately adapted to each body type. Creating a pneumoperitoneum is similar for robotic and non–robotic-assisted laparoscopic procedures. We insert a bladed 12-mm trocar (Ethicon, Somerville, NJ) with the direction of blade in the midline. This blade orientation is necessary because the fascia is further incised vertically at the end of the case to properly retrieve the final specimen. In obese patients, it is always better to use a long cannula for the camera arm trocar. This will help prevent inadvertent port dislodgment resulting from the frequently extreme pitch and yaw movements of the camera arm. A 30-degree lens is used for peritoneoscopy and for visualizing the anterior abdominal wall during placement of secondary ports. Two 8-mm ports are placed, one on each side 8 to 10 cm from the midline and about 2.5 cm below the level of the umbilicus. These are the *robotic ports* for the working arms of the robot. A 5-mm *suction port* is introduced between the camera port and the 8-mm port on the right side. A 12-mm port is placed in the midaxillary line on the right side about 1.5 inches superior to the iliac crest. Another 5-mm port is introduced symmetric and contralateral to the 12-mm port. These are the *assistant ports* (Figure 6–1).

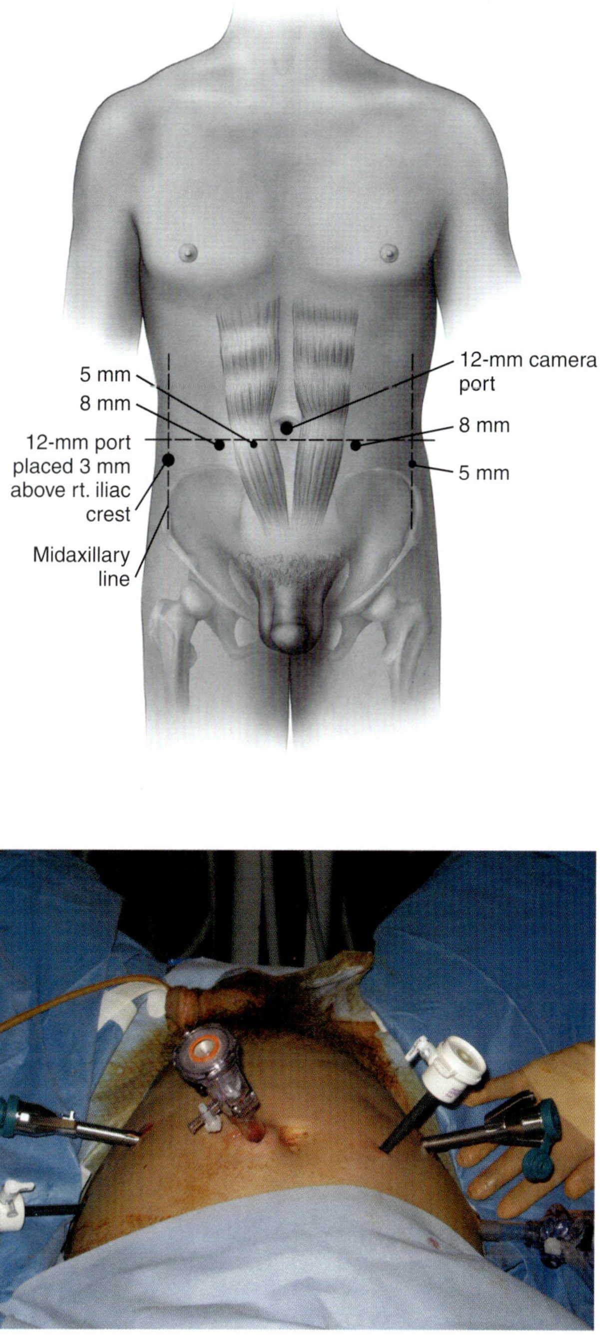

FIGURE 6–1 Port placement.

DOCKING THE ROBOT

Before docking the robot at the patient, the assistant should make sure that the camera arm is vertically straight and flexed with the second joint toward the left side of the patient. For a right-handed surgeon at the console, the dominant robotic arm (right arm) moves more than the nondominant arm. The distance between the posts of the first and third joint should be equal to about two fists. This distance invariably establishes the floor position of the robot tower core. With this ideal arrangement, the distance from the center column of the robot to the edge of the table is usually from 50 to 60 cm. This careful tower positioning helps in obtaining an ergonomically similar position of the robotic arms, mimicking that of human arms during open surgery.

LENS CHOICE

We use a 30-degree lens angled upward for initial bladder and prostate mobilization. This is followed by a 0-degree lens for defatting the anterior surface of the prostate, exposing the endopelvic fascia, taking the initial dorsal venous complex (DVC) bunching suture, taking the proximal bladder neck suture by bimanual pinch, and performing posterior and anterior apical prostate dissection and the vesicourethral anastomosis. A 30-degree lens angled downward is used for the bladder neck incision, seminal vesicle and vasa dissection, control of the prostate pedicles, and neurovascular bundle dissection. On average, there are four lens changes in a typical procedure.

CURRENT TECHNIQUE

Our present technique reflects our current understanding of trizonal neural architecture, compensatory maneuvers to operate in a visually rich 3D platform, and our protocol for selecting patients for nerve sparing and wide excision. Overall, this approach could be either transperitoneal or extraperitoneal. The retropubic space is developed and the anterior surface of the prostate, endopelvic fascia, apex, and prostatovesical junction is defatted, and important landmarks such as puboprostatic ligaments, arcus tendineus, and prostatovesical junction are identified.

Development of Space of Retzius

We place a camera through the 12-mm camera port and perform laparoscopy with a 30-degree lens angled downward. Adhesiolysis is performed if required. The cecum and sigmoid colon are mobilized. The medial umbilical ligament, urachus, vas deferens, and internal ring are identified and used as landmarks for further dissection. The vas is seen coursing laterally to the internal ring and is divided medial to the internal ring and lateral to the medial umbilical ligaments. The incision is deepened, and fat and areolar tissue teased away until the transversalis fascia is seen. The external iliac vein is identified, and dissection is carried down to the anterior pelvic ramus. We keep the dissection medial to the epigastric vessels.

An identical dissection is carried out on the opposite side. The two vertical incisions are then joined across the midline in an inverted U-shaped manner above the pubis (Figure 6–2). The incision is deepened, and the pubic arch completely exposed. While dropping the bladder, integrity of the posterior transversalis fascia should not be breached and fat covering endopelvic fascia and anterior surface of the prostate is dissected. Adherence to these principles is important to provide adequate surgical exposure during robotic prostatectomy. This is particularly true in difficult cases such as obesity, narrow pelvis, large prostate, previous pelvic or inguinal surgery, salvage surgery, or any combination of these.

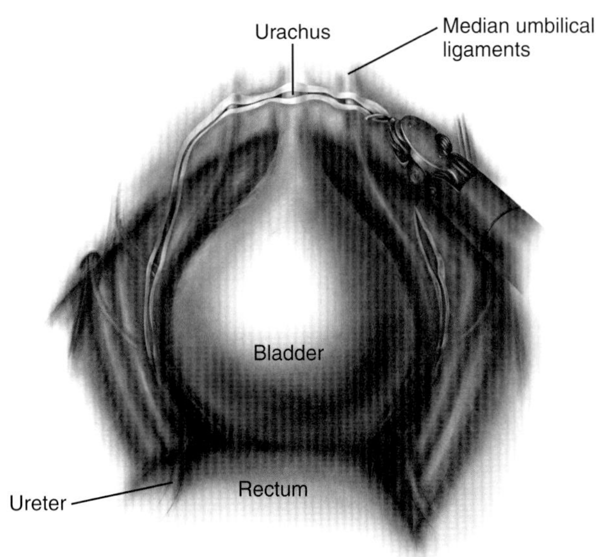

FIGURE 6–2 U-shaped incision for dropping the bladder.

Exposure of Apex and Endopelvic Fascia

Once the pubic arch is seen, fat is cleared to reveal the glistening fibers of the endopelvic fascia. The fat near the apex of the prostate is also cleared to reveal the puboprostatic ligaments and the DVC. We do not tackle the DVC now but rather toward the end just before urethral transection when the prostate is mobile. The endopelvic fascia is now opened sharply using the sharp tip of the multijointed robotic scissors. A single downward stroke is used to make a distal incision in the fascia limited to the proximal third of the prostate and cautery is avoided (Figure 6–3*A* and *B*). The levator fascia is swept off the lateral surface of the prostate. The distal limit of the incision is the sickle-shaped extension of the puboprostatic ligaments, which are preserved by avoiding lateral dissection. The fibers of the levator ani are seen below the incision. The lateral attachments of the apex are partially freed at this stage. At the end of this step of dissection, the intact puboprostatic ligaments are seen in continuity with the fascia on either side (Figure 6–3*C*).

Bladder Neck Transection

The subtle and gradual transition of bladder to prostate makes the clear identification of prostatovesical junction difficult. There is a strategic area located anteriorly where a mucosal tube joins the bladder mucosa to the urethra. This tube is usually superficial and covered by a thin layer of detrusor apron and the proximal extension of dorsal venous complex. Once a back bleeding stitch has been placed in the midprostate and another suture bunches up the veins on the bladder side, development of this anterior plane is easy and without much bleeding. We call this technique the *bimanual bladder neck pinch* for identification of anterior bladder neck.[11] This part of the dissection is performed with a 30-degree lens angled downward. We place a stitch with 0 Vicryl on the anterior surface of the prostate proximal to the puboprostatic ligaments to prevent back bleeding and also for traction (Figure 6–4*A*). Another bunching stitch is placed in the bladder superficially for traction. Using robotic forceps and scissors, the prostate is trapped on both sides and pulled proximally and medially with gentle distal traction on the Foley catheter until the prostatovesical junction is easily identified (Figure 6–4*B*). The left-sided assistant pulls the prostatic traction suture to the foot of the patient. The surgeon provides firm countertraction with the da Vinci forceps. The surface is scored to precisely mark the prostatovesical junction anteriorly. The anterior bladder neck is then incised in a curvilinear manner. We use a Maryland bipolar forceps and hot shears with 1:1 scaling for adequate coagulation of the bleeders. The dissection is deepened until the Foley catheter is seen (Figure 6–4*C*).

Identification of the Foley catheter ensures that the anterior bladder neck has been incised appropriately. The catheter is delivered out of the bladder. The Foley balloon is deflated

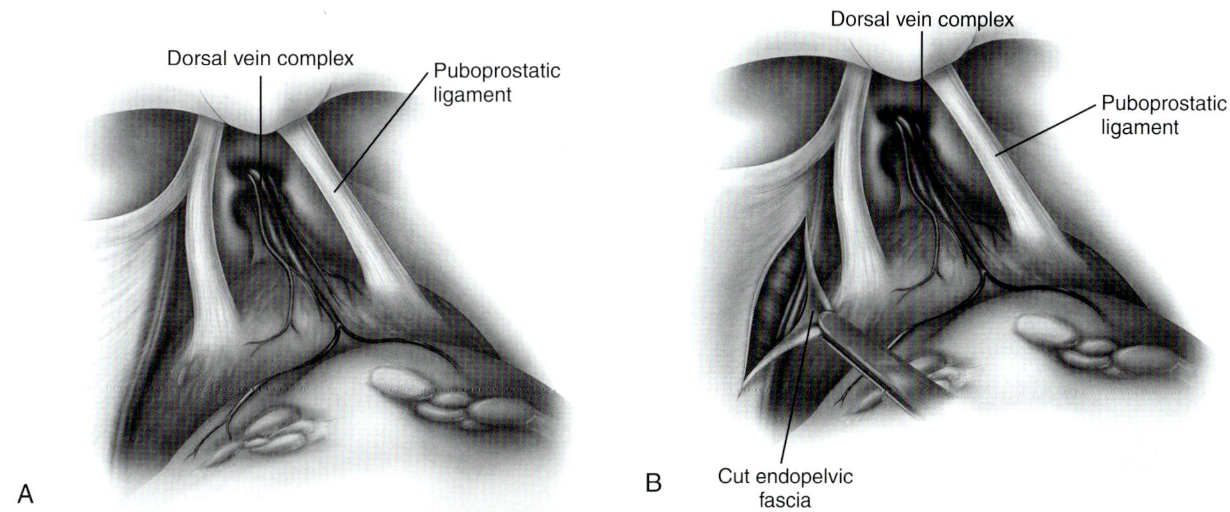

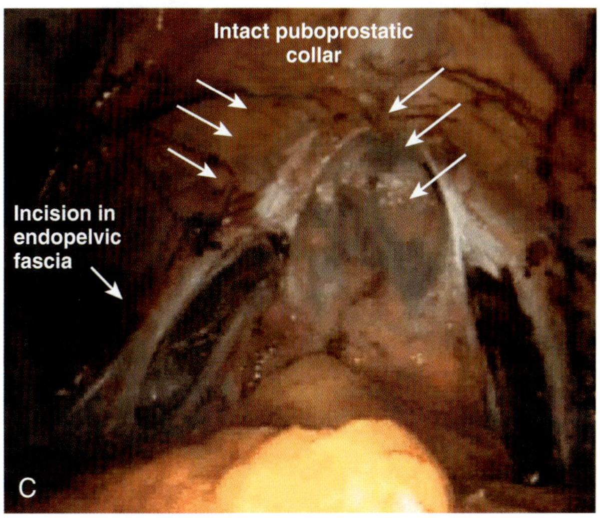

FIGURE 6–3 *A*, Fat near pubic arch cleared to reveal the endopelvic fascia (EPF). *B*, Limited distal incision in the left endopelvic fascia sparing the puboprostatic ligaments (PPLs). *C*, Bilateral incisions in the EPF with intact puboprostatic collar.

now, and the left-side assistant grasps the tip of the catheter with firm anterior traction. The anterior bladder neck incision is widened laterally with cautery in the fibrofatty plane between bladder and prostate. With traction on the shaft of the catheter, the exact location for the posterior incision becomes visible and the mucosa of the posterior bladder neck is now incised precisely. Every precaution is taken to preserve the anatomic bladder neck as far as is possible and avoid injury to the ureteric orifices. The posterior incision is modified according to the size and configuration of the prostate. The incision is deepened, keeping tangential to the prostate and avoiding any undermining into the substance of the prostate. Vertical downward dissection also protects against inadvertent undermining of the trigone or buttonholing of the bladder. Brisk bleeding from fibromuscular tissue at this at this stage is a warning that dissection may have extended into the prostate. The catheter is now withdrawn into the urethra, and the left-sided assistant retracts the posterior prostatic base anteriorly. We then develop a plane behind the posterior wall of the bladder neck that exposes the retrotrigonal layer.[12]

Seminal Vesicle and Vas Dissection

Anatomically, the vas and seminal vesicles are enclosed in a space bound by the retrotrigonal layer anteriorly, neurovascular tissue and prostatic pedicle laterally, rectum and Denonvilliers' fascia posteriorly, trigone and bladder base superiorly, and prostatic base inferiorly. Both the vas and seminal vesicles have their own sheaths and blood supply. The vesiculodeferential artery, a branch of the superior vesical artery along with a few branches of the inferior vesical artery, supplies the seminal vesicles near its tip.

We start the dissection by opening the retrotrigonal layer and exposing the anterior surface of the vasa (Figure 6–4*D*). Although the vas and seminal vesicles are relatively attached near the prostate, they are slightly separate proximally under the trigone. Therefore, we develop a plane within the perivasal sheath and isolate the vasa proximally. The vasa are grasped, and surrounding vessels are controlled with 5-mm surgical clips. The proximal vasa are clipped with Hemolok clips and divided.

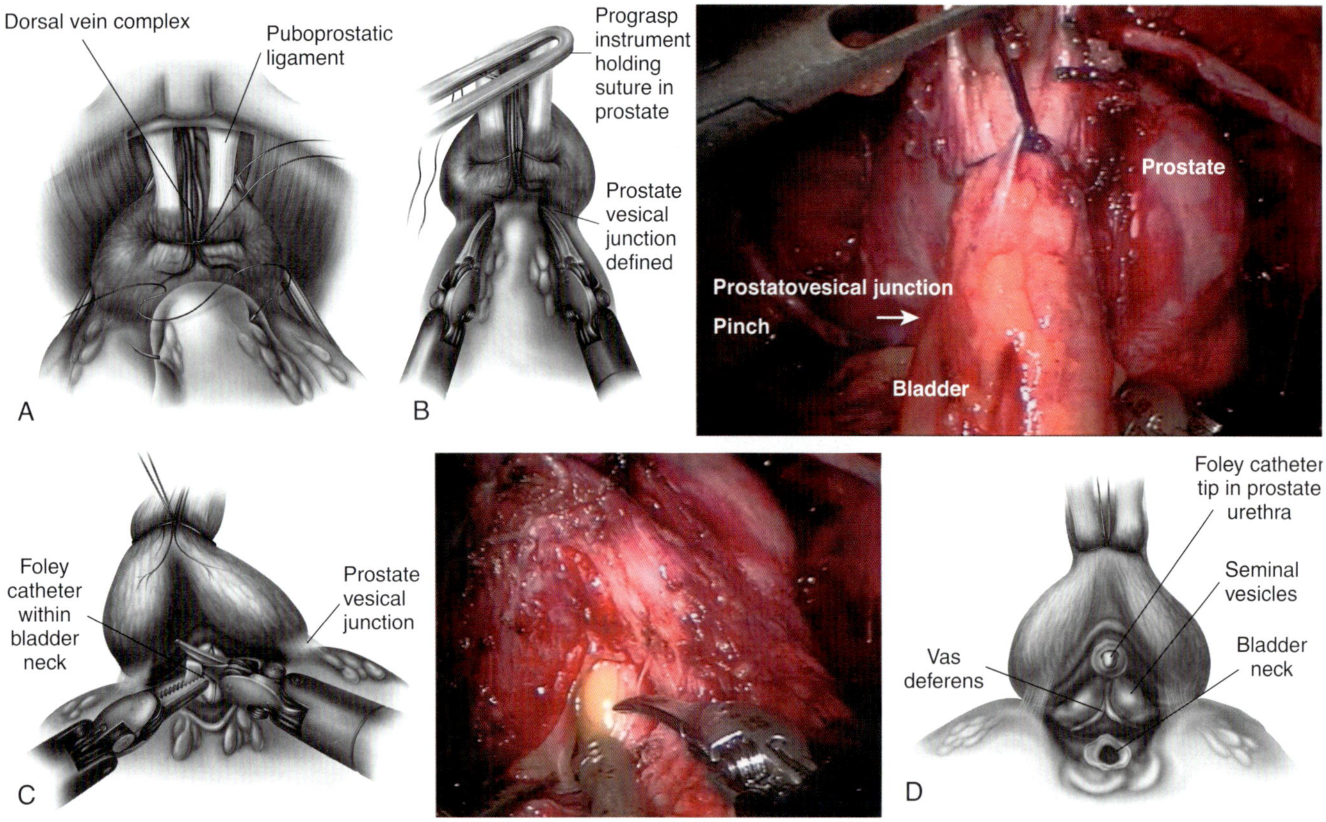

FIGURE 6–4 *A,* Traction suture on the prostate. *B,* The bladder neck pinch. *C,* Anterior bladder neck transaction and urethra incised—Foley catheter seen within. *D,* Posterior bladder neck transected and both seminal vesicles in view.

We have noted that the seminal vesical sheath surrounds the vesicles and most of the vessels travel through the sheath. Medially, the plane is quite avascular and easy to develop. Therefore, we start the dissection by developing this medial avascular plane and extracting the vesicles from this sheath. As we come close to the tip, the seminal vesicular blood supply is bunched together as a pedicle and controlled using a 5-mm locking clip. Laterally, several vessels and the PNP are located within 5 to 10 mm from the surface of the vesicles and are in danger of getting thermally damaged or crushed in large clips, thus temporarily or permanently affecting recovery of erectile function. Therefore, this part of the dissection is performed athermally by developing small pedicles and controlling them with 5-mm surgical clips or suturing them close to the surface of the seminal vesicle. Electrocautery is avoided. Both seminal vesicles and vasa are lifted up to expose the posterior surface of the prostate (Figure 6–5).

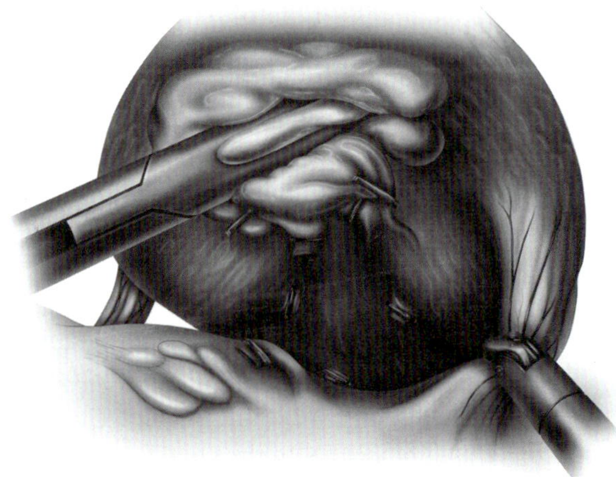

FIGURE 6–5 Dissection of right seminal vesicle (SV). Left SV dissected and left vas clipped.

Separation of Prostate from Rectum

We have noted in our anatomic dissections that there are communicating nerve fibers, which cross over to the other side at various levels through the layers of Denonvilliers' fascia. These fibers are most marked distally where they form a distal plexus behind the apex and membranous urethra. It is often written in colorectal literature that to preserve sexual function during rectal surgery, Denonvilliers'

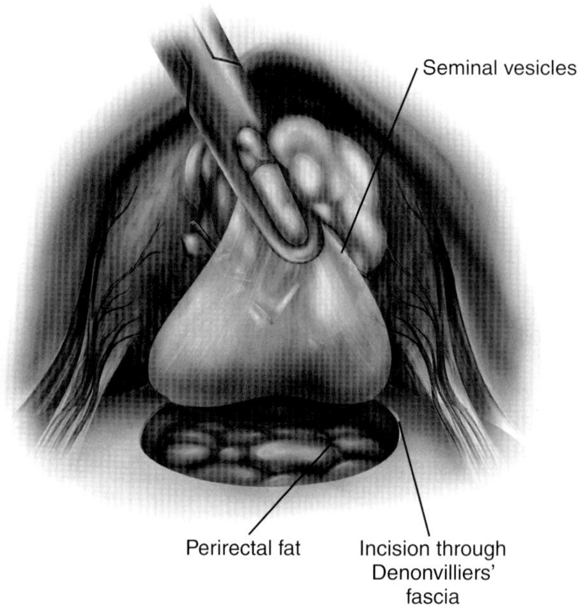

FIGURE 6–6 U-shaped incision in Denonvilliers' fascia in high-risk cases.

fascia should be left in the body because autonomic nerves run superficially through its layers. It is a conventional dogma in prostatic surgery that the Denonvilliers' fascia must be excised in every patient (even in early T_{1C}) undergoing radical prostatectomy. This may have been a safe oncologic principle in the pre–prostate-specific antigen (PSA) era when cancers were relatively more advanced locally at diagnosis. However, in the current era of early diagnosis, in patients with low-risk disease who are candidates for nerve sparing, a partial thickness of Denonvilliers' fascia can be left behind over the rectum without compromising oncologic safety. We always excise the fascia in patients who are not candidates for nerve sparing and have an abnormal DRE, suspicion of extracapsular extension on endorectal magnetic resonance imaging (MRI), high-volume cancer (>2 positive cores or >22% cancer in each core), Gleason score of 7 or more, and apical cancers. In these patients, traction is applied over both vasa and seminal vesicles, and an inverted U-shape incision is made over the base of the prostate and continued on the prostatic undersurface. Care should be taken to leave both layers of the Denonvilliers' fascia on the specimen and expose the prerectal fat. This dissection is continued distally to the apex (Figure 6–6). The oncologic results of our strategy are presented in the next section.

Lateral Pedicle Control

The prostatic pedicle includes arteries and veins entering the prostate and is intermixed with proximal neurovascular plate. There are two distinct components: (1) medial, supplying the base of the seminal vesicles and prostate, and (2) lateral, entering the prostate at its base on the posterior lateral aspect. The lateral component is the predominant pedicle whose shape, thickness, and width vary based on the anatomic variations and size of the prostate. Differentiating the prostatic pedicle from the proximal neurovascular plate and the predominant neurovascular bundles often presents a challenge to the surgeon. Sometimes a plane is readily apparent between the prostatic pedicle and nerve bundle, and at other times, a plane is created with the robotic forceps and then selective clipping or ligation of the prostatic vessels is performed (Figure 6–7). The key is to stay close to the prostate, dissect the vessels in small packets, identify them entering the prostate, and control them athermally with small clips and individual pedicle controls. Electrocautery and mass ligature are avoided. The orientation, size, and extent of the pedicle vary significantly depending on prostate anatomy and cancer-induced neovascularization. Hence, sufficient time should be invested to gently free the prostate base.

Traction on the vas and seminal vesicles will cause the prostatic pedicles to become more prominent. With the prostate lifted upward, the medial pedicle is identified and controlled close to the prostate using a clip. We then focus on the lateral pedicles. Starting medially we develop two to four small pedicles close to the prostate and control them with 5-mm clips. This exposes the undersurface of the prostate and gently separates the PNP from the dissection zone. We now switch to a 0-degree lens to visualize the entire posterior surface of the prostatic capsule and superficial layers of Denonvilliers' fascia. A slight contralateral traction exposes the few remaining vessels entering the prostate, which are then clipped and cut.

Release of Neurovascular Bundles

When the prostate is freed from the vascular pedicle, it becomes more mobile and can be rotated to expose the neurovascular triangle, which is a potential avascular triangle bounded posteriorly by the Denonvilliers' fascia, laterally by the levator fascia, and medially by prostatic capsule covered by prostatic fascia (Figure 6–8*B*).[13] Once this triangular space springs open, the rest of the dissection appears very elegant and is done by pushing the prostate away from the bundles. If this is done athermally using clips, tissues are not coagulated or desiccated and natural tissue texture is preserved (Figure 6–8*A*).

Depending on the preoperative estimation of the extent of cancer, we develop a plane very close to the prostate (just on the prostatic capsule—aggressive nerve sparing/intrafascial) or close (outside the prostatic fascia but within the lateral pelvic fascia, which is safe nerve sparing—most commonly performed/interfascial) or far from the prostate (leaving a few medial layers of lateral pelvic fascia on the specimen—partial/incremental nerve sparing). The extent of the

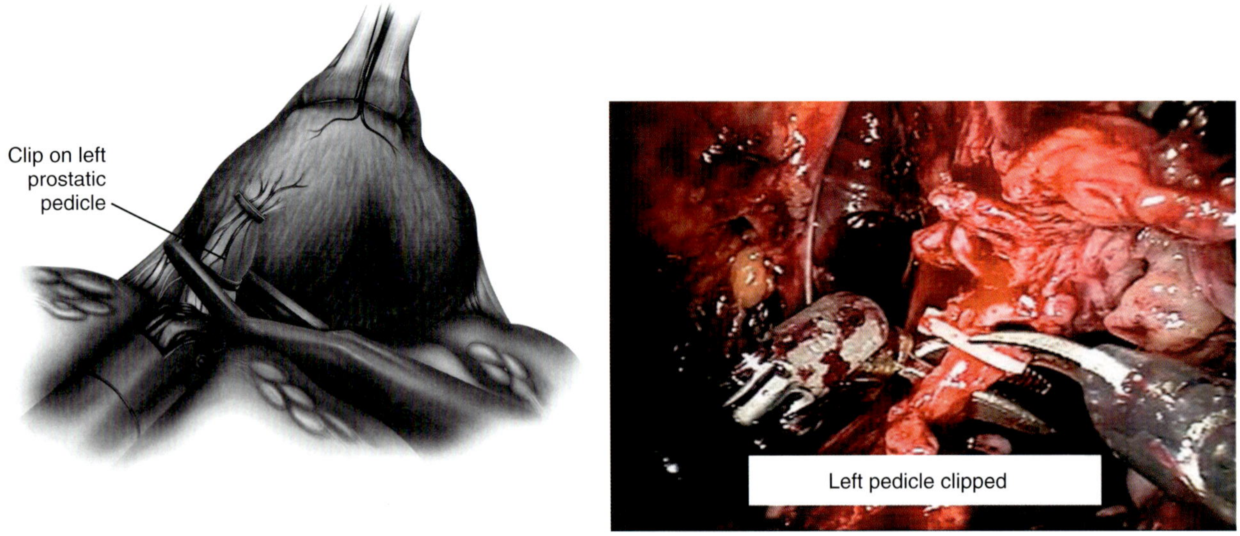

FIGURE 6–7 Control of left lateral pedicle.

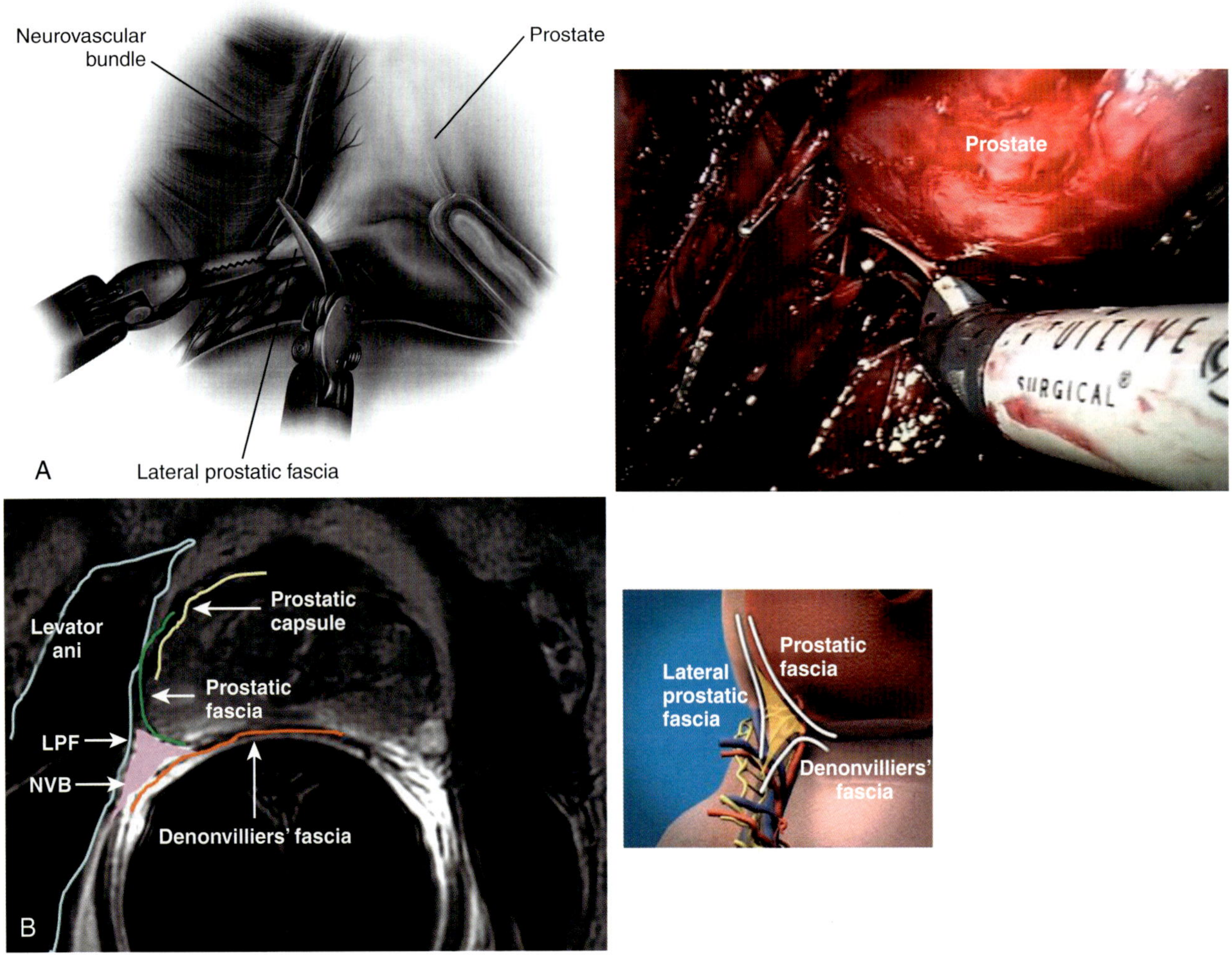

FIGURE 6–8 *A*, Release of left neurovascular bundle. *B*, Neurovascular triangle bounded posteriorly by Denonvilliers' fascia, laterally by levator fascia, and medially by prostatic fascia.

preserved fascia (and enclosed nerves) is well described in elegant articles by Menon and associates (veil of Aphrodite).[14] They recommend that the incision be quite anterior to handle those nerve fibers that are deviated anteriorly while destined to continue as cavernous nerves beyond the pelvic hiatus.

Thus, in the trizonal approach, we incorporate the anterior incision as recommended by Menon and associates. In addition, in appropriate cases, we preserve the retroapical plexus by leaving distally a layer of superficial Denonvilliers' fascia. These two modifications maximize preservation of accessory nerves responsible for sexual function.

Trizonal Nerve Preservation

Our trizonal approach described herein minimizes damage to all three neural zones, including the PNP, the PNB, and the accessory pathways. Obviously, the extent of nerve sparing and the plane of dissection depend on the extent, location, and proximity of cancer to the capsule of the prostate.

Antegrade versus Retrograde and Synchronous Nerve Preservation

In robotic surgery, neurovascular bundles (NVB) are usually released antegradely; that is, dissection continues distally (as described earlier). In patients with large prostates or wide prostatic pedicles and in patients with apical variations, we release the bundles retrogradely and continue proximally up to the pedicles. Next, we approach the release antegradely until the prostate is attached to the body only through a clearly defined pedicle, which is controlled and prostate released.

Apical Dissection, Dorsal Vein of the Prostate Ligation, and Urethral Transection

With the prostate freed all around, we embark on distal dissection of the apex. Apical dissection is the most critical step in robotic prostatectomy. Dissection at this point will have a profound impact on the three important outcomes of this surgery: apical margin, continence, and sexual function. There are significant anatomic variations in prostatic shape and its relationship to the distal sphincter complex, nerves, and urethra. Variations in shape can significantly affect the level of membranous urethral transaction. Unrecognized variations could result in either apical positive margins or loss of significant urethral length.

Traction is exerted on the prostate, and the DVC is sutured with 0 Vicryl. The suture is passed over the dorsal vein and underneath the puboprostatic ligaments on the right and then brought out on the left over the dorsal vein and underneath the ligament (Figure 6–9*A*). Two or three such throws are taken and then tied. Thus, the DVC is sutured, taking every precaution to avoid including the puboprostatic ligaments and always taking cognizance of the rhabdosphincter and the neural branches for continence. The prostate is held under proximal traction, and using the Endowrist round-tip scissors, the DVC and the anterior urethra are cut proximal to the puboprostatic ligaments (Figure 6–9*B*). The posterior urethra is then cut, ensuring dissection and separation of the neurovascular bundles and taking cognizance of the accessory pathways posteriorly, that is, the posterior plexus. Care is taken to leave as long a urethral stump as possible without compromising cancer control. The arcus tendineus, the lateral leaflet of the endopelvic fascia, and the preserved puboprostatic ligaments on either side form a collar of tissue around then urethral stump left behind after prostatectomy. Frozen sections are then taken from the margins of the urethral stump and sent for analysis.

Almost the entire neurovascular tissue converges to the apex, and the distal and posterior plexus can be damaged during urethral transection and anastomosis. The visual angles are changed several times to allow identification of both bundles and their relationship with the sphincter.

Total Anatomic Restoration of the Continence Mechanism

Posterior Reconstruction

We use a combination of two techniques, the Pagano suture[15] and the Rocco technique,[16] for posterior reinforcement, which is performed prior to urethrovesical anastomosis. A 2-0 Vicryl suture is placed across the posterior bladder neck, 3 cm from the everted edge of the bladder neck, and this is tied down reinforcing the bladder neck. This imbrication procedure probably serves to prevent opening of the bladder neck as the bladder is filled. Using the same suture, the posterior median raphe is joined proximally to the residual Denonvilliers' fascia, and this is now fixed to the posterior bladder wall, the aim being to restore the functional and anatomic length of the urethral sphincter (Figure 6–12*C*).

Urethrovesical Anastomosis

Urethrovesical anastomosis is performed in a continuous running fashion in a manner described previously by Van Velthoven et al.[17] and Menon et al.[18] Two 9-inch 3-0 Monocryl sutures on an RB needle are used, one dyed and the other undyed. Their tails are tied extracorporeally using 10 knots. The anastomosis is begun with the dyed suture and proceeds in a clockwise direction, with the posterior wall secured first (Figure 6–11). The first throw is taken at the 4 o'clock position in the posterior bladder neck from the outside-in and continued in the urethra inside-out. After the first three sutures, the suture is locked thrice, bringing the bladder down to the urethra and forming the posterior plate. The anastomosis is continued in a clockwise manner until the 11 o'clock position, where it is held under traction either by the assistant or by inserting the needle into the pelvic side wall.

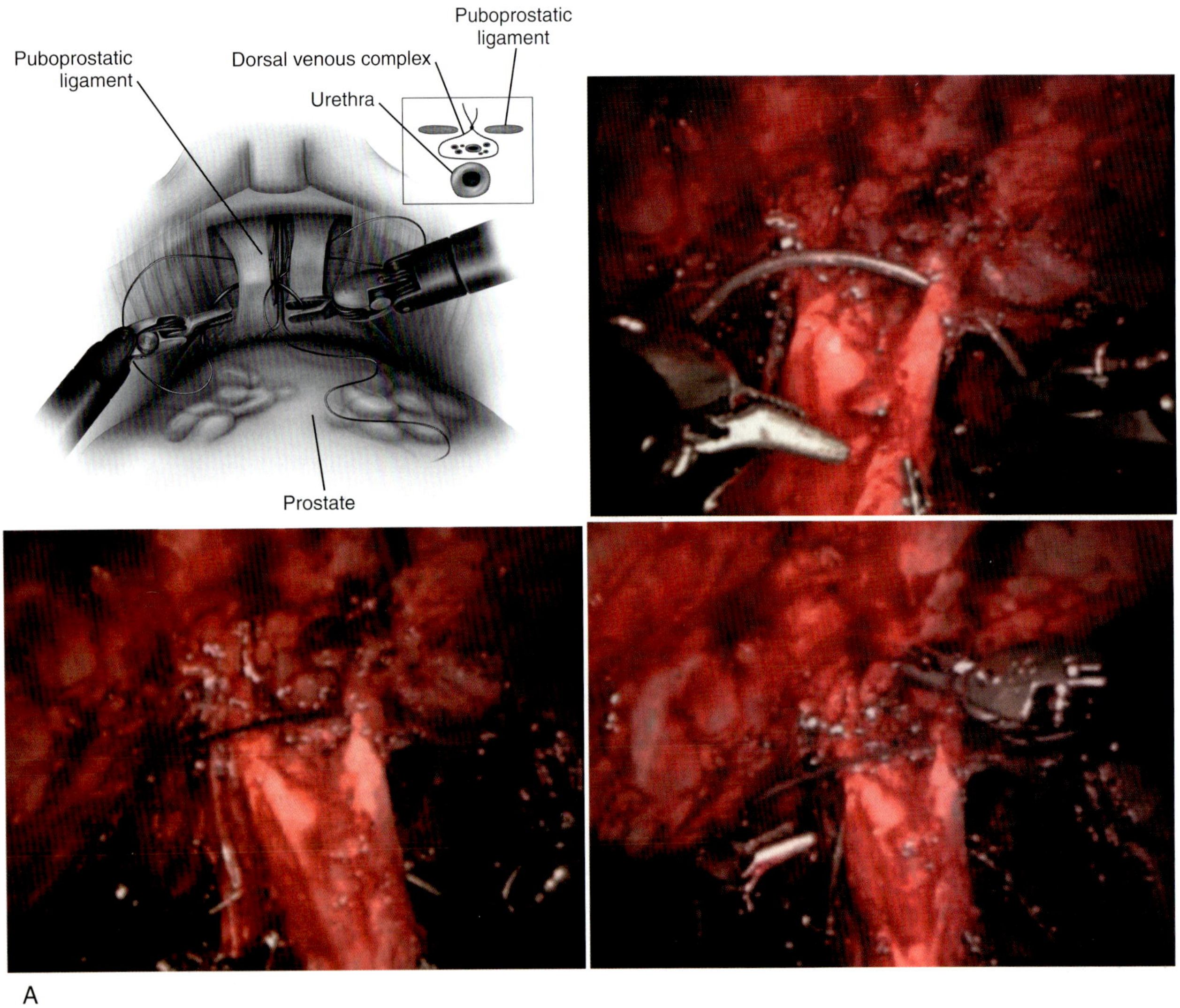

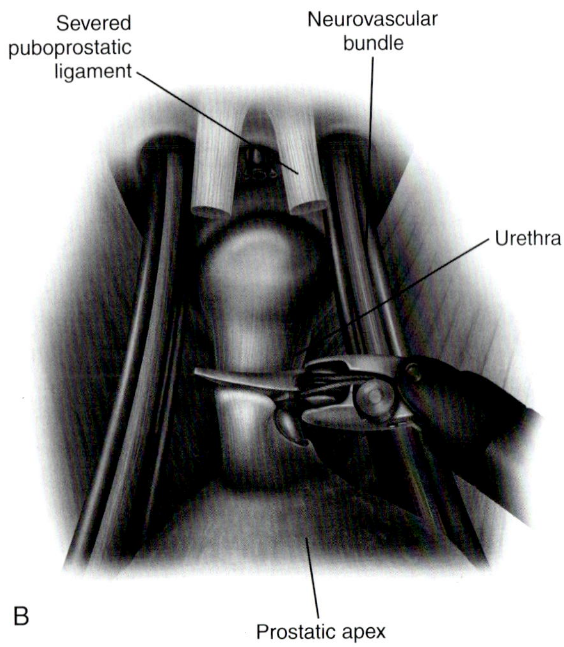

FIGURE 6–9 *A*, Dorsal venous complex. Stitch is taken sparing the puboprostatic ligaments. Needle is passed from midline laterally below the right puboprostatic ligament. The needle is passed posterior to the dorsal venous complex anterior to urethra from right to left. The needle is passed from lateral to medial below the left puboprostatic ligament. *B*, Urethral transection.

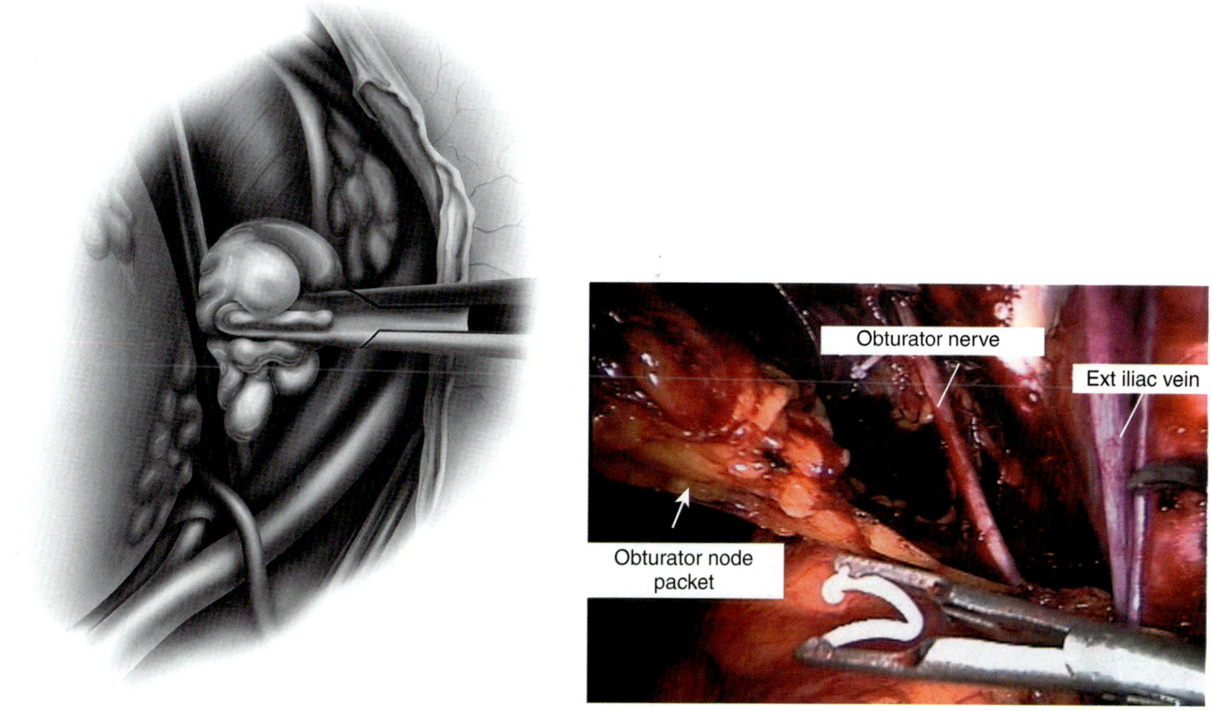

FIGURE 6–10 Right pelvic lymphadenectomy, obturator packet dissected.

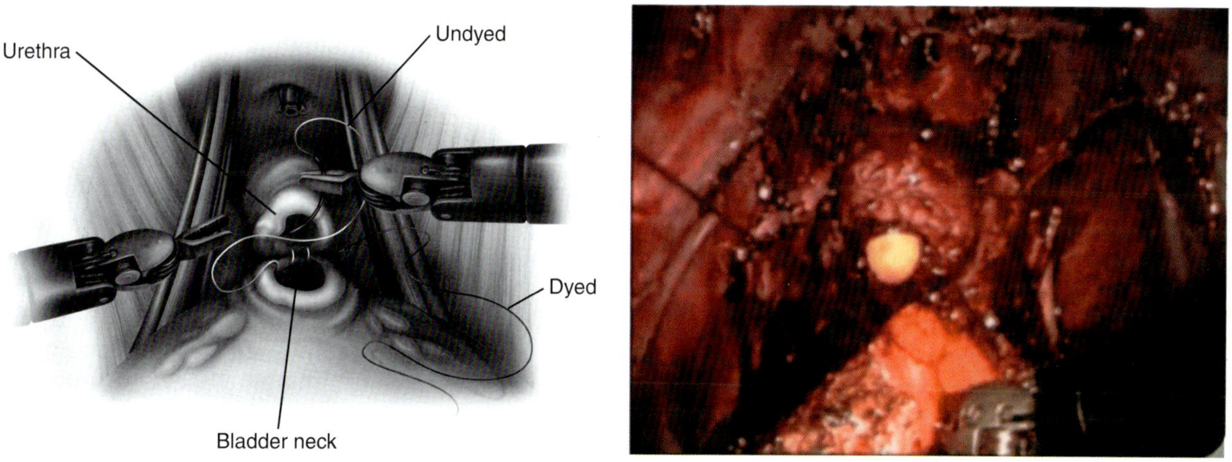

FIGURE 6–11 Urethrovesical anastomosis begun of the posterior wall.

Now the rest of the anastomosis is completed with the undyed suture in an anticlockwise manner. It is first passed outside-in on the urethra and inside-out on the bladder at the 4 o'clock position and continued up to the 11 o'clock position, where it meets the dyed suture. The needles are cut off, and the two ends tied together with multiple knots. During the entire anastomosis, the right-sided assistant plays an important role by pulling the catheter in and out as required to expose the urethral mucosa. The average time for the anastomosis is 12 minutes (range, 8–15 minutes).

Anterior Reconstruction

Our aim is to disturb the anatomy of the continence mechanism as little as possible with preservation and restoration of the puboprostatic collar. We avoid dissection lateral to the puboprostatic ligaments and preserve the arcus tendineus, which is the lateral support to the urethra. The puboprostatic ligaments are left intact until just before urethral transection. This helps protect the puboperinealis muscle, which offers hammock-like posterior support to the urethra, where

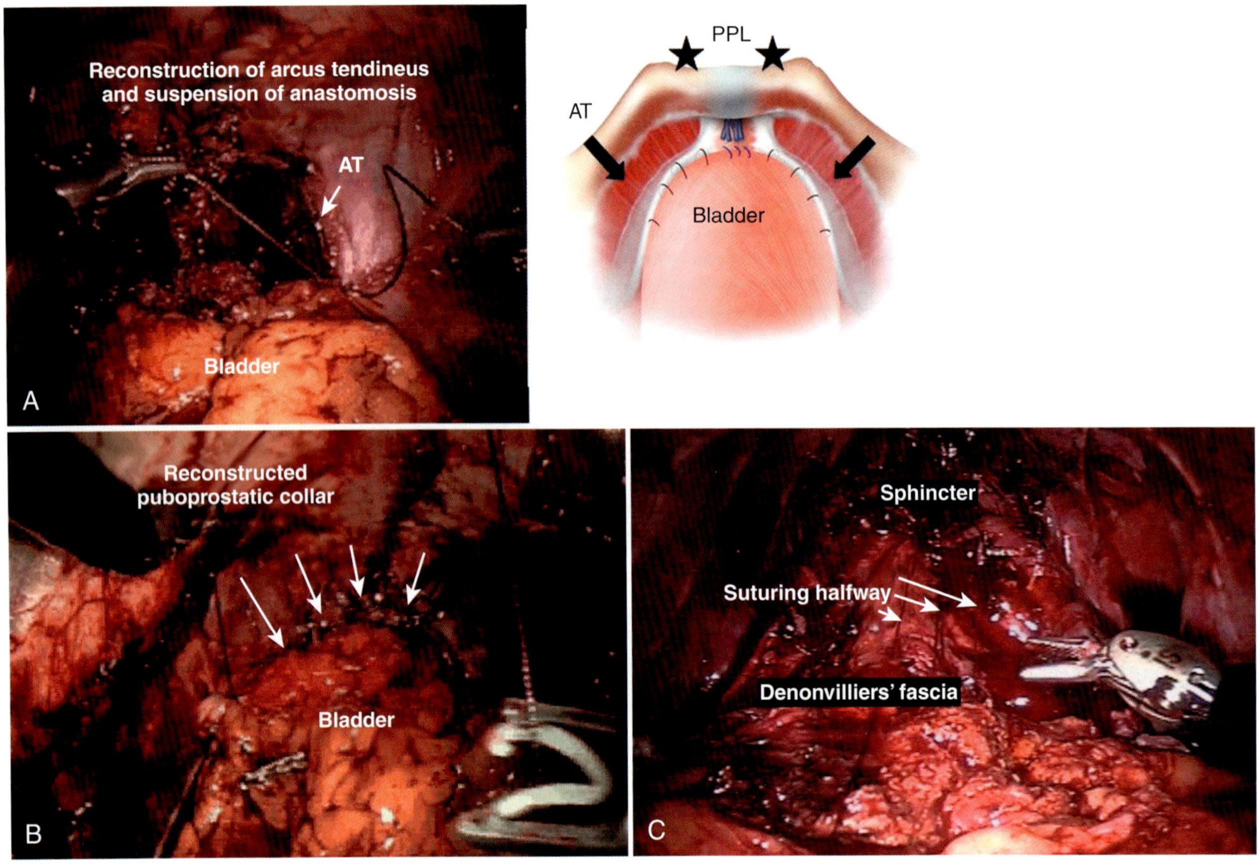

FIGURE 6–12 *A*, Reattachment of arcus tendineus (AT) to the bladder. *B*, Final picture of the reconstructed puboprostatic collar after arcus tendineus reattachment and suspension of anastomosis. *C*, Rocco stitch posteriorly suturing the dorsal median raphe to the Denonvilliers' fascia, fixing the sphincter posteriorly. PPL, puboprostatic ligament.

the sphincter is deficient.[19] Reattachment of the puboprostatic ligaments to the bladder restores anterior support.

The reconstruction of the arcus tendineus and suspension of anastomosis is achieved by using a running suture starting at the proximal aspect of the bladder neck.[20] Three continuous tacking sutures using 2-0 Vicryl on an RB1 needle are taken on either side between the puboprostatic collar left behind and the bladder (Figure 6–12*A* and *B*). The suturing approximates distal bladder and vesicourethral anastomosis to arcus tendineus, puboprostatic ligaments, and puboperinealis muscle and midline connective tissue on either side. The aim is to restore periurethral support. The average time taken for the anterior and posterior reconstruction is about 10 to 12 minutes.

BILATERAL PELVIC LYMPHADENECTOMY

Pelvic lymphadenectomy is performed with a 0-degree lens. The retroperitoneal fat is cleared from the anterior surface of the external iliac vein. The external iliac vessels are cleared of fatty tissue and lymph nodes. Dissection proceeds posteriorly until the obturator nerve, inferiorly until the femoral canal, and superiorly until the common iliac bifurcation. Extended pelvic lymphadenectomy is performed in patients with T_3 cancers, high-volume cancers, PSA more than 10 ng/mL, and Gleason score of 8 or higher. All fibrofatty tissue is removed posteriorly until the floor of the obturator fossa and medially until the side wall of bladder, and three nodal packages, that is, external iliac, internal iliac, and obturator, are labeled separately.

SPECIMEN RETRIEVAL AND PORT CLOSURE

An EndoCatch device is deployed from the right-side 12-mm port just after the prostate is isolated. The string attached to the endobag is left hanging outside the right-side assistant port. After the console procedure is complete, the long thread of the endobag is held with endoscopic grasping forceps and fed back through the right-side assistant port into the camera port under direct vision; the string is then taken out of the abdomen through this camera trocar. The paraumbilical camera port incision is then enlarged, depending on the volume of the prostate, and the specimen bag is removed. Because most of the ports are self-dilating, the paraumbilical camera port is the only port requiring fascial closure. An indwelling 18-French Foley catheter is inserted, and leakage is checked with instillation of 200 mL of saline. A 14-French Jackson-Pratt drain is left in to suck out any irrigation fluid that may have accumulated in the upper abdomen because of the Trendelenburg position.

INTRAOPERATIVE EXAMINATION OF THE SPECIMEN

Intraoperative examination of the specimen aids in decision making regarding handling of the NVB. In patients with high-grade cancers, with a preoperative endorectal MRI report of suspicious capsular penetration, or who demonstrate poorly developed planes between prostatic and lateral pelvic fascia, we remove the specimen immediately after apical transection. In all other cases, we remove it following anastomosis and examine the specimen. The examination is done by close inspection and palpation for its shape, apical contour, nodularity, indurations near posterior or lateral surface, and any iatrogenic violation of specimen integrity. Intraoperative frozen sections are taken of suspicious areas, and if the frozen section report or findings of palpation suggest involvement of NVB with cancer, we place clips on the bundles near the base and at the apex and excise them widely to ensure adequate oncologic control.

RESULTS

A total of 215 patients were operated on between January and December 2005 by the author (AT). The mean age of the patients was 60 years, and serum PSA was less than 10 ng/mL in 92.5% of patients. The majority of patients had a Gleason score of 6 (72.6%), and 4.7% patients had a Gleason score of 8 or higher. Using predescribed criteria, 182 patients (85%) underwent a bilateral nerve sparing using our trizonal-athermal technique, 24 patients (11%) underwent either an incremental nerve sparing (17 patients [7.9%]) or a nerve excision, advancement and end-to-end anastomosis (7 patients [3.1%]), and another 9 patients (4%) underwent wide excision.

Approximately 47% of patients had a Gleason score of 6 or less. Capsular invasion was seen in 36 patients (17%), perineural invasion in 104 (48%), and high-grade prostatic intraepithelial neoplasia (PIN) in 55 (26%). Surgical margins were positive in 14 (6.5%). The most common location of positive surgical margins was apical (25% of all positives). The overall PSA recurrence was seen in 7%.

We defined continence as the use of "0 pads" or a "security liner." Using this definition, our continence rates at 1 year were 92%. Following the introduction of the anterior reconstruction technique of continence, the continence rates at 1 year were 97%. Of patients who were preoperatively potent (sexual health inventory in men [SHIM] score >22) and who had nerve-sparing surgery, 80% were able to have an erection firm enough to have an intercourse or were actively having sexual intercourse at 1 year of follow-up (see Figure 6-11).

CONCLUSIONS

We have described the athermal robotic technique of robotic prostatectomy and have introduced the concept of trizonal nerve preservation. We have described a new anatomic technique for restoration of the continence mechanism. The oncologic and functional results with this technique are promising.

REFERENCES

1. Jemal A, Siegel R, Ward E, et al: Cancer statistics, 2007. CA Cancer J Clin 57:43–66, 2007.
2. Walsh PC: Radical prostatectomy for localized prostate cancer provides durable cancer control with excellent quality of life: a structured debate. J Urol 163:1802–1807, 2000.
3. Han M, Partin AW, Pound CR, et al: Long-term biochemical disease-free and cancer-specific survival following anatomic radical retropubic prostatectomy. The 15-year Johns Hopkins experience. Urol Clin North Am 28:555–565, 2001.
4. Chang SS, Peterson M, Smith JA Jr: Intraoperative nerve stimulation predicts postoperative potency. Urology 58:594–597, 2001.
5. Tewari A, Takenaka A, Mtui E, et al: The proximal neurovascular plate and the tri-zonal neural architecture around the prostate gland: importance in the athermal robotic technique of nerve-sparing prostatectomy. BJU Int 98:314–323, 2006.
6. Walsh PC, Lepor H, Eggleston JC: Radical prostatectomy with preservation of sexual function: anatomical and pathological considerations. Prostate 4:473–485, 1983.
7. Walsh PC: Anatomic radical prostatectomy: evolution of the surgical technique. J Urol 160:2418–2424, 1998.
8. Menon M, Hemal AK: Vattikuti Institute prostatectomy: a technique of robotic radical prostatectomy: experience in more than 1000 cases. J Endourol 18:611–619, 2004.
9. Menon M, Tewari A, Peabody J: Vattikuti Institute prostatectomy: technique. J Urol 169:2289–2292, 2003.
10. D'Amico AV, Whittington R, Malkowicz SB, et al: Biochemical outcome after radical prostatectomy, external beam radiation therapy, or interstitial radiation therapy for clinically localized prostate cancer. JAMA 280:969–974, 1998.

11. Tewari A, Rao SR: Anatomical foundations and surgical maneuvers for precise identification of the prostatovesical junction during robotic radical prostatectomy. BJU Int 98:833–837, 2006.
12. Tewari A, El-Hakim A, Rao SR, et al: Identification of the retrotrigonal layer as a key anatomic landmark during robotic assisted radical prostatectomy. BJU 98:829–832, 2006.
13. Tewari A, Peabody JO, Fischer M, et al: An operative and anatomic study to help in nerve sparing during laparoscopic and robotic radical prostatectomy. Eur Urol 43:444–454, 2003.
14. Kaul S, Bhandari A, Hemal A, et al: Robotic radical prostatectomy with preservation of the prostatic fascia: a feasibility study. Urology 66:1261–1265, 2005.
15. Moinzadeh A, Shunaigat AN, Libertino JA: Urinary incontinence after radical retropubic prostatectomy: the outcome of a surgical technique. BJU Int 92:355–359, 2003.
16. Rocco F, Carmignani L, Acquati P, et al: Restoration of posterior aspect of rhabdosphincter shortens continence time after radical retropubic prostatectomy. J Urol 175:2201–2206, 2006.
17. Van Velthoven RF, Ahlering TE, Peltier A, et al: Technique for laparoscopic running urethrovesical anastomosis: the single knot method. Urology 61:699–702, 2003.
18. Menon M, Tewari A, Peabody JO, et al: Vattikuti Institute prostatectomy, a technique of robotic radical prostatectomy for management of localized carcinoma of the prostate: experience of over 1100 cases. Urol Clin North Am 31:701–717, 2004.
19. Myers RP, Cahill DR, Kay PA, et al: Puboperineales: muscular boundaries of the male urogenital hiatus in 3D from magnetic resonance imaging. J Urol 164:1412–1415, 2000.
20. Tewari AK, Bigelow K, Rao S, et al: Anatomic restoration technique of continence mechanism and preservation of puboprostatic collar: a novel modification to achieve early urinary continence in men undergoing robotic prostatectomy. Urology 69:726–731, 2007.

CHAPTER 7

Ketan K. Badani • Michael J. Fumo • Mani Menon

Vattikuti Institute Prostatectomy (VIP) Technique and Current Analysis of Results

INTRODUCTION

Robotic radical prostatectomy has exploded in popularity in the United States among both practitioners and patients who continue to seek the benefits of this procedure. The robotic system offers several advantages over standard laparoscopy. Prominent among these are wristed movement of the robotic arms allowing six degrees of freedom (two more than laparoscopy), three-dimensional visualization, elimination of physiologic hand tremor with a sophisticated filtering system, and magnification for superior visualization of tissues. Given these advantages, we have developed a technique named the Vattikuti Institute prostatectomy (VIP) and have shown that it can overcome the steep learning curve of laparoscopic radical prostatectomy (LRP) for those with minimal laparoscopic skills and have further shown that it does provide superior outcome in cancer control, continence, and potency, rivaling the best open and LRP series.[1–4] At present, we have performed more than 2000 VIP procedures, the largest series in the world.

INDICATIONS FOR SURGERY

Robotic radical prostatectomy follows the tenets of traditional anatomic radical prostatectomy for the treatment of patients with localized adenocarcinoma of the prostate.[5] Our patents undergo a thorough preoperative evaluation, including serum prostate-specific antigen (PSA), international prostate symptom score (IPSS), sexual health inventory in men (SHIM), and incontinence questionnaire. Obesity is not a contraindication to this approach; however, in patients with morbid obesity (body mass index of ≥35), the perceived difficulty level has increased significantly during the operation. Previous abdominal surgery alone is also not an exclusion criterion. Multiple surgeries with the possibility of numerous adhesions or a hostile abdomen should give the surgeon pause to consider the best approach. Approximately one third of our patients had previous abdominal surgery. Need for a limited lysis of adhesions is commonplace, yet not restrictive to the robotic portion if done correctly. Surprisingly, in 5% to 10% of patients, adhesions are seen even in the absence of previous abdominal surgery. Operative position should be taken into account for patient screening, because the steep Trendelenburg position with a thoracic wrap and relative dehydration intraoperatively may exclude patients with cardiac and pulmonary comorbidities from this approach.

TECHNIQUE OF VIP

Preparation

Patients are admitted the day of surgery and receive deep venous thrombosis prophylaxis (heparin 5000 IU subcutaneously) and antibiotic prophylaxis (third-generation cephalosporin) preoperatively. Sequential compression devices are placed on the patient as well. The abdomen is shaved from the nipple to the groin. Bowel preparation is not deemed necessary. However, we do recommend a laxative or suppository the night prior to surgery to decompress the lower intestines.

Surgical Team

The VIP team includes one console-side surgeon along with two patient side assistants. One assistant is a physician; the other may be a physician, a physician's assistant (PA), or a registered nurse (RN). The operating surgeon is not scrubbed, and the patient side assistants place the ports, suction, and present the operative field to the console surgeon. The team should have some members facile with laparoscopy.

Patient Positioning

General endotracheal anesthesia is mandated given the laparoscopic nature of the surgery as well as the patient's positioning. An orogastric tube is also placed for the duration of the case and removed at the time of extubation. The patient is placed in a supine, modified lithotomy position with the arms at the sides of the body to avoid the risk of brachial plexus injury. This will then be transferred to a steep Trendelenburg position. Care is taken to adequately pad the pressure points and lower extremities. An 18-French Foley catheter is inserted in the sterile field, and the bladder is drained.

Port Placement

We perform VIP through a transperitoneal approach. Proper port placement is imperative for adequate robotic access to the pelvis. Three ports are required for the robotic arms and two to three ports for the assistants. Throughout our series, we have performed surgeries using a left-side and right-side assistant as part of our residency training process, thus necessitating three assistant ports; however, the procedure can just as easily be completed with only a right-side assistant, thus decreasing the number of assistant ports to two.

A pneumoperitoneum is created with a Veress needle introduced through a left periumbilical puncture. After raising initial pressures to 15 to 20 mm Hg for the placement of ports, the Veress needle is replaced with a 12-mm trocar and a 30-degree laparoscope is inserted to transilluminate the abdominal wall. The rest of the ports are then placed under direct vision starting with the two 8-mm metal trocars for robotic arms, which are placed 3 to 5 cm below the level of the umbilicus, lateral to the rectus muscle on either side. Next, a 12-mm trocar is placed in the midaxillary line, 2.5 cm above the right iliac crest for the right-side assistant. A 5-mm trocar is placed between the camera port and the right-side robotic port, and a second 5-mm trocar is then placed in left iliac fossa 5 cm above and lateral to the anterior superior iliac spine. It is important to remember that the position of each trocar insertion may vary from patient to patient as the anatomy of port placement varies based on height, weight, and previous operations.

Mobilization of Bladder—Creation of the Extraperitoneal Space

The remainder of the operation is performed in the extraperitoneal space. With the camera aimed 30 degrees up, an inverted U-incision is made using the cautery hook so that the horizontal part of the incision is high enough on the anterior wall of the abdomen to preclude injury to the bladder and each vertical limb is located lateral to the medial umbilical ligament extending to the vasa on both sides (Figure 7–1). This dissection is performed in the avascular plane involving the dissection of adipose and loose areolar tissue. The first landmark visualized is the pubic bone, and dissection is completed laterally on either side, anteriorly

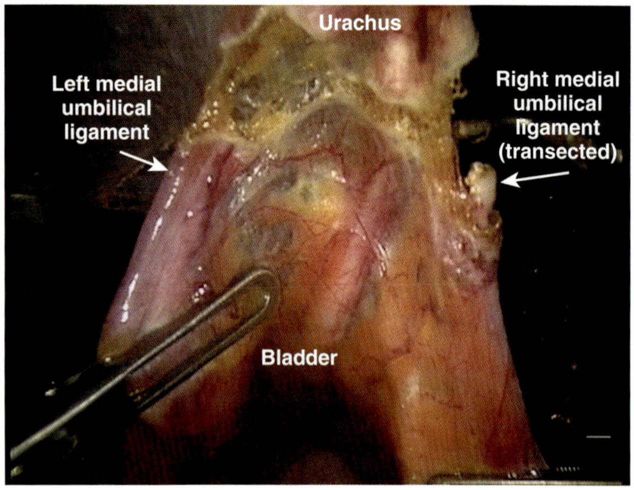

FIGURE 7–1 Mobilization of bladder—creation of the extraperitoneal space.

and completely exposing the endopelvic fascia bilaterally. This approach allows the bladder, prostate, and bowel to fall posteriorly, facilitating retraction during the posterior dissection.

Incision of the Endopelvic Fascia and Exposure of the Prostatic Apex

Incision of the endopelvic fascia and exposure of the prostatic apex is not necessary, because we routinely do not incise the endopelvic fascia, if an extensive nerve-sparing technique is to be performed. For standard nerve-sparing procedures and for those who are novice at the technique, incision of the endopelvic fascia allows for identification of the prostatic contour, location of neurovascular bundle and pedicle, and identification of the dorsal venous complex. The 0-degree lens with a 1:3 scaling is used. The endopelvic fascia is incised at the point at which it reflects over the pelvic side wall, thus exposing the levator ani muscle, which can then be gently dissected laterally to expose the lateral surfaces of the prostate (Figure 7–2). The incision is then extended toward the apex of the prostate to expose the dorsal vein, the urethra, and the striated urethral sphincter. The puboperinealis muscle covers the urethra and is the most anteromedial component of the levator ani; it has a special role in the urinary continence mechanism.[6] It is dissected bluntly from the apex of the prostate, thus exposing the urethra.

Dorsal Vascular Complex Ligation

Ligation of the dorsal vascular complex can be performed at two distinct points of the operation: either immediately after the endopelvic fascia is opened or after the urethra is transected. If performed after incision of endopelvic fascia, a 6-inch 0-braided polyglactin suture on a CT-1 taper needle

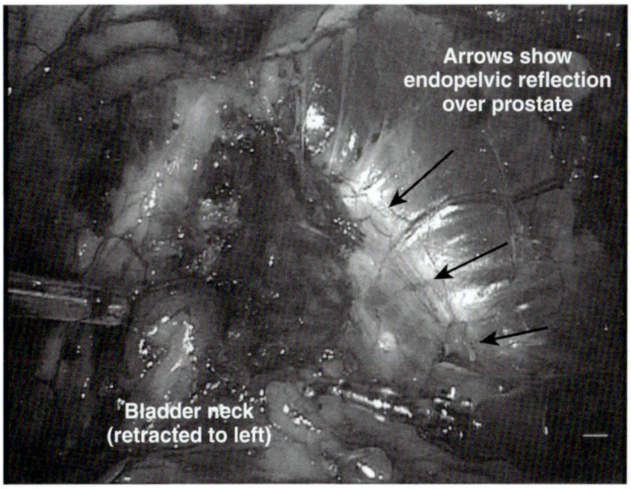

FIGURE 7–2 Reflection of prostate over endopelvic fascia with bladder retracted to the left.

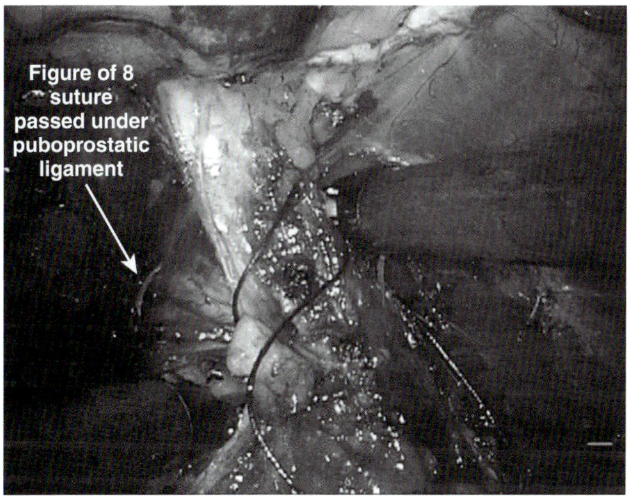

FIGURE 7–3 Dorsal venous stitch placed under puboprostatic ligaments.

is used to ligate the deep dorsal vein located behind the puboprostatic ligaments while attempting to exclude the puboprostatic ligaments (Figure 7–3). Technically, this is performed by passing the needle under the dorsal vein from one side to the other and then grasping it from the contralateral side and passing it above the dorsal vein complex and under the puboprostatic ligaments. If control of the complex is performed after transection of the urethra, a 2-0 polyglactin suture on a RB-1 needle is used in a running fashion to include the entire complex.

Dissection and Division of Bladder Neck

Dissection and division of the bladder neck is one of the more difficult steps of the VIP because there is no specific anatomic landmark. We use a 30-degree angled lens directed downward for the bladder neck dissection. The identification of the bladder neck can be very difficult given that only visual cues are used to find the prostatovesical junction. The patient side assistant will grasp the bladder and provide taut traction cephalad to expose this area. The movements of an inflated balloon inside the bladder may also aid in this maneuver. There is a shiny, smooth pad of fat that helps demarcate the prostatovesical junction. Starting laterally with a hook, gentle blunt dissection is used to find the area where the shiny prevesical fat ends and to make an incision there, which is then duplicated on the contralateral side. Both lateral incisions are then joined horizontally, thus dividing the anterior bladder neck in the midline. As the dissection is carried down, the catheter should be encountered, and after deflating the balloon, the tip of the Foley catheter can be delivered through this opening (Figure 7–4). The tip of the Foley catheter can then be grasped by an assistant and retracted upward to help visualize the rest of the dissection as the posterior wall of the bladder neck is divided. Great care must be taken at this point to localize and avoid the ureteral openings to avoid damage and to maintain a clear, wide detrusor margin for subsequent vesicourethral anastomosis. The posterior mucosa is divided sharply and precisely with cautery, and a plane is carried along the prostate and detrusor muscle until the anterior layer of Denonvilliers' fascia is encountered. The fascia is incised exposing the vasa and seminal vesicles (Figure 7–5).

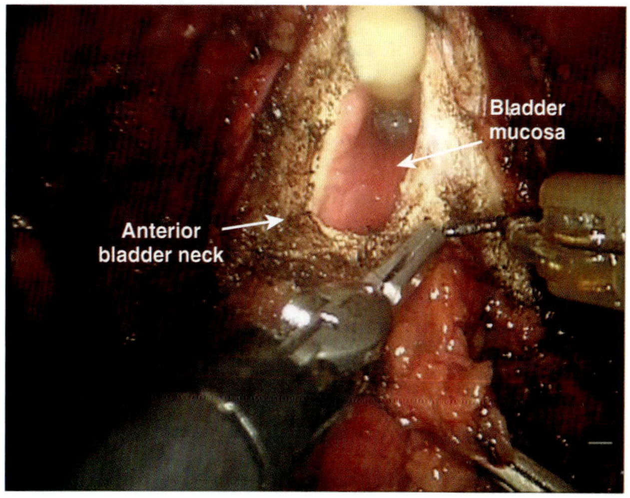

FIGURE 7–4 Incision of bladder neck with cephalad retraction of bladder.

Posterior Dissection

The lens is kept at the 30-degree downward direction. The vas deferens should be divided individually before commencing with the dissection of the seminal vesicles. The vasa are retracted upward, and the seminal vesicles are skeletonized using a combination of blunt and sharp dissection with the aid of retraction from the assistants. Attempts

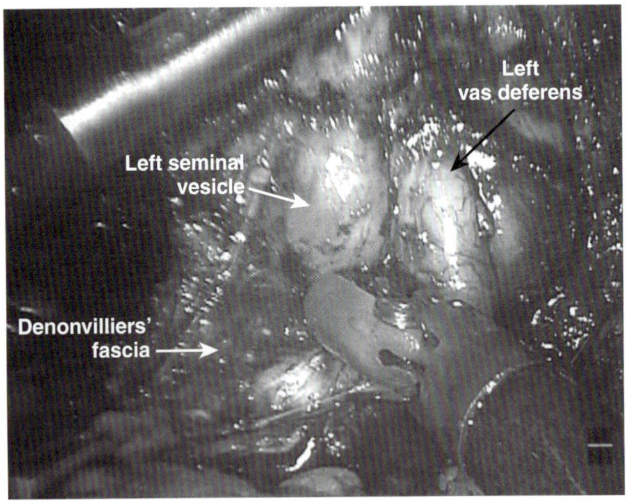

FIGURE 7–5 Exposure of seminal vesicles and posterior Denonvilliers' fascia.

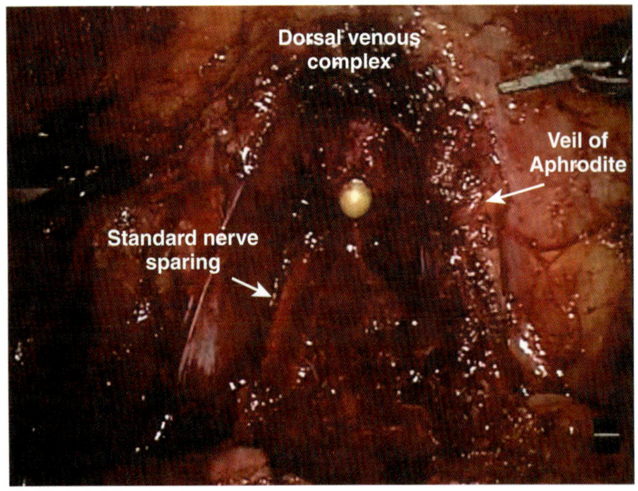

FIGURE 7–6 After removal of specimen, left-side standard nerve-sparing technique and right-side veil of Aphrodite technique.

should be made to use minimal electrocautery to avoid heat or electrical injury to the neurovascular bundles. Both seminal vesicles are freed circumferentially. Optionally, both tips of the seminal vesicles may be left in situ for optimal preservation of potency in selected low-risk patients. The seminal vesicles and vas are now used as a leverage point to retract the entire prostate upward, thus exposing the prostatic pedicles.

A transverse incision is performed with the articulated scissors through the thick layers of Denonvilliers' fascia to develop a plane between rectum and prostate. Once the fascia is open, the prerectal fat will appear posteriorly and the plane of dissection should leave the posterior most layers of Denonvilliers' fascia on the rectum. We believe that this will minimize the likelihood of rectal injury. This dissection is carried down to the apex of the prostate.

Control of Lateral Prostatic Pedicles and Preservation of the Neurovascular Bundles

The robotic arms are equipped with a pair of articulated scissors and bipolar forceps. The packet of tissue containing the neurovascular bundles is freed by incising the lateral pelvic fascia anteromedially and parallel to the neurovascular bundles between the prostatic venous plexus and the prostatic capsule. The posterolateral surface of the prostate is sharply cleared by dropping a layer of fascia, fat, nerves, and blood vessels from the base and working toward the apex. Most of the dissection occurs in a relatively avascular plane, such that the neurovascular bundles can be freed from the prostate laterally, easily requiring only minimal cautery use. Once the lateral pedicles have been isolated, Hem-o-lock clips (Weck, Research Triangle Park, NC) are applied close to the prostate. The bundle is divided sharply on both sides, thus exposing a relatively avascular plane for the rest of the dissection. Minimal bipolar cautery is used as the neurovascular bundles are bluntly freed posterolaterally from the capsule (Figure 7–6). If the endopelvic fascia has not been opened previously, it can easily be accomplished at this point to facilitate the dissection.

As the development of our approach has evolved, we have made some important technical modifications. One of the most important is an attempt to spare the accessory penile and cavernosal nerves, which may course along the side of the prostate. Animal and human studies suggest that there may be accessory cavernosal nerves that run underneath the lateral pelvic fascia on the anterolateral surface of the prostate.[7] These nerves may be physiologically relevant in erectile function. Given the improved vision and robotic manipulation, it is feasible to dissect this lateral fascia free of the prostate. We have developed an atraumatic technique of dissection of the neurovascular bundles and lateral prostatic fascia. In young patients without significant risk for extraprostatic extension, the lateral periprostatic fascia is preserved, creating a veil of tissue, named the "veil of Aphrodite" (Figures 7–6 and 7–7).

We have recently further refined our technique of nerve preservation in select patients with low-risk disease by extending our sparing of the previously described atraumatic veil of Aphrodite lateral prostatic fascia to the anterior surface of the prostate. A plane of tissue between the dorsal venous tributaries and the prostate anteriorly can be developed after lateral fascia has been reflected. We named the anterolateral peri-prostatic fascia sparing surgery the "super VIP."

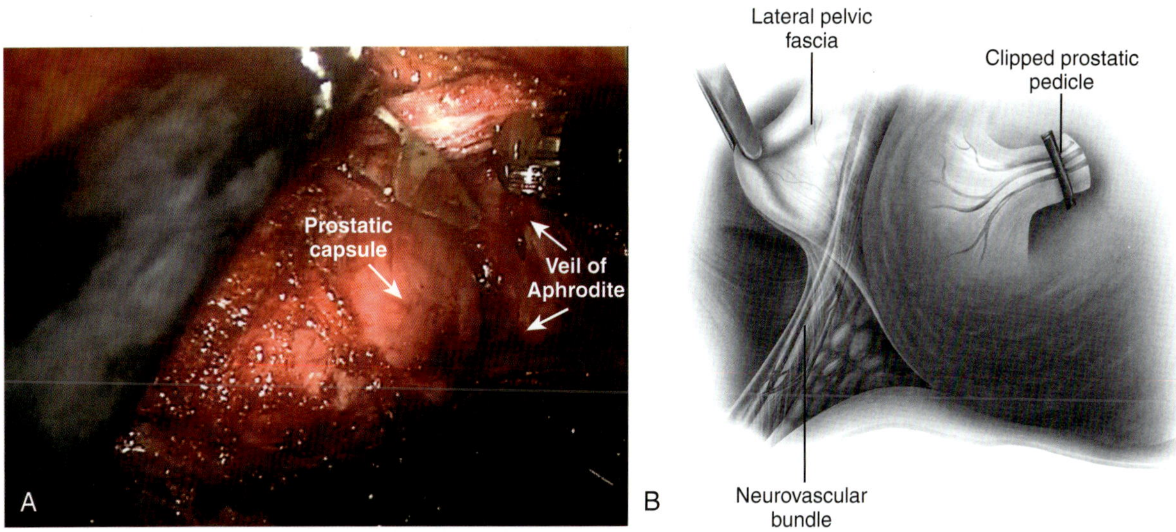

FIGURE 7–7 Development of lateral prostatic fascia-sparing plane.

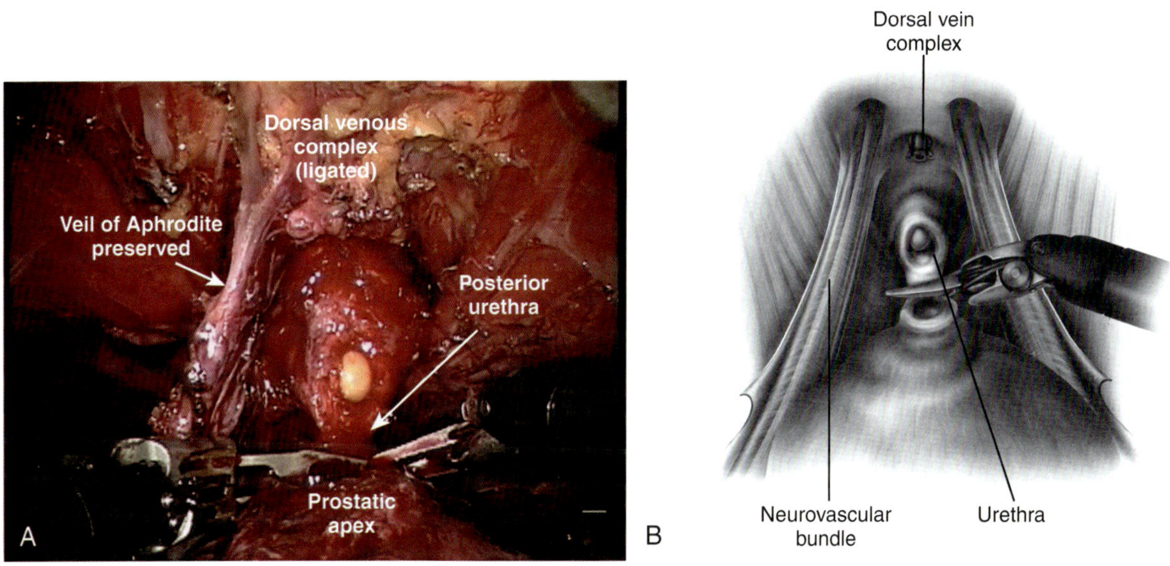

FIGURE 7–8 Incision of posterior urethra.

Incision of Dorsal Vascular Complex and Urethra

We now change to the 0-degree lens. The prostate is retracted cephalad by the patient side assistant exposing the dorsal venous complex. The puboprostatic ligaments are incised, and the previously ligated dorsal venous complex is now divided with scissors proximal to the puboprostatic ligaments using a combination of sharp and blunt dissection until the urethra is encountered. If a dorsal venous stitch has not been placed previously, a combination of bipolar cautery and the pneumoperitoneum allows for continued visualization to complete transection of the urethra. A stitch can then be placed to control the complex after transection of the urethra is completed.

The urethra should now be the last connection remaining to the prostate. Great care is taken to preserve as much urethral stump as possible to facilitate anastomosis. With the anterior urethral wall divided, the catheter is retracted out, and care is taken to ensure that the neurovascular bundles have been freed laterally such that the last remaining tissue, posterior urethral wall, and the rectourethralis muscle can be sharply incised (Figure 7–8). The specimen is then placed in a specimen retrieval bag and set aside during the remainder of the operation.

Parietal Biopsies

Given the constraints of the anatomic dissection and individual consideration, we believe in biopsies at the margins. Parietal biopsies from the anterior, posterior, and lateral margins of the urethra, as well as from the bladder neck and neurovascular bundle, are sharply excised and sent for frozen section when indicated. In the rare instance that cancer is found in the frozen specimen, additional tissue is removed from the corresponding location.

Lymphadenectomy

Lymphadenectomy is performed with a 0-degree lens and occasionally a 30-degree lens directed downward for proximal dissection, especially at the bifurcation of common iliac vessel. The nodal package will be lifted off the anterior surface of the external iliac vessels medially. Starting at the medial border of the external iliac vein, the nodal packet is cleaned medially and careful dissection continues along its inferior border until the obturator nerve is identified. The obturator nerve serves as the inferior margin of dissection. This nodal package contains the external iliac and the obturator nodes (Figure 7–9). The accessory obturator veins should be avoided because they are often present and need to be clipped or cauterized if encountered. Each nodal package is retrieved through the 12-mm assistant port.

Vesicourethral Anastomosis

We use a running anastomosis[8] tying together the tails of two 3-0 poliglecaprone 25 (monofilament) sutures (one dyed and one undyed for ease of identification during anastomosis) on an RB-1 needle (Ethicon, USA). The total length of the suture varies according to the diameter of the bladder neck, and it may be anywhere from 15 to 20 cm as required. A 0-degree laparoscopic lens is used with two Endowrist large-needle drivers. The anastomosis is begun by passing the needle outside in at the 4 or 5 o'clock position on the bladder neck and inside out on the urethra. After two or three throws on the urethra and three to four throws on the bladder to create an adequate posterior base, the suture is doubly locked and bladder is cinched down against the knot of the sutures lying on the posterior surface of the bladder. The anastomosis is continued clockwise to the 9 o'clock position on the bladder. The suture is then turned into the bladder in such a way that it runs inside out on the bladder and outside in on the urethra to continue further up to the 11 or 12 o'clock position. Then the suture (dyed) is pulled cephalad toward the left lateral side of the pelvis and maintained under traction by an assistant. Subsequently, the anastomosis is started on the right side of the urethra with the undyed end, passing it outside in on the urethra and then inside out on the bladder, from the point where the anastomosis was started and continuing counterclockwise to the point where the other suture is met. The needle of the dyed end is cut off, and the free dyed end and undyed ends are tied together with several knots. The urethral catheter is used throughout the anastomosis as a guide in showing the urethral mucosa and finally is advanced into the bladder just before tying the sutures (Figure 7–10).

Retrieval of Specimen and Closure of Ports

The specimen is extracted via the umbilical port with extension of the semicircular incision as needed. Fascial closure is performed only at this incision given its size. Because small noncutting trocars are used for all ports except the umbilical site, these other ports are closed with subcuticular skin sutures only. A Jackson-Pratt drain is left extending into the pelvis from one of the 5-mm ports.

CURRENT ANALYSIS OF RESULTS

To date, we have performed more than 2000 robotic radical prostatectomies using the VIP technique.

The operating time (Veress needle to skin closure) ranged from 70 to 160 minutes. Port placement and specimen

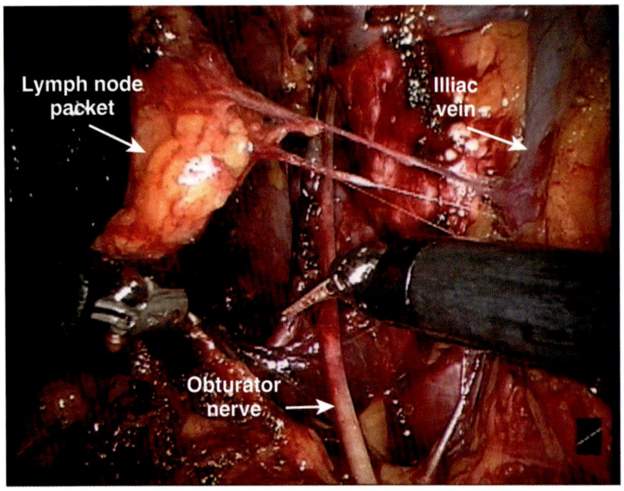

FIGURE 7–9 Right-side pelvic lymph node dissection.

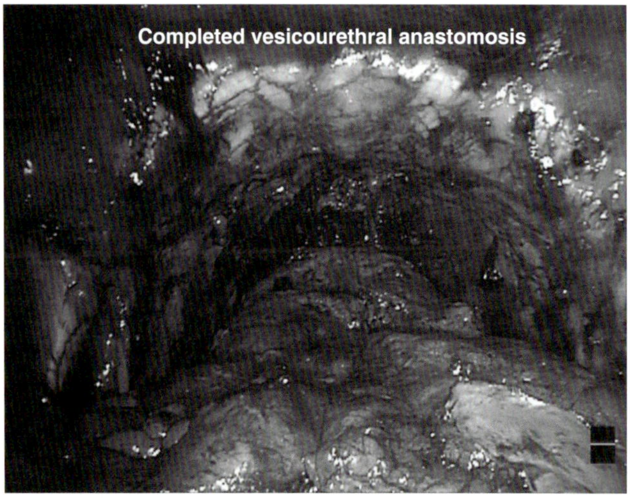

FIGURE 7–10 Completed watertight vesicourethral anastomosis.

retrieval took approximately 20 to 40 minutes, leaving an actual robotic console (dissection) time of 90 to 100 minutes. Estimated blood loss ranged from 50 to 250 mL. No patient required an intraoperative transfusion, and none provided autologous blood preoperatively. More than 95% of patients were discharged within 24 hours of hospital stay. Those who stayed longer were for social reasons (3%) and ileus (2%).[9] Body mass index did not show a statistical difference in our series for operative time, blood loss, and hospital stay for normal weight and obese patients.

Total continence, defined as using no pad at all, was achieved in 96% of patients at a follow-up of 6 months. At the time of catheter removal, 50% of patients were found to be continent (requiring no pad at all or just one liner for security).[9]

Potency

During our initial series of the robotic program, we found that at a follow-up of 6 months, 82% of preoperatively potent patients younger than 60 years had a return of some sexual function and 64% were able to achieve erections sufficient for intercourse. We have recently described a technique to preserve the prostatic fascia that appears to enhance the quality of nerve preservation during robotic prostatectomy, named the veil of Aphrodite.

We performed a prospective study comparing selected patients undergoing prostatic fascia preserving against those with standard nerve sparing techniques. At 12-month follow-up, 74% of control patients (standard nerve sparing) and 97% of study patients (prostatic fascia sparing) were able to achieve erections sufficient for intercourse with or without phosphodiesterase-5 inhibitors[10] (Figure 7–11).

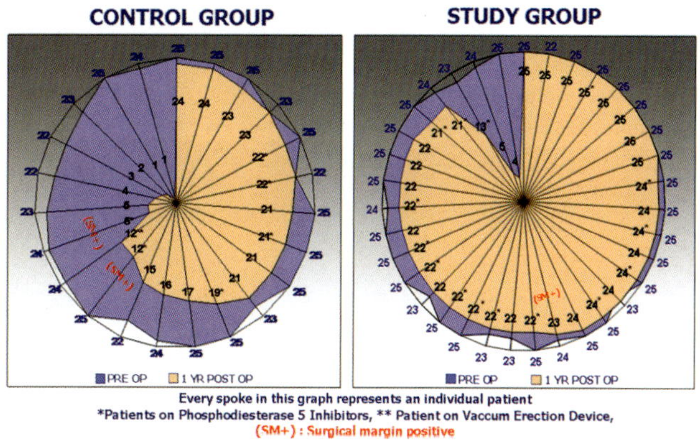

FIGURE 7–11 Potency outcome after enhanced nerve sparing versus conventional nerve sparing robotic prostatectomy at 1 year. *(From Menon M, Kaul S, Bhandari A, et al: Potency following robotic radical prostatectomy: a questionnaire based analysis of outcomes after conventional nerve sparing and prostatic fascia sparing techniques. J Urol 174:2291–2296, 2005.)*

CONCLUSION

It is clear that oncologic outcome is the most important factor in treating prostate cancer, and all approaches to radical prostatectomy have shown established results in this regard. As a result, secondary outcomes are becoming an extremely important factor in decision making by patients. The robotic approach has proved to be a superior approach to prostate cancer surgery, with all the benefits of minimally invasive surgery, improved continence, potency, and easy translation from open experience to robotic skills.

REFERENCES

1. Schuessler WW, Schulam PG, Clayman RV, et al: Laparoscopic radical prostatectomy: Initial short term experience. Urology 50:854–857, 1997.
2. Tewari A, Peabody J, Sarle R, et al: Technique of daVinci robot–assisted anatomic radical prostatectomy. Urology 60:569–572, 2002.
3. Patel VR, Tully AS, Holmes R, et al: Robotic radical prostatectomy in the community setting—the learning curve and beyond: initial 200 cases. J Urol 174:269–272, 2005.
4. Ahlering TE, Eichel L, Edwards RA, et al: Robotic radical prostatectomy: a technique to reduce pT2 positive margins. Urology 64:1224–1228, 2004.
5. Walsh PC: Anatomic radical prostatectomy: evolution of the surgical technique. J Urol 160:2418–2424, 1998.
6. Steiner MS: The puboprostatic ligament and the male urethral suspensory mechanism: an anatomic study. Urology 44:530–534, 1994.
7. Tewari A, Peabody JO, Fischer M, et al: An operative and anatomic study to help in nerve sparing during laparoscopic and robotic radical prostatectomy. Eur Urol 43:444–454, 2003.
8. Menon M, Hemal AK, Tewari A, et al: The technique of apical dissection of the prostate and urethrovesical anastomosis in robotic radical prostatectomy. BJU Int 93:715–719, 2004.
9. Menon M, Tewari A, Peabody J, et al: Vattikuti Institute prostatectomy, a technique of robotic radical prostatectomy for management of localized carcinoma of the prostate: experience of over 1100 cases. Urol Clin North Am 31:701–717, 2004.
10. Menon M, Kaul S, Bhandari A, et al: Potency following robotic radical prostatectomy: a questionnaire based analysis of outcomes after conventional nerve sparing and prostatic fascia sparing techniques. J Urol 174:2291–2296, 2005.

CHAPTER 8

András Hoznek • Laurent Salomon • Clément-Claude Abbou

Extraperitoneal Laparoscopic Robotic-Assisted Radical Prostatectomy

INTRODUCTION

Initial development of laparoscopic radical prostatectomy (LRP) was based on the experience of a few surgeons with transperitoneal laparoscopic access to the prostate and seminal vesicles.[1–3] Transperitoneal LRP was successfully introduced in routine clinical practice in France following the pioneering work of Gaston and Piéchaud in 1998 (unpublished series). The transperitoneal approach became predominant worldwide and was considered the gold standard of laparoscopic prostatectomy.

However, many teams have later reported that opening of the peritoneal cavity is not indispensable and that primary transperitoneal access to the seminal vesicles should not be considered the key of laparoscopic prostatectomy anymore.[4–7] A growing number of centers worldwide developed their technique of extraperitoneal laparoscopic prostatectomy, and many of them have definitively abandoned the transperitoneal approach.[6–13]

However, both of these techniques are difficult to learn and teach because of the inherent limitations of laparoscopic surgery.

Feasibility and reproducibility of robotic-assisted LRP has also been described,[14–18] but mostly with transperitoneal approach. Telerobotics provides technical features such as three-dimensional vision, increased robotic instrument maneuverability, and physiologic tremor filtering. These factors are thought to provide an ergonomic environment for the surgeon that simplifies performance of complex laparoscopic tasks. Unfortunately, obligatory close proximity of the laparoscopic ports with transperitoneal robotic radical prostatectomy (RP) can create interference between the robot and conventional instruments used by the assistant.[17]

Given our favorable results with conventional extraperitoneal LRP, we first described the feasibility of the extraperitoneal approach using the da Vinci robotic system on an initial series of four patients.[19]

MATERIALS AND METHODS

da Vinci Robotic System

The da Vinci robotic system is an integrated computer-based system consisting of two interactive robotic arms, a camera arm, and a remote control with three-dimensional vision capability. The da Vinci robot uses instruments with six degrees of freedom that provide the same flexibility as the human wrist. Interchangeable instruments recommended for robotic RP include the hook electrocautery, round-tip scissors, Cadiere forceps, large-needle drivers, and the Prograsp forceps with additional grasping force specifically developed for robotic RP. The working robotic arms are attached to reusable 8-mm trocars, and the camera is placed through a standard 12-mm laparoscopic port. For optimal robot function and to minimize the risk of collisions, the angle created by the camera port and each working robotic port should be obtuse and the distance between the camera port and each working port should be at least one handbreadth. With telerobotic surgery, the motions of the surgeon at the remote control unit are replicated by the robotic arms placed inside the patient. Tactile feedback is not available with da Vinci; therefore, an increased reliance on visual inputs is required. During telerobotic surgery, an assistant surgeon is scrubbed at the operating table. The assistant is first responsible for obtaining access to the operating field and for placing all trocars. The assistant performs a variety of important robot-related tasks, including alignment and exchange of instruments on the robotic arms. Furthermore, the assistant performs operative maneuvers with conventional instruments, including tissue countertraction, hemostasis, hemoclip application, suction, and assistance during suturing. Most important, the scrubbed assistant is available in the event that an emergent conversion would be required.

Surgical Technique

The patient was placed supine on the operating table. After general anesthesia was established, a nasogastric tube was placed, both arms were tucked beside the torso, and the legs were abducted to permit perineal access during the procedure. A 20-French Foley catheter was sterilely inserted.

A midline 3-cm incision was made transversally 1 cm inferior to the umbilicus. The subcutaneous tissue was divided down to the anterior rectus fascia. The anterior rectus fascia was then incised transversally to identify the inner borders of the rectus muscles separated by the linea alba. The index finger was introduced medially under the rectus muscle and along the posterior rectus sheath (Figure 8–1*A*). A blunt finger dissection was performed to create a space extending superiorly from the level of the skin incision to the lateral border of the rectus muscle. This space is limited caudally by the arcuate line of Douglas, posteriorly by the posterior rectus sheath, anteriorly by the posterior fibers of the rectus muscle, and medially by the linea alba. The same step was performed on the other side. At this stage, two spaces were created under each rectus muscle and separated by the linea alba.

The linea alba was then incised in contact with the anterior rectus fascia. The disruption of linea alba is continued by the index finger as far as possible toward the symphysis pubis. At the end of the blunt finger dissection, a large preperitoneal space is created (Figure 8–1*B*).

A Hasson cannula (Bluntport; US Surgical) was placed, and insufflation commenced at 18 mm Hg. With the use of blunt dissection with a conventional laparoscope, a midline "tunnel" in the Retzius space was developed to the pubis. If available, space creation is greatly facilitated at this stage with a balloon dilatator.

Additional ports were subsequently positioned. For patients 1 to 3, laparoscopic ports were placed as superior as possible in the Retzius space to replicate port placement previously used for transperitoneal robotic RP.[14] For patient 4, the working robotic ports were placed 4 cm more distal (Figure 8–2). The patient was placed in a 15- to 20-degree Trendelenburg position, and insufflation pressures were reduced to 12 mm Hg. The robot was positioned at the foot of the operating table and aligned.

During the procedure, the assistant was on the patient's right side using conventional laparoscopic ports (see Figure 8–2). The surgeon used a Prograsp instrument on the left robotic arm and hook electrode on the right arm during lymph node dissection. The assistant used a suction/irrigator and conventional laparoscopic instruments (graspers, bipolar cautery, clip appliers). The same robotic instruments were used initially during laparoscopic RP. The superficial dorsal vein was identified, coagulated, and divided. The endopelvic fascia was incised bilaterally with the hook electrode, and the levator musculature was swept laterally. Dissection was performed to identify the dorsal vein complex and the puboprostatic ligaments. Before the dorsal vein complex was ligated, the assistant retracted the prostate posteriorly while the puboprostatics were partially released with the hook electrode. The hook electrode was then removed from the right robotic arm, and a large-needle driver was placed on the robotic arm. The assistant introduced a No. 2 Vicryl suture on a 26-mm needle into the surgical field. During ligation of the dorsal vein complex, the assistant rotated the prostate to facilitate identification

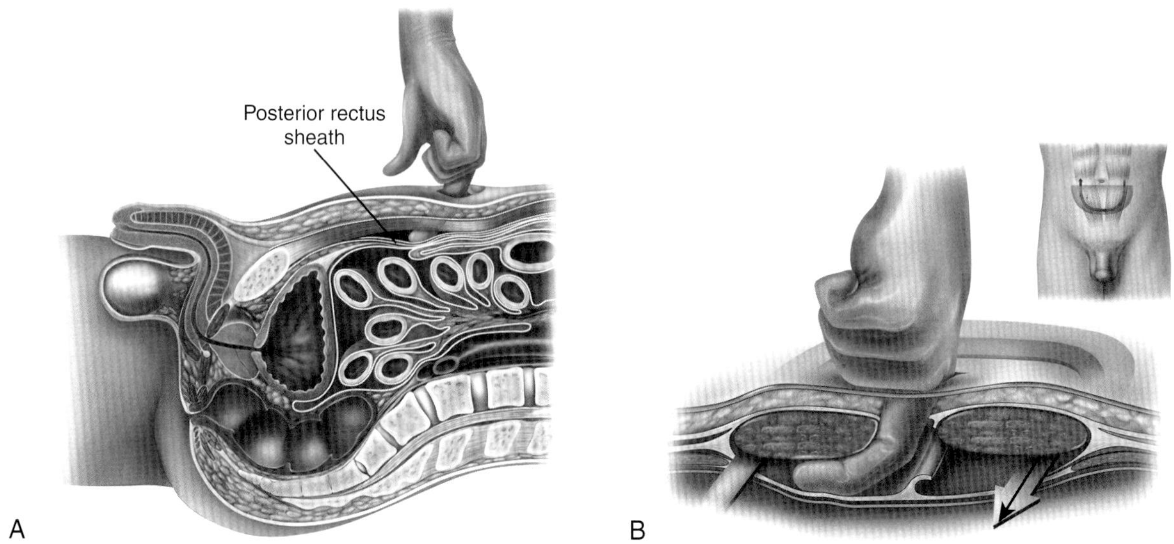

FIGURE 8–1 Creation of the extraperitoneal working space.

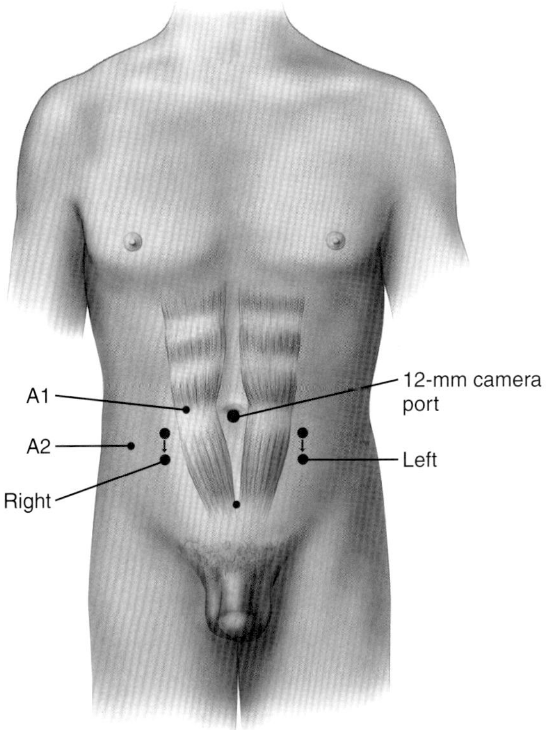

FIGURE 8–2 Trocar placement *(marked dots)* during extraperitoneal telerobotic laparoscopic radical prostatectomy illustrating more distal placement of right (R) and left (L) robotic working trocars in comparison to placement of the robotic working trocars with the transperitoneal approach *(unmarked dots)*. A1, assistant port; A2, assistant port; Left, left extraperitoneal working robotic port; Right, right extraperitoneal working robotic port.

of the plane between the dorsal vein complex and urethra. Using the same suture, a second knot was placed at the bladder neck for retraction.

Bladder neck transection was then performed with the hook electrode. The assistant retracted the prostate anteriorly with a locking grasper and retracted the bladder posteriorly with the suction/irrigator. After the bladder neck was opened anteriorly, the Foley catheter was maneuvered through the opening and grasped by the assistant and retracted anteriorly. The bladder neck was incised circumferentially with no attempt to spare the bladder neck.

Dissection was continued in the midline to release the anterior Denovilliers' fascia. The surgeon then used the hook electrode and the Prograsp forceps to free the seminal vesicles and the vas deferens. At the distal tip of the seminal vesicle, careful dissection was performed and hemostasis was attained with clips rather than cautery to avoid damage to the neurovascular bundles. As the seminal vesicles and the vasa were freed, these structures were grasped by the assistant and retracted anteriorly. In this manner, incision of the posterior layer of the Denonvilliers' fascia was facilitated with the hook electrode. Dissection was then performed toward the apex of the prostate in the midline.

Control of the prostatic pedicles was now performed. The assistant placed tension on the pedicles by retraction of the prostate to the contralateral side. Dissection was performed using the hook electrode, and hemostasis was secured with clips placed by the assistant. When a nerve-sparing procedure was performed, the hook electrode was exchanged for robotic scissors that were used to incise the prostatic fascia and thereby release the neurovascular bundles.

The robotic scissors were used to transect the dorsal vein complex. The assistant retracted the prostate in an anterior cranial direction. The urethra and rectourethralis were then divided with robotic scissors. The specimen was placed in an EndoCatch bag by the assistant. The assistant then placed the prostate on the left side of the Retzius space cephalad to the spermatic cord.

A running vesicourethral anastomosis was then performed with a 3-0 Vicryl suture on a {5/8} circle tapered needle, as previously described.[20,21] The large-needle driver was again placed on the right robotic arm, and a Cadiere forceps was placed on the left robotic arm. During the anastomosis, important roles of the assistant were to push the bladder toward the urethral stump and to provide constant tension on the suture between subsequent needle placements. After finishing the anastomosis, the catheter balloon was inflated to 15 mL. A Jackson-Pratt drain was positioned through the assistant's lateral 5-mm working trocar. The prostate was removed via the infraumbilical port, and the wounds were closed in two layers with Vicryl fascial sutures, except the remaining 5-mm suprapubic site, which was closed only with an intradermal running suture.

PUBLISHED SERIES

In our initial series, no difficulties were noted when developing the extraperitoneal space.[22] All additional steps were successfully performed with telerobotics. More distal placement of the robotic ports appeared to improve the feasibility of the extraperitoneal approach. The peritoneum acted as a natural bowel retractor, and the distal port placement facilitated use of the assistant ports. Mean operative time was 274 minutes (range, 124 to 360 minutes). Mean catheterization time and hospital stay were 2.7 and 5.3 days, respectively. A positive margin was observed in one patient, and pathologic stage was pT2 in three patients and pT3 in one patient. No postoperative complications or open conversions were observed.

More recently, these ergonomic advantages were confirmed on a larger series of 154 consecutive patients.[23] Esposito et al. used a fourth robotic arm and found that this decreased reliance on highly trained laparoscopic assistants, provided efficient traction and exposure, and allowed a more natural patient position during the operation with smaller degree of Trendelenburg.

The largest experience was reported by Joseph et al.,[24] who treated 325 patients with da Vinci robot-assisted extraperitoneal LRP. Average total operative time was 130 minutes (range, 80 to 480 minutes), mean blood loss was 196 mL, and 1.3% of patients required blood transfusion. Ninety-six percent of patients were discharged from the hospital within 8 to 23 hours of surgery. Pathologic stage was pT2a, pT2b, pT3a, and pT3b in 18%, 63%, 14%, and 5% of patients, respectively. The surgical margin was positive in 5% of pT2a, 11.1% of pT2b, 37.1% of pT3a, and 27.3% of pT3b cases.

COMMENT

The extraperitoneal approach for telerobotic laparoscopic RP was successfully performed in a growing number of centers worldwide.[22–25] A favorable byproduct of the extraperitoneal approach may be improved port placement for robotic RP. With the transperitoneal technique, all ports are placed essentially on a horizontal umbilical line to facilitate dissection of the seminal vesicles and vas deferens in the pouch of Douglas and to facilitate takedown of the urachus. Although we found a higher trocar insertion was feasible with the extraperitoneal approach, distal trocar placement appeared more efficacious. More distal port placement is possible because the extraperitoneal approach permits direct access to the Retzius space and obviates urachal takedown. Joseph et al.[24] use a very similar trocar geometry when performing extraperitoneal robotic prostatectomy. The ergonomic advantage is threefold: increasing the working area between laparoscopic and conventional ports, reducing the likelihood of instrument collisions, and increasing access to the perineum. In addition, the extraperitoneal approach does not adversely impact laparoscopic geometry, possibly because the telerobotic instruments restore two degrees of freedom not present with conventional laparoscopy.

In addition to benefits for robotic prostatectomy, the extraperitoneal approach also provides other advantages.[8,10,11,13,26–28] Access creation in the case of a previously operated abdomen is safer. Postoperative ileus is less frequent. Fluid collections (e.g., anastomotic leak, hematoma) are easier to manage. This latter observation is important, especially for those who have limited laparoscopic experience. With direct access to the Retzius space, the peritoneum also functions as a natural type of bowel retractor, thereby preventing bowel displacement into the surgical field. In our experience, the size of the extraperitoneal space can easily approximate the size of the actual working space used during the transperitoneal approach. In addition, the extraperitoneal approach better approximates the steps of open retropubic RP.

CONCLUSION

The extraperitoneal approach for da Vinci–assisted LRP is a viable alternative. The extraperitoneal robotic approach, using a more distal port placement, appears to permit better access to the prostate and a more coordinated approach between the surgeon and assistant; however, additional clinical experience is warranted. If technical advantages can be proved in a larger series of patients, the extraperitoneal approach could ultimately become the approach of choice for robotic and nonrobotic LRP.

REFERENCES

1. Schuessler WW, Vancaillie TG, et al: Transperitoneal endosurgical lymphadenectomy in patients with localized prostate cancer. J Urol 145:988–991, 1991.
2. Kavoussi LR, Schuessler WW, Vancaillie TG, et al: Laparoscopic approach to the seminal vesicles. J Urol 150(2 pt 1):417–419, 1993.
3. Guillonneau B, Vallancien G: Laparoscopic radical prostatectomy: the Montsouris technique. J Urol 163:1643–1649, 2000.
4. Bollens R, Vanden Bossche M, Roumeguere T, et al: Extraperitoneal laparoscopic radical prostatectomy. Results after 50 cases. Eur Urol 40:65–69, 2001.
5. Stolzenburg JU, Do M, Pfeiffer H, et al: The endoscopic extraperitoneal radical prostatectomy (EERPE): technique and initial experience. World J Urol 20:48–55, 2002.
6. Hoznek A, Antiphon P, Borkowski T, et al: Assessment of surgical technique and perioperative morbidity associated with extraperitoneal versus transperitoneal laparoscopic radical prostatectomy. Urology 61:617–622, 2003.
7. Dubernard P, Benchetrit S, Chaffange P, et al: Prostatectomie extra-péritonéale rétrograde laparoscopique (P.E.R.L) avec dissection première des bandelettes vasculo-nerveuses érectiles. Technique simplifiée—à propos de 100 cas. Prog Urol 13:163–174, 2003.
8. Bollens R, Roumeguere T, Quackels T, et al: Extraperitoneal laparoscopic radical prostatectomy: Brussels technique. Contemp Urol (in press).
9. Ruiz L, Salomon L, Hoznek A, et al: Comparison of early oncologic results of laparoscopic radical prostatectomy by extraperitoneal versus transperitoneal approach. Eur Urol 46:50–54, 2004.
10. Stolzenburg J, Truss M, Bekos A, et al: Does the extraperitoneal laparoscopic approach improve the outcome of radical prostatectomy? Curr Urol Rep (in press).
11. Eden CG, King D, Kooiman GG, et al: Transperitoneal or extraperitoneal laparoscopic radical prostatectomy: does the approach matter? J Urol 172(6 pt 1):2218–2223, 2004.
12. Brown JA, Rodin DM, Lee B, et al: Laparoscopic radical prostatectomy and body mass index: an assessment of 151 sequential cases. J Urol 173:442–445, 2005.
13. Brown JA, Rodin D, Lee B, Dahl DM: Transperitoneal versus extraperitoneal approach to laparoscopic radical prostatectomy: an assessment of 156 cases. Urology 65:320–324, 2005.
14. Abbou CC, Hoznek A, Salomon L, et al: Laparoscopic radical prostatectomy with a remote controlled robot. J Urol 165(6 pt 1):1964–1966, 2001.

15. Binder J, Kramer W: Robotically-assisted laparoscopic radical prostatectomy. BJU Int 87:408–410, 2001.
16. Pasticier G, Rietbergen JB, Guillonneau B, et al: Robotically assisted laparoscopic radical prostatectomy: feasibility study in men. Eur Urol 40:70–74, 2001.
17. Rassweiler J, Frede T, Seemann O, et al: Telesurgical laparoscopic radical prostatectomy. Initial experience. Eur Urol 40:75–83, 2001.
18. Menon M, Tewari A, Baize B, et al: Prospective comparison of radical retropubic prostatectomy and robot-assisted anatomic prostatectomy: the Vattikuti Urology Institute experience. Urology 60:864–868, 2002.
19. Gettman MT, Hoznek A, Salomon L, et al: Laparoscopic radical prostatectomy: description of the extraperitoneal approach using the da Vinci robotic system. J Urol 170(2 pt 1):416–419, 2003.
20. Hoznek A, Salomon L, Rabii R, et al: Vesicourethral anastomosis during laparoscopic radical prostatectomy: the running suture method. J Endourol 14:749–753, 2000.
21. Van Velthoven RF, Ahlering TE, Peltier A, et al: Technique for laparoscopic running urethrovesical anastomosis: the single knot method. Urology 61:699–702, 2003.
22. Gettman MT, Hoznek A, Salomon L, et al: Laparoscopic radical prostatectomy: description of the extraperitoneal approach using the da Vinci robotic system. J Urol 170(2 pt 1):416–419, 2003.
23. Esposito MP, Ilbeigi P, Ahmed M, et al: Use of fourth arm in da Vinci robot-assisted extraperitoneal laparoscopic prostatectomy: novel technique. Urology 66:649–652, 2005.
24. Joseph JV, Rosenbaum R, Madeb R, et al: Robotic extraperitoneal radical prostatectomy: an alternative approach. J Urol 175(3 pt 1):945–950, 2006.
25. Wolfram M, Brautigam R, Engl T, et al: Robotic-assisted laparoscopic radical prostatectomy: the Frankfurt technique. World J Urol 21:128–132, 2003.
26. Abreu SC, Gill IS, Kaouk JH, et al: Laparoscopic radical prostatectomy: comparison of transperitoneal versus extraperitoneal approach. J Urol 167(4 suppl):19, 2002.
27. Cathelineau X, Cahill D, Widmer H, et al: Transperitoneal or extraperitoneal approach for laparoscopic radical prostatectomy: a false debate over a real challenge. J Urol 171(2 pt 1):714–716, 2004.
28. Hoznek A, Menard Y, Salomon L, Abbou CC: Update on laparoscopic and robotic radical prostatectomy. Curr Opin Urol 15:173–180, 2005.

CHAPTER 9

Joseph A. Smith, Jr.

Principles of Open Radical Prostatectomy: Applied to Robotic-Assisted Laparoscopic Prostatectomy

INTRODUCTION

There are a number of different surgical procedures, both within and outside of the discipline of urology, wherein multiple surgical approaches can be used. Depending on the incision, the method of dissection, and the instrumentation, each can have its particular advantages and proponents. Radical nephrectomy, for example, can be performed through a subcostal, midline abdominal, flank, or thoracoabdominal incision. Furthermore, either hand-assisted or pure laparoscopic approaches with or without robotic surgery can be applied. All of these different approaches have a role, and each has its particular merits. None has such dominant advantages that it has become widely adopted as the only reasonable approach to be used for radical nephrectomy.

Many of these same observations apply to radical prostatectomy. For more than 50 years, both a retropubic and a perineal approach have been used for radical prostatectomy, and there are still ongoing debates, both formal and informal, over the merits of each approach. Radical perineal prostatectomy can be performed via either a subsphincteric or suprasphincteric approach, and either a retrograde or antegrade dissection of the prostate can be used through the retropubic route. More recently, laparoscopic prostatectomy has entered mainstream clinical practice and the use of robotic assistance is expanding rapidly.

As with other operations, it seems unlikely that any single technique for radical prostatectomy will become so dominant and accepted that others will be eliminated. The goal of the operation, that is, complete removal of the prostate and its investing fascia, can be accomplished by various methods. The preference of an individual surgeon is often dependent on training and experience as well as equipment availability. Nonetheless, the same surgical principles and anatomic considerations apply regardless of surgical approach. Skills learned with one approach are partially transferable to another. Furthermore, some situations make one approach preferable over another, and conversion to another approach is sometimes required. Therefore, the surgeon performing radical prostatectomy ideally is experienced and familiar with multiple approaches.

Virtually all practicing clinical urologists have learned the technique for open radical prostatectomy during residency, and most incorporate at least some experience with open radical prostatectomy into their clinical practice. On the other hand, few practitioners currently have had the opportunity to become adept at robotic-assisted laparoscopic prostatectomy during residency. Therefore, adoption of laparoscopic prostatectomy into clinical practice, with or without robotic assistance, requires acquisition of new surgical skills. This chapter outlines some of the considerations that must be undertaken in transitioning from a practice focused predominantly on open radical prostatectomy to one which actively incorporates robotic-assisted laparoscopic prostatectomy (RALP).

WHY MAKE A TRANSITION FROM OPEN TO ROBOTIC PROSTATECTOMY?

Undoubtedly, the motivation to learn RALP for many urologists is a need to respond to marketing pressures and patient demands. In addition, although there are some valid potential advantages for RALP, population-based studies continue to show a substantial risk of at least some degree of incontinence in patients undergoing radical retropubic prostatectomy (RRP). In most series, positive margins occur in up to one-third of patients and erectile dysfunction occurs in the majority. Even in expert hands, only half of patients eventually achieve good continence and erectile function and remain tumor free.[1] Thus, there is substantial room for improvement in the results achieved with RRP.

The potential for improvement with RALP is based primarily on the well-documented superb visualization and precision of instrumention. Furthermore, there is minimal bleeding to obscure the operative field.[2] The small surgical incisions and minimally invasive approach may facilitate patient recovery and return to activity. There are legitimate patient benefits, then, that can be pursued with RALP.

PATIENT SELECTION

With a few exceptions, patients who are candidates for open radical prostatectomy are also eligible for RALP. Patients ideally suited for radical prostatectomy are those with biopsy-proven and apparently localized carcinoma of the prostate. When radical prostatectomy is contemplated in a patient with a suspicion of extracapsular extension, RALP can still be appropriate. Just as a precise dissection can be performed adjacent to the prostatic capsule, the margins can be extended laterally and away from the prostate just as well with RALP as with an open approach.

Although it is wise early in a surgeon's experience to choose ideal candidates, obesity is not a contraindication to RALP.[3] We have performed RALP in patients weighing up to 400 pounds, and long trocars that adapt to the robotic equipment are available. A prior history of an inguinal herniorrhaphy with mesh may make a laparoscopic approach even more desirable than a retropubic approach because an incision traversing the mesh is not required.[4] The bladder can be satisfactorily dissected from the mesh via the laparoscopic approach. Prior transurethral prostatectomy can create a large bladder neck with either an open or a laparoscopic approach but does not preclude either.

A large prostate size is also not necessarily a contraindication to RALP.[5] We have satisfactorily performed the procedure in men with prostate volumes exceeding 150 mL. A large median lobe can be easily dissected with RALP. With a small prostate, accurate identification of the prostatic apex can be somewhat difficult with an open approach but seems to be less of a problem with RALP.

Previous surgery in the perivesical space such as partial cystectomy, ureteral reimplant, or ureterolithotomy can make mobilization of the bladder difficult. In these circumstances, we have preferred an open surgical approach. In addition, previous intraperitoneal surgery performed through an infraumbilical incision can also be problematic, especially sigmoid colon resection. An extraperitoneal approach for robotic prostatectomy can be performed under these circumstances, but the working space is more limited.[6–8] Prior appendectomy does not usually create significant difficulties. An umbilical hernia, whether repaired by prior surgery or not, probably best mandates placement of the umbilical trocar with a peritoneal cutdown approach. Repair of the umbilical hernia can be incorporated into closure of the camera port site after extraction of the surgical specimen.

TECHNICAL CONSIDERATIONS

For a surgeon accustomed to a retropubic approach to the prostate, the initial view achieved with laparoscopy is somewhat different, especially with an intraperitoneal approach. The peritoneum must be incised and the space of Retzius developed. However, once this space has been entered and the bladder satisfactorily mobilized, the anterior view of the prostate becomes quite familiar. Dissection and exposure of the endopelvic fascia and superficial dorsal vein is identical. Some surgeons perform RRP by initially incising the prostatovesical junction and dissecting antegrade. More commonly, however, the next step in an open surgical procedure is dissection of the prostatic apex and retrograde mobilization of the prostate. With RALP, retrograde mobilization is very difficult because the steep camera angle limits visualization over the lip of the prostatic apex. An antegrade dissection, then, is used with RALP.[9]

Because the surgeon is unable to feel the tissue with RALP, many open surgeons are concerned that anatomic identification of the prostatovesical junction and bladder neck may be difficult. Some advocate pulling of the catheter so that the Foley balloon identifies the junction. However, if the surgical field is prepared correctly, identification of the bladder neck becomes an easy step.

Visualization of the prostatic contour can be readily achieved by dissecting the fatty tissue completely away from the lateral margins of the prostate and the endopelvic fascia. A suture placed on the anterior portion of the prostate is not necessary to control back bleeding because division of the dorsal vein complex is the final step in the procedure. However, a suture placed anteriorly on the prostate near the bladder neck bunches some of the preprostatic fatty tissue and shows the prostatic contour well. The fat at the prostatovesical junction can be dissected, and this allows ready visualization of the bladder neck.

Once the anterior bladder neck is incised, the trigone and posterior bladder neck are easily visualized. If there is any concern about the location of the ureteral orifices, indigo carmine should be administered. A large median lobe can be lifted anteriorly to expose the posterior bladder neck (Figure 9–1). Complete incision through all of the detrusor muscle of the posterior bladder neck brings the dissection directly on top of the seminal vesicles and vasa differentia. Some surgeons, especially those trained primarily in laparoscopy, prefer a Montsouris approach for dissection of the seminal vesicles.[9] This allows entry into a tissue plane familiar to surgeons experienced with radical cystectomy by initially incising the peritoneum overlying the pouch of Douglas and identifying the tip of the seminal vesicle first. However, we have found this additional dissection to be unnecessary and have preferred direct visualization of the seminal vesicles after dividing the posterior bladder[10] (Figure 9–2). The small arteries that supply the seminal vesicles and vasa are usually identified and controlled with limited application of cautery or clips.

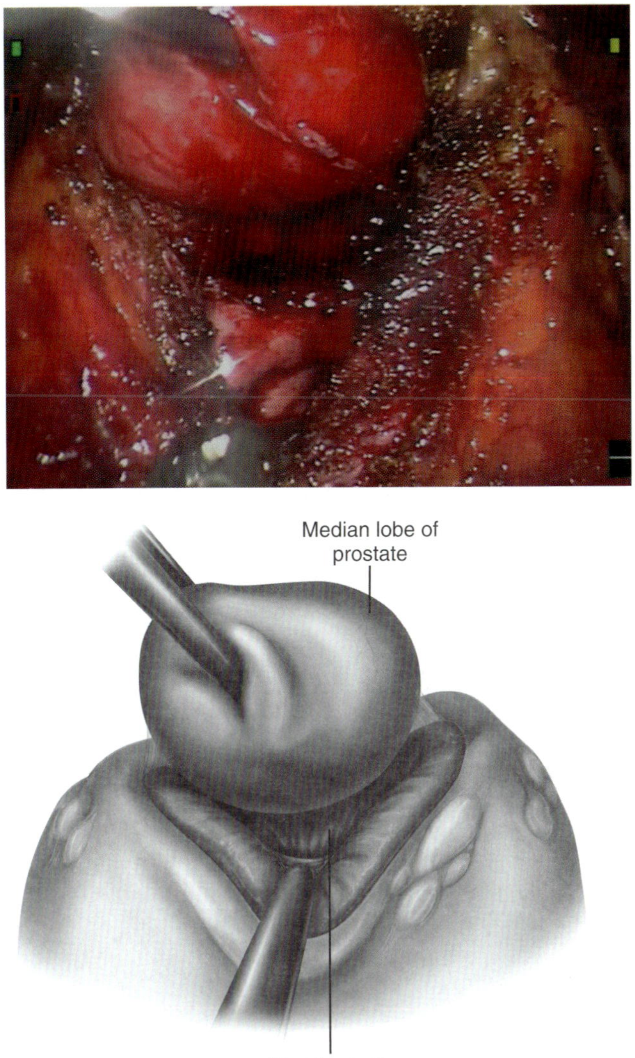

FIGURE 9–1 The anterior bladder has been incised. The graspers lift a large median lobe anteriorly. This allows visualization of the posterior bladder and trigone so that the posterior incision can be made distal to the ureteral orifices.

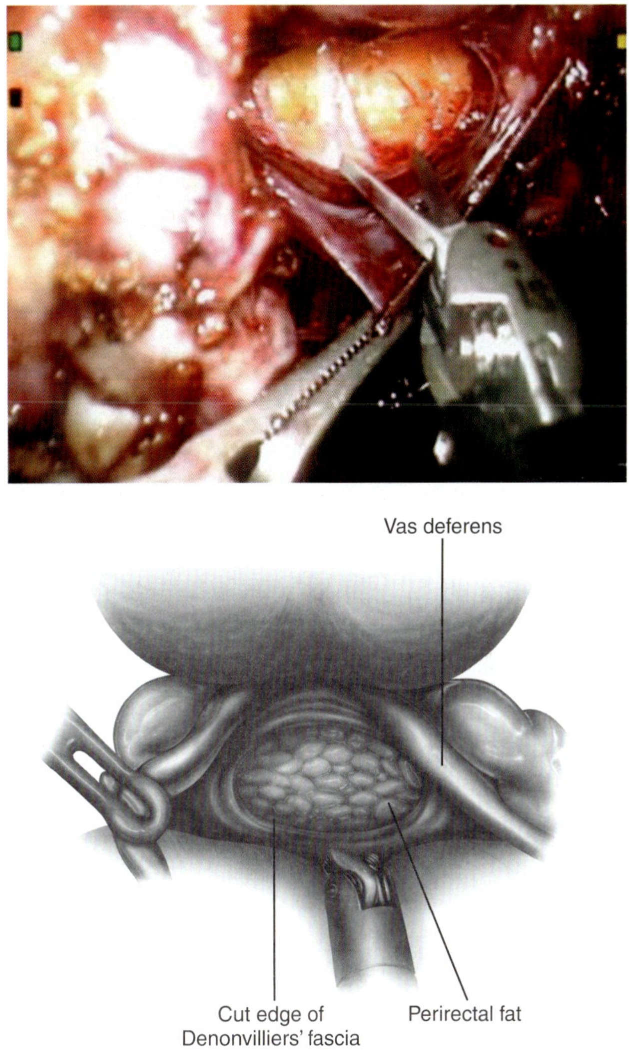

FIGURE 9–2 The bladder neck has been completely divided, exposing the anterior surface of the seminal vesicles and vasa deferentia. The prostate is being lifted anteriorly. The graspers hold the left vas deferens.

Complete dissection all the way to the tip of the seminal vesicles often is easier with RALP than with RRP.

The next key step is sharp incision of Denonvilliers' fascia. This is, again, a maneuver that may be unfamiliar via this approach for a surgeon experienced with RRP. Fear of entry into the rectum may cause the surgeon to incise the tissue too close to the base of the seminal vesicles and create an entry into the prostatic tissue. Rectal injury is best avoided by complete, sharp incision of Denonvilliers' fascia. The perirectal fat is readily visible, and the rectum can be dissected completely off of the posterior prostate all the way to the prostatic apex.

Various methods have been described for control of the vascular pedicles.[9,10] Many surgeons use bipolar electrocautery. However, even though there may be less tissue spread and nerve damage with bipolar compared with monopolar electrocautery, any method that generates heat can cause nerve damage. Therefore, we have simply used Weck clips to control the pedicle. This allows division of the pedicle tissue using cold scissors and avoids the application of any thermal energy (Figure 9–3).

A key aspect of surgical judgment is deciding how much hemostasis is required in dissecting the neurovascular bundle. Achieving perfect hemostasis by whatever method risks damage to the nerves within the bundle, and active bleeding obscures the operative field, especially with the magnified view used with RALP. Again, small clips are useful for substantial bleeding vessels, but for the most part, the neurovascular bundle can be completely separated from the prostate using sharp dissection alone. The modest bleeding that occurs is not usually enough to interfere with a precise dissection. As with open surgery, we prefer to initiate the separation of the lateral prostatic fascia along the greater curvature of the prostate. Although we have not been convinced that there are significant nerves present along the anterior part

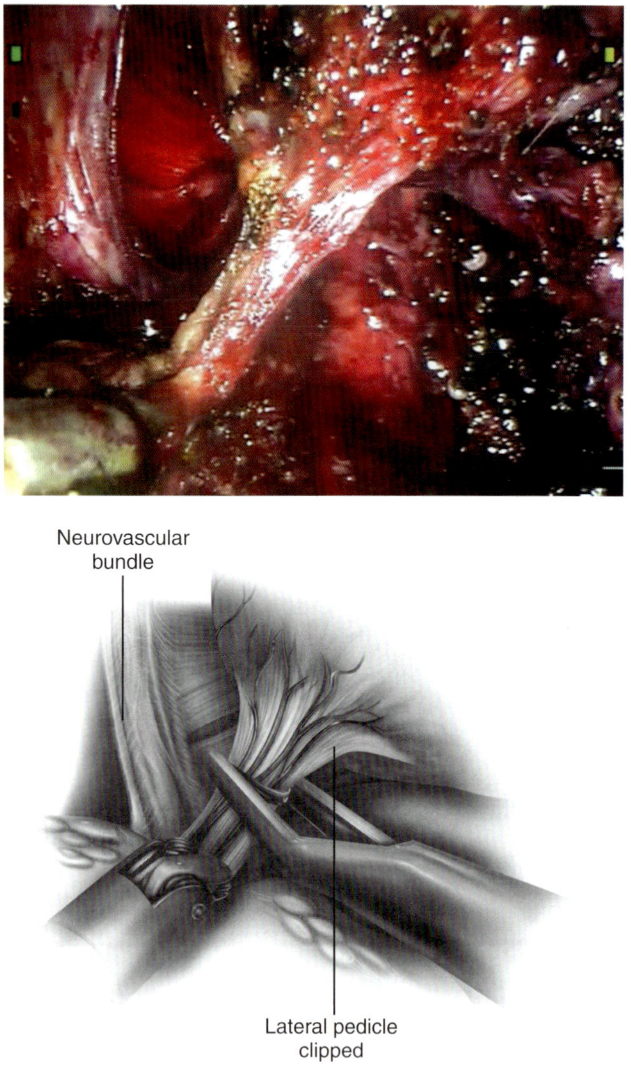

FIGURE 9–3 The left prostatic pedicle is isolated so that the vessels can be controlled with hemoclips. The prostate gland is lifted anteriorly and to the right. The preserved neurovascular bundle is visible just lateral to the pedicle.

of the prostate, division of the fascia at this level allows an edge for grasping far enough away from the neurovascular bundle itself to prevent crush injury.

Division of the dorsal vein complex and urethra is the final step before placement of the prostate in an entrapment bag. Considerations of whether or not to incise the puboprostatic ligaments are independent of surgical approach. We prefer to leave the entire dorsal vein complex and puboprostatic ligaments intact and encircle them with a hemostatic suture. This tissue is then divided sharply, exposing the prostatic apex. The prostatourethral junction should be well visualized and incised distal to the prostate (Figure 9–4). Care should be taken to avoid incision into a posterior lip of prostatic tissue, which can extend behind the urethra.

With open radical prostatectomy, use of a running suture is technically very difficult, whereas with RALP a running suture is preferable (Figure 9–5). If necessary, a racket handle

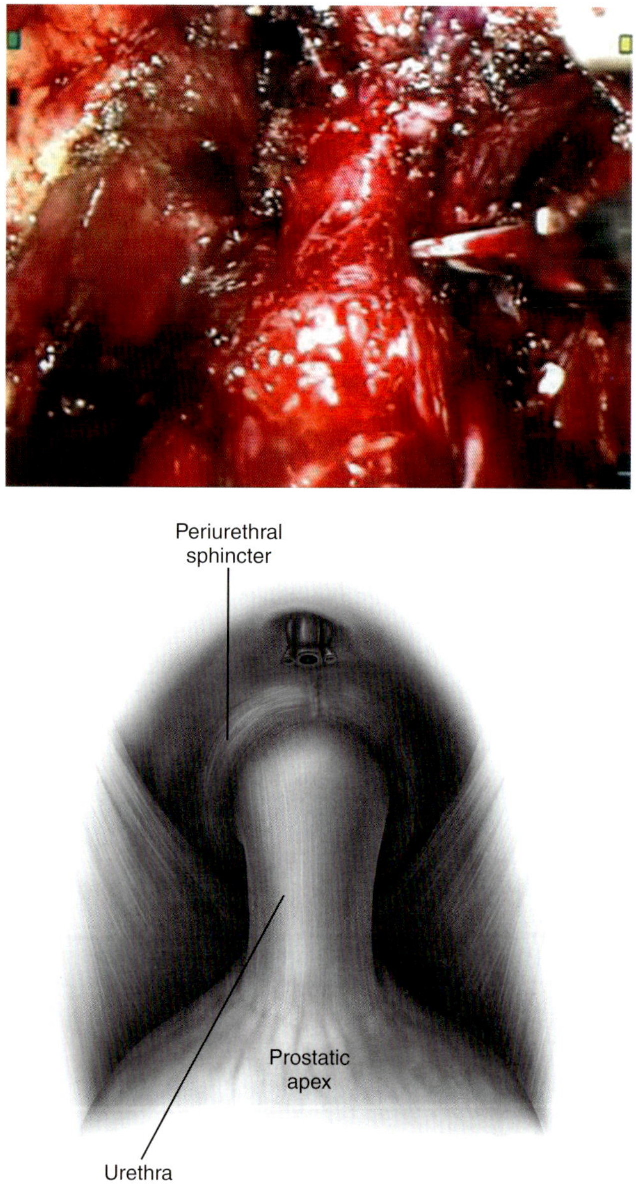

FIGURE 9–4 The dorsal vein complex has been divided, exposing the prostatic apex and the urethra.

closure of the bladder neck can be performed with RALP. This can be either posterior or anterior based. However, unlike with RRP, we have typically used an anterior racket handle closure with RALP because the posterior bladder is most easily displaced toward the urethra as the sutures are tied.

POSTOPERATIVE CARE

The postoperative care pathway we use for radical prostatectomy is identical, regardless of whether an RALP or RRP is performed.[11] The only difference is in the use of prophylactic anticoagulation. Our standard pathway for RRP includes perioperative low-molecular-weight heparin as prophylaxis for thromboembolic complications.[12] There is at least some

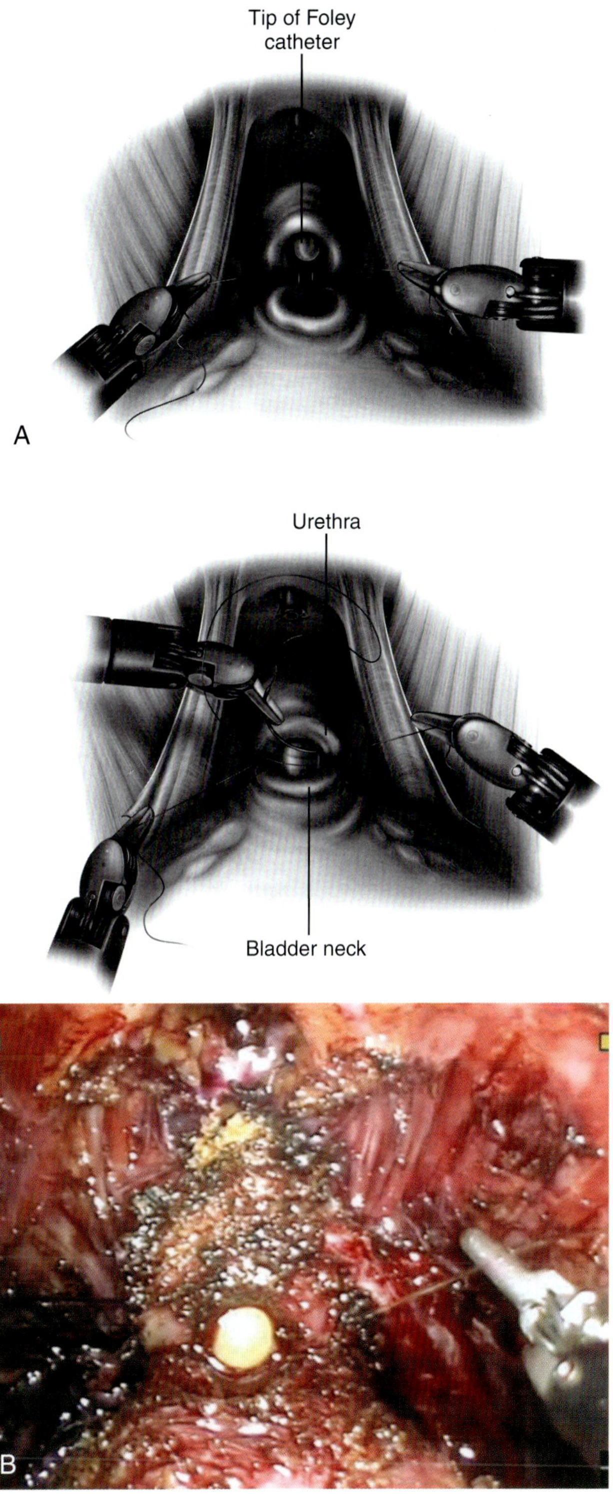

FIGURE 9–5 *A*, A running, single knot suture is used for the anastomosis. The sutures have been partially placed and careful tension on the sutures approximates the posterior bladder neck to the urethra. *B*, The running anastomosis is almost complete. The remaining anterior sutures are being placed and the catheter position shows that the posterior urethra is in good approximation.

information to suggest that thromboembolic complications are less common after RALP. Furthermore, because there is less postoperative tamponade of the operative site with RALP, we have had some concerns about a risk of postoperative bleeding. Therefore, in the patients undergoing RALP, we use early ambulation and pneumatic surgical compression devices as prophylaxis.

We keep both patient groups NPO (nothing by mouth) on the actual day of surgery. It has been our observation that many patients are quite thirsty when they return to their room after surgery and consume large amounts of fluids. Withholding oral intake until the first postoperative morning and quickly advancing the diet allows a target discharge date of postoperative day 1 in almost 90% of both RALP and RRP patients.

We also used similar instructions on return to activity for both patient groups. Even though the surgical incisions are small with RALP, there is a risk of hernia, especially at the umbilical port site, if strenuous activity is resumed too quickly. Therefore, although we allow patients to drive a car after a couple of weeks, those patients undergoing RRP and RALP are advised against any strenuous activity for 1 month after surgery.

The duration of catheterization after surgery is largely a matter of surgeon philosophy. Early catheter removal can be accomplished with either the interrupted suture technique used with RRP or the running anastomosis with RALP.[13] However, a cystogram must show no evidence of extravasation, and some patients will require reinsertion of a catheter because of inability to void if catheter removal is performed within a week of surgery. Routinely waiting 7 to 10 days after surgery has allowed us to avoid routine performance of a cystogram and fewer than 1% of patients require catheter reinsertion because of inability to void.

COMPARATIVE OUTCOMES

The most important parameters that will ultimately determine the role of RALP are the patient-related outcomes.[14] Often, surgeons quote the data from large-volume centers of excellence as if they were their own. However, population-based studies clearly show results that fall far short of the best reported in the literature.[15–17] The often-repeated statement that, with experience, moderate volume surgeons may more readily achieve reproducible results with RALP compared with RRP may contain an element of truth.[18] The visualization and equipment may "level the playing field" once sufficient experience has been achieved.

POSTOPERATIVE PAIN

RRP can be performed through a limited infraumbilical incision. However, many open surgeons routinely use epidural catheters or patient-controlled analgesia postoperatively.

These methods are not used on our clinical pathway, and many patients report pain of less than 3 on a 10-point Likert scale with RRP. This does limit the potential for significant improvement in postoperative pain with RALP. Our prospective series has shown no statistically significant difference in patient-reported pain postoperatively and no difference in narcotic use.[19] Again, it is important to emphasize that the failure to demonstrate a difference is because of the low pain scores in both patient groups.

THE LEARNING CURVE

Because RALP requires acquisition of a new skill set, there is a learning curve even for a surgeon with expertise and extensive experience with open radical prostatectomy.[20,21] Regardless of the procedure, surgical learning never reaches a complete plateau, but the so-called learning curve becomes less steep with experience. There is the potential for adverse patient outcomes during a learning curve for RALP.

Minimal bleeding and a precise dissection of the prostatic apex can usually be accomplished during an initial experience with RALP. Most patients then quickly achieve good urinary control even in the hands of a relatively inexperienced surgeon performing RALP.[22] As with open surgery, identification and dissection of the neurovascular bundle is a more advanced skill. Rectal injury can occur even in the hands of an experienced surgeon but is a greater risk when identification and dissection of Denonvilliers' fascia may be less technically satisfying.

The vesicourethral anastomosis can be difficult for the novice robotic surgeon. Consequently, a technically poor anastomosis with a potential for urinary extravasation exists. When the operation is performed through an intraperitoneal approach, urinary ascites and prolonged ileus may result.

The most concerning patient compromise that results from the surgeon's learning curve is a higher incidence of positive margins.[23–26] Virtually every surgical series has shown a decrease in positive margins as surgical experience is gained. This phenomenon is not unique to RALP and likely applies to RRP, although there are few studies documenting this.

FROM OPEN TO ROBOTIC PROSTATECTOMY: SURGEON CONCERNS

Open surgeons have voiced several recurrent concerns voiced about RALP. Often, these concerns are used as arguments to support an open approach, but they are also issues that must be considered by any surgeon who is considering transforming a predominantly open radical prostatectomy practice to one that uses RALP. The following discussion addresses some of these issues.

Lack of Tactile Feedback

With many operations, surgeons rely heavily on tissue palpations and the information gained from tactile feedback. The surgeon may be able to feel blood vessel pulsations and tissue induration. In addition, blunt finger dissection can be a useful maneuver. With radical prostatectomy, many open surgeons prefer to feel the tissue around the neurovascular bundle to decide how widely to dissect. Once the proper posterior plane is entered, blunt finger dissection can quickly and effectively mobilize the rectum from the prostate. Because there is no tactile feedback with RALP, this is often put forward as a limitation of the procedure.

The value of palpation to determine tumor extent along the neurovascular bundle is grossly overstated. Significant extraprostatic tumor extension, especially posteriorly and posterolaterally, is evident on the preoperative rectal examination. Gross extracapsular extension along the neurovascular bundle would likely be recognizable then preoperatively. The open surgeon really relies on visual cues to determine how easily the neurovascular bundle separates and whether a wider dissection should be performed.

The magnification available with RALP enhances visualization. Some open surgeons have adopted the wearing of higher-power surgical loupes in recognition of the value of operative field magnification. Furthermore, visual observation of tissue compressibility and tensile strength served as a good substitute for actual tissue palpation. Future generations of surgical robots likely will incorporate haptic feedback. In the meantime, however, loss of the ability to actually palpate the tissue during radical prostatectomy introduces very little, if any, compromise in the ability to perform the procedure.

Identification of the Bladder Neck

With RRP, the final step in the removal of the prostate typically is separation of the prostate from the bladder neck. Because the dissection is otherwise complete at this point, anatomic identification of the bladder neck often is relatively straightforward. An isolated positive margin at the bladder neck with RRP is a relatively unusual occurrence, both because of the relative infrequency of tumor in this portion of the prostate and because of the ability to dissect in the proper tissue planes.

With RALP, division of the bladder neck is one of the first steps of surgery. The overlying and surrounding perivesical and periprostatic fatty tissue can obscure the landmarks, and palpation to identify the prostatovesicular junction is not possible. Pulling on the Foley catheter to identify the balloon gives only a gross estimation of the prostatovesicular junction.

Identification of the proper anatomic location for incision in the bladder is facilitated by thorough dissection of the

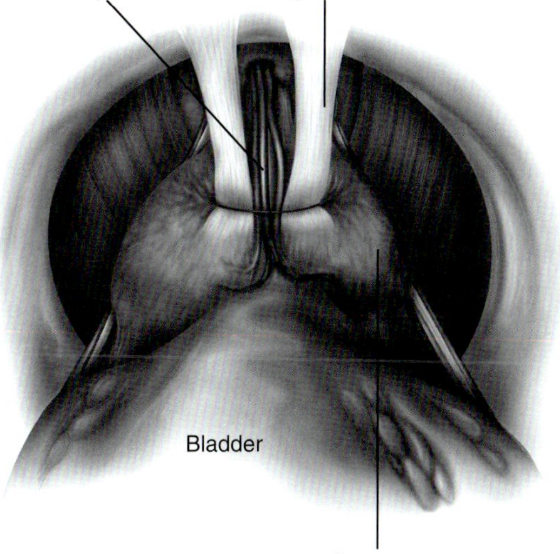

FIGURE 9–6 The endopelvic fascia has been excised bilaterally. A suture has been placed anteriorly on the prostate to bunch the dorsal vein complex. Removal of some of the perivesical fat allows good visualization of the prostatic contour so that this can be followed at the base to identify the bladder neck.

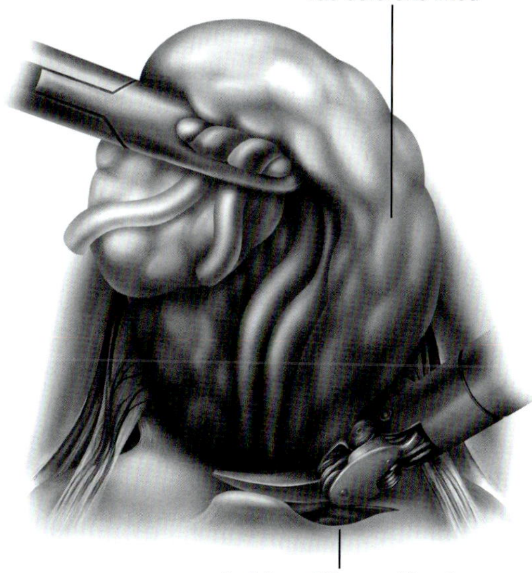

FIGURE 9–7 The vasa deferentia and seminal vesicles have been dissected free and are being lifted anteriorly. The grasper is holding Denonvilliers' fascia, which has been incised. The exposed fat lies just anterior to the rectum.

perivesical and periprostatic fat, especially that overlying the proximal portion of the endopelvic fascia. Placement of a suture on the anterior surface of the prostate can bunch the dorsal vein complex to allow good identification of the prostate. The contour of the prostate at the bladder neck is readily visible, and the anatomic junction of the prostate with the bladder can be determined (Figure 9–6). Initial entry into the bladder anteriorly can ensure that no prostatic tissue has been left at the bladder neck and allow direct visualization of the trigone and posterior bladder neck for a precise anatomic dissection. With experience, identification of the bladder neck becomes no more difficult with RALP than with RRP.

Rectal Injury

Most reported series of either RALP or pure laparoscopic prostatectomy include at least some cases of rectal injury in the initial experience.[27,28] In addition, rectal injury occurs occasionally even in the hands of a highly experienced open or robotic surgeon. With RRP, rectal injury typically occurs near the prostatic apex during an attempt to identify the proper plane of dissection posterior to Denonvilliers' fascia and after division of the prostatorectal fascia (rectourethralis muscle). With RALP, rectal injury is best avoided by complete mobilization of the rectum from the posterior surface of the prostate prior to division of the urethra. A well-defined layer of Denonvilliers' fascia is evident after the seminal vesicles have been dissected free and lifted anteriorly (Figure 9–7). It is best to incise this tissue layer sharply and to extend the incision laterally to the level of the neurovascular bundles. The prerectal fat plane is readily evident, and dissection along the posterior prostate mobilizes the rectum completely. In performing almost 1000 robotic-assisted laparoscopic prostatectomies, we have had a single rectal injury.

Use of Thermal Energy along the Neurovascular Bundle

Nerves, especially the small fibers typically present in the neurovascular bundle, are highly sensitive to thermal injury.[29] Suction devices for evacuation of blood from the operative field are more effective with open surgery. Furthermore, small clips or ties can be placed around perforating vessels from the neurovascular bundle. Even though there is excellent hemostasis with RALP because of the pneumoperitoneum, relatively small amounts of blood can obscure the magnified operative field. Different methods have been described for control of the vascular pedicle to the prostate and for dissection along the neurovascular bundle. Often, bipolar electrocautery is used because there is less tissue spread of the energy and less potential damage to adjacent nerves. Use of harmonic scalpels has also been described. However, it is best to avoid any thermal injury near the neurovascular bundle, and this can be accomplished with RALP.

In our hands, use of a Weck clip has been the best approach for control of the vascular pedicle. Separation of the

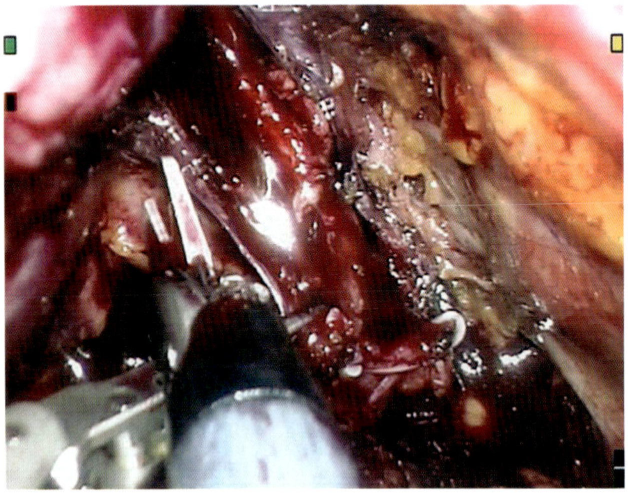

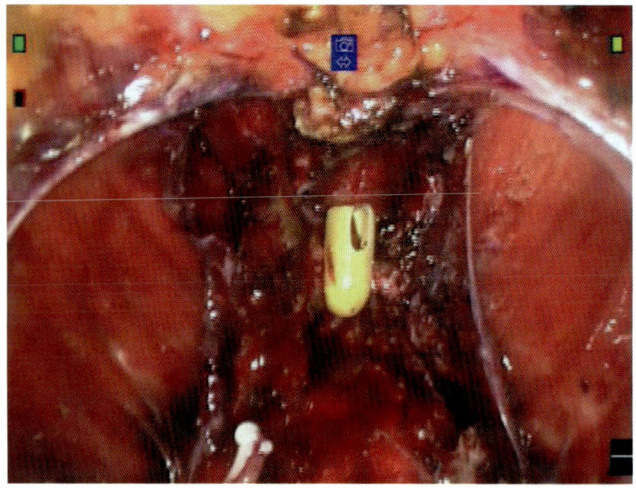

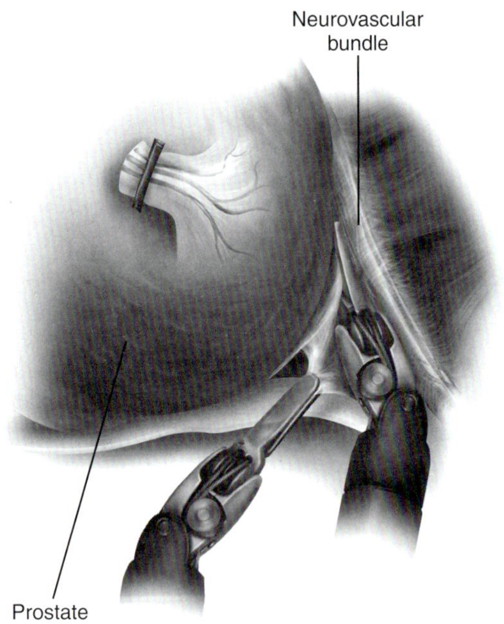

FIGURE 9–8 The neurovascular bundle is being separated from the right side of the prostate. The robotic scissors are being used to develop this plane, and cautery energy is avoided.

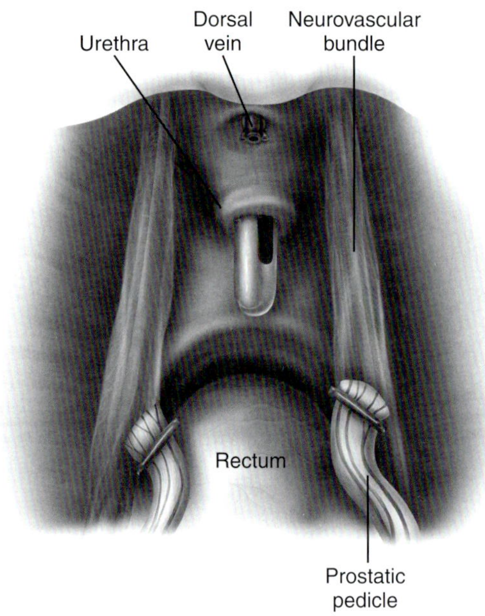

FIGURE 9–9 The prostate has been removed and placed in an entrapment bag. The catheter tip shows the cut urethra, and the clips on the pedicle are seen. The preserved neurovascular bundles are visible bilaterally.

neurovascular bundle from the posterolateral prostate can then be accomplished sharply (Figure 9–8). Small clips can be used to control identifiable perforating vessels. Placement of small hemostatic sutures in the neurovascular bundle can also be performed robotically. This does require instrument change out, but very precise suture placement, which limits damage to the underlying nerves, can be accomplished (Figure 9–9).

An important aspect of surgical judgment with radical prostatectomy is the determination of how much bleeding is permissible. With RRP, there is substantial tamponade of bleeding along the neurovascular bundle once the vesicourethral anastomosis is complete and the extraperitoneal tissues collapse. With RALP, especially via an intraperitoneal approach, an opposite phenomenon is possible. When the pneumoperitoneum is released, venous bleeding may ensue and there is free communication with the entire peritoneal cavity. Nonetheless, clinically significant postoperative bleeding is an extremely unusual phenomenon with RALP and attempts to achieve total hemostasis may be counterproductive because damage to the neurovascular bundle could occur.

EXAMINATION OF THE SURGICAL SPECIMEN

Inspection of the surgical specimen once the prostate is removed can provide helpful information. Gross violation of the surgical capsule may be evident, and areas where tumor seems to extend near the margin may be identifiable. The prostate is placed in an entrapment bag after removal with RALP. It is then extracted after completion of the anastomosis and as a final step prior to closure.

Although there is some value in immediate examination of the surgical specimen, this rarely results in modification of the surgical procedure. Frozen section analysis of the prostate specimen and excision of additional tissue at the site of a positive margin is not usually fruitful. The excised tissue rarely shows carcinoma and can result in interruption of the neurovascular bundle or overzealous removal of tissue from the urethra. However, if a surgeon believes that immediate examination of a surgical specimen is important, this can be performed with RALP. The camera port site can be enlarged, and the specimen extracted. The fascia can then be partly closed to allow reintroduction of the camera and completion of the anastomosis.

MANAGEMENT OF UNEXPECTED FINDINGS

The ability to recognize anatomic variations or manage intraoperative complications is an important aspect of surgery. RALP conveys this ability to the surgeon just as readily as open surgery. The superb visualization may allow identification of accessory pudendal arteries much more readily. Identification of accessory vessels is reported much more commonly with RALP or laparoscopic prostatectomy than with open surgery, with the difference being attributable simply to a better ability to visualize these vessels. Preservation of accessory pudendal arteries may contribute to improved continence and potency and is almost always feasible robotically (Figure 9–10). Typically, the vessels perforate the genitourinary diaphragm just lateral to the dorsal vein complex. Cystoscopy to identify an enlarged median lobe is not required to select patients suitable for RALP. Just as with open surgery, a large median lobe can be identified and managed intraoperatively. After the anterior bladder is incised, the median lobe becomes evident and can be grasped and lifted anteriorly. Incision through the posterior bladder neck is then performed.

If the neurovascular bundle does not separate readily from the prostate, consideration must be given to wider resection. Wide resection around the prostate can be accomplished robotically just as with open surgery.

Rectal injuries can occur with either open or robotic prostatectomy. Likewise, intraoperative closure of a recognized rectal injury can be performed robotically.[28,29] It is important to visualize the full extent of the injury and to perform a multilayered closure. A pelvic drain is placed postoperatively. If the adequacy of technical closure of the defect is suspect, the same principle applies as with open surgery: A temporary diverting colostomy should be performed.

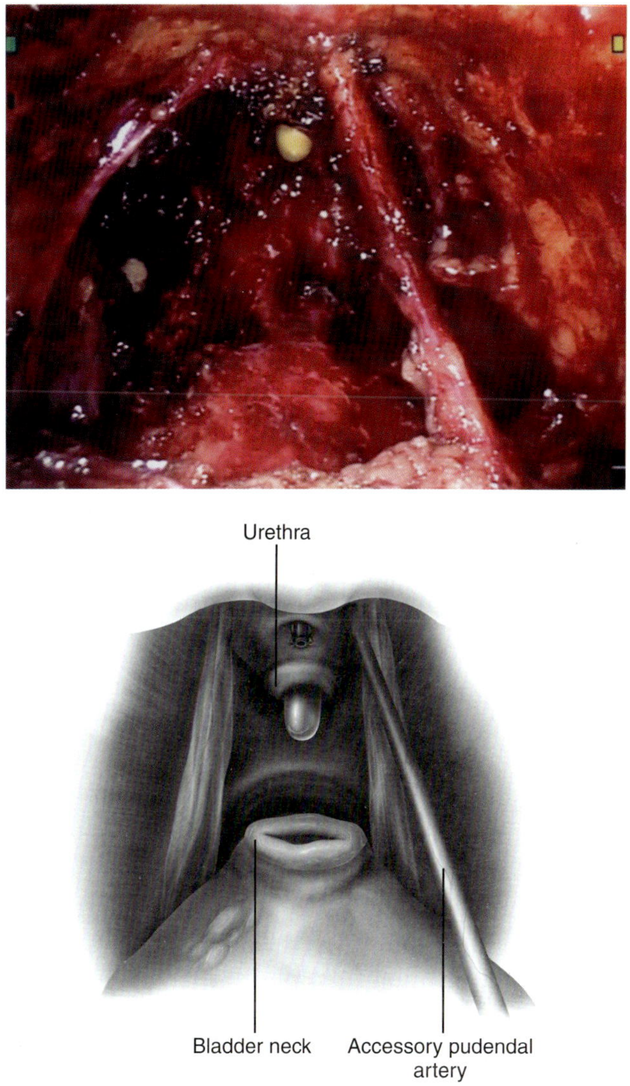

FIGURE 9–10 A large accessory pudendal artery is visible on the right side. This pierces the genitourinary diaphragm just at the prostatic apex. Identification and preservation of accessory arteries may be important for maintaining penile blood flow and avoiding incontinence and erectile dysfunction.

SUMMARY

Many of the principles familiar to surgeons who perform open prostatectomy are applicable to RALP. There are some differences in the anatomic approach and sequence of the surgical dissection. The superb visualization with RALP overcomes the problems associated with lack of tactile feedback. Mechanical manipulation of the robotic arms requires acquisition of new skills for most open surgeons, but robotic assistance facilitates suturing and other aspects of the surgery that can be quite difficult with pure laparoscopy. The skills for both approaches are partially complementary, and a surgeon skilled in both techniques has the greatest flexibility.

REFERENCES

1. Saranchuk JW, Kattan MW, Elkin E, et al: Achieving optimal outcomes after radical prostatectomy. JCO 23:4146–4151, 2005.
2. Farnham S, Webster TM, Herrell SD, et al: Intraoperative blood loss and transfusion requirements for robotic-assisted prostatectomy versus radical retropubic prostatectomy. Urology 67:360–363, 2006.
3. Brown JA, Rodin DM, Lee B, et al: Laparoscopic radical prostatectomy and body mass index: an assessment of 151 sequential cases. J Urol 173:442–445, 2005.
4. Erdogru T, Teber D, Frede T, et al: The effect of previous transperitoneal laparoscopic inguinal herniorrhaphy on transperitoneal laparoscopic radical prostatectomy. J Urol 173:769–772, 2005.
5. Singh A, Fagin R, Shah G, et al: Impact of prostate size and body mass index on perioperative morbidity after laparoscopic radical prostatectomy. J Urol 173:552–554, 2005.
6. Cthelineau X, Cahill D, Widner H, et al: Transperitoneal or extraperitoneal approach for laparoscopic radical prostatectomy: a false debate over a real challenge. J Urol 171:714–716, 2004.
7. Erdogru T, Teber D, Frede T, et al: Comparison of transperitoneal and extraperitoneal laparoscopic radical prostatectomy using match-pair analysis. Eur Urol 46:312–319, 2004.
8. Brown JA, Rodin D, Lee B, et al: Transperitoneal versus extraperitoneal approach to laparoscopic radical prostatectomy: an assessment of 156 cases. Urology 65:320–324, 2005.
9. Guillonneau B, Vallancien G: Laparoscopic radical prostatectomy: the Montsouris technique. J Urol 13:1643–1649, 2000.
10. Menon M, Tewari A, Peabody JO, et al: Vattikuti Institute prostatectomy, a technique of robotic radical prostatectomy for management of localized carcinoma of the prostate: experience of over 1100 cases. Urol Clin North Am 31:701–717, 2004.
11. Smith JA Jr: Robotic-assisted laparoscopic prostatectomy: an assessment of its contemporary role in the surgical management of localized prostate cancer. Am J Surg 188:63S–67S, 2004.
12. Holzbeierlein JM, Peterson M, Smith JA Jr: Radical prostatectomy and collaborative care pathways. Semin Urol Oncol 8:60–65, 2000.
13. Nadu A, Salomon L, Hoznek A, et al: Early removal of the catheter after laparoscopic radical prostatectomy. J Urol 166:1662–1664, 2001.
14. Smith JA Jr: Outcome after radical prostatectomy depends upon surgical technique but not approach. Curr Urol Rep 3:179–181, 2002.
15. Dindo D, Demartines N, Clavien PA: Classification of surgical complications: a new proposal with evaluation in a cohort of 6336 patients and results of a survey. Ann Surg 240:205–213, 2004.
16. Fowler JF Jr, Barry MF, Lu-Yao G, et al: Patient-reported complications and follow-up treatment after radical prostatectomy. The national Medicare experience: 1988-1990 (updated June 1993). Urology 42:622–629, 1993.
17. Geary ES, Dendinger TE, Freiha FS, et al: Incontinence and vesical neck strictures following radical retropubic prostatectomy. Urology 45:1000–1006, 1995.
18. Catalona WJ, Carvalhal GF, Mager DE, et al: Potency, continence and complication rates in 1,870 consecutive radical retropubic prostatectomies. J Urol 162:433–438, 1999.
19. Webster T, Herrell SD, Chang SS, et al: Robotic-assisted radical prostatectomy versus radical retropubic prostatectomy: a prospective assessment of postoperative pain. Urology 66:105–107, 2005.
20. Martina GR, Giumelli P, Scuzzarella S, et al: Laparoscopic extraperitoneal radical prostatectomy B learning cure of a laparoscopy-naive urologist in a community hospital. Urology 65:959–963, 2005.
21. Guillonneau B, Vallancien G: Laparoscopic radical prostatectomy: the Montsouris experience. J Urol 163:418–422, 2000.
22. Herrell SD, Smith JA Jr: Robotic-assisted laparoscopic prostatectomy: what is the learning curve? Urology 66:105–107, 2005.
23. Ahlering TE, Eichel L, Edwards RA, et al: Robotic radical prostatectomy: a technique to reduce pT2 positive margins. Urology 64:1224–1228, 2004.
24. Brown JA, Garlitz C, Gomella LG, et al: Pathologic comparison of laparoscopic versus open radical retropubic prostatectomy specimens. Urology 62:481–486, 2003.
25. Guillonneau B, ed-Fettouh, Baumert H, et al: Laparoscopic radical prostatectomy: oncological evaluation after 1,000 cases at Montsouris Institute. J Urol 169:1261–1266, 2003.
26. Rassweiler J, Schulze M, Teber D, et al: Laparoscopic radical prostatectomy with the Heilbronn technique: oncological results in the first 500 patients. J Urol 173:761–764, 2005.
27. Guillonneau B, Gupta R, el-Fettouh H, et al: Laparoscopic management of rectal injury during laparoscopic radical prostatectomy. J Urol 169:1694–1696, 2003.
28. Katz R, Borkowski T, Hoznek A, et al: Operative management of rectal injuries during laparoscopic radical prostatectomy. Urology 62:310–313, 2003.
29. Ong AM, Su LM, Varkarakis I, et al: Nerve sparing radical prostatectomy: effects of hemostatic energy sources on the recovery of cavernous nerve function in a canine model. J Urol 1772:1318–1322, 2004.

CHAPTER 10

Lee R. Schachter • Melissa R. Kaufman • S. Duke Herrell

Establishment of a Robotic Prostatectomy Program

INTRODUCTION

Robotic-assisted or computer-assisted surgical technology has already had a major impact in multiple surgical disciplines. Although a variety of surgical specialties, such as cardiac, thoracic, general, and gynecologic surgery, have described potential uses for robotic-assisted surgical systems, in no other surgical discipline has the impact of robotic operative technology been as rapidly adapted, researched, and placed into widespread clinical use as in urologic surgery. A renewed interest in harnessing the potential benefits of laparoscopic minimally invasive approaches for prostate cancer surgery arose with the reintroduction of laparoscopic radical prostatectomy as a viable option in the late 1990s. This interest, coupled with the difficult learning curve and skill set needed for such advanced extirpative and reconstructive oncologic surgery, created a fertile ground for the introduction of robotic-assisted technology. The design elements of the robotic surgery systems, including "wristed" technology with degrees of freedom lacking in current laparoscopic instrumentation, three-dimensional (3D) vision, surgeon control of the camera, and multiple arm functions provided some potential advantages even for skilled laparoscopic surgeons. As a result of these advantages, along with widespread interest and marketing from both academic and community urologists and their patients, the number of robotic surgical systems (da Vinci) in use has increased from 100 in 2002 to more than 300 in 2005 (www.intuitivesurgical.com).

The methodology of establishment of a "successful" robotic prostatectomy surgical program is therefore a very timely and important subject for urologists and hospital systems throughout the world. This chapter introduces and discusses many of the key factors to consider when establishing a successful robotic prostatectomy program in the context of establishment of a urologic surgery robotics program and an institutional-wide robotic surgery program.

BACKGROUND

To date, no other specialty has seen as rapid and far-reaching impact from the advent of robotic surgery as urology. In 1994, the AESOP robot (Computer Motion, Goleta, CA) became the first surgical robotic assistant approved for human use,[1] allowing surgeon camera control and movement via voice command to augment performance of many different urologic laparoscopic procedures. In 1997, the da Vinci robotic surgical system was approved for human use. The first robotic-assisted laparoscopic prostatectomy (RALP) was performed by Binder and Kramer in 2000.[2] Subsequently, the U.S. Food and Drug Administration (FDA) approved the da Vinci robot for performance of RALP in May 2001. By 2003, more than 800 RALPs had been performed in the United States, and by 2004, this number had grown to more than 8000, with an expected continued increase.[3]

Successful development of a robotic surgery program includes the evaluation of several factors prior to system acquisition. The initial unit cost, maintenance agreement, and disposable instrument costs of robotic surgery are substantial and must be weighed against the benefits to the patient and the institution. A market analysis including survey of the internal surgical services and surgeons who will use the robotic technology, procedures for which it will be used, and the local and regional health care markets is essential. In addition, one must consider the operating room (OR) requirements, training, credentialing, and performance outcomes related to robotics and their impact on the program and institution.[4]

COSTS

The initial outlay to purchase a da Vinci robot is approximately $1.3 million. Annual maintenance costs run $100,000 to $130,000, and per case instrument costs can vary from $400 to greater than $1600.[3] These are tangible financial costs of initiating a robotic surgery program. The auxiliary costs associated with developing a new program are significant and can be more difficult to anticipate. These include adaptation of existing OR facilities, training of physicians and surgical teams, and marketing. Training, in particular, requires significant paid time for employees. Typically, a number of surgeon and team training sessions at a training center are included with system purchase. Delays in training will set back the initiation of the entire program; therefore, time and funds must be budgeted prior to acquisition of the technology. After program initiation, increased operative times during the surgeons' learning curve experience will not be offset by increased reimbursement, thereby escalating the initial costs of performing robotic procedures. Reimbursement is not greater at this time for robotic surgery. With experience, operative times typically rapidly decline, thereby making the robotic procedure less costly, but time equivalency with open surgery can be difficult to achieve, especially for expert open surgeons. A urologic program or practice and the associated institutions must be able to absorb these increased relative costs of the program to be successful.

BENEFITS

There are many perceived benefits to robotic surgery, especially for radical prostatectomy. For the patient, these advantages potentially include reduction in blood loss, transfusion rate, hospitalization time, catheterization time, and perioperative complications and the potential for improved oncologic outcomes, continence rates, and potency. RALP may provide for wider availability of a minimally invasive procedure and has been promoted to offer other potential benefits, including smaller incisions, less pain, less hospitalization time, shorter convalescence, and less time to get back to work. Although a reduction in blood loss and transfusion rate has been shown consistently in RALP, some of the other benefits mentioned are controversial. For example, postprostatectomy patients at our institution are managed on a common clinical pathway and discharged on postoperative day 1 whether they had their surgery performed via standard open radical retropubic prostatectomy (RRP) or with RALP.[5] Foley catheter removal is in a comparable amount of time (7–10 days). It is still too early in our experience and ongoing validated outcome data evaluation to make a definitive statement about oncologic outcomes, continence rates, and potency preservation. Finally, although the incisions for the robotic prostatectomy are smaller than for open surgery, the marked reduction in pain noted for many laparoscopic procedures, such as with nephrectomy, has been more controversial when evaluated for prostate procedures. Several early series noted a marked reduction in pain; however, in our prospective evaluation using standardized pathways and validated pain scale instruments for both procedures, no difference in mean pain score was found. Both procedures result in a mean pain score below 4, indicating the procedure is typically well tolerated, as would be expected for lower abdominal surgeries and incisions.[6]

There are potential advantages for an institution to undertake development and expansion of a robotic prostatectomy and urologic surgery program. Patients want to sense that they are receiving state-of-the-art care using the latest technology. Patients are increasingly savvy in seeking out large amounts of information on procedures and surgeons via media and the Internet. A robotic surgery program provides a marketing opportunity to reach this demographic and encourage them to seek care at a particular hospital. Thus, even if they have an unrelated problem that does not require a robotic surgical procedure, they may be attracted to a hospital known to have this technology. This is an intangible benefit, the potential significance of which may be revealed in the initial market analysis. A dedicated marketing and advertising strategy may need to be in place to capture this opportunity. Media coverage, including spotlights in the local and regional news, will enhance visibility of the program and the institution as a whole. In addition to attracting more patients through self-referral, there is also the potential to attract additional referrals from community and regional physicians who want their patients to have access to this care but who are unable to access the technology locally. Also, as robotic technology has spread into many areas and become available at an institution, other institutions may add the technology just to maintain market share. A robotic surgery program also has the potential to attract well-trained surgeons and, at academic institutions, to aid recruitment of residents and/or fellows. In 2001, a survey of general surgery residents found that 57% had a very high interest in robotic surgery, yet only 20% had access to a robot. Today, in urologic surgery, both of these numbers would likely be increased.[7]

Finally, there are potential advantages for the surgeon. These include 3D visualization, improved dexterity, greater surgical precision, increased range of motion, tremor reduction, motion scaling, and improved ergonomics and comfort. The da Vinci provides a steady, tireless, magnified, 3D view that is controlled directly by the surgeon. The surgeon manipulates both the camera and two to three additional instrumented arms. The da Vinci Endowrist technology has seven degrees of freedom with which to operate the instruments. The instruments' movements are directed by the surgeon's own fingers, hands, and wrists (Figure 10–1), innately making it feel far closer to open rather than standard pure laparoscopic surgery. With these advantages, the robotic surgical system has been purported to and seemingly does allow even laparoscopically naïve surgeons to adapt to performing even complex laparoscopic surgeries such as the radical prostatectomy.[8,9]

MARKET ANALYSIS

As mentioned previously, market analysis is an important component of robot program development because of equipment expense coupled with no defined reimbursement increase for the robot than for a similar open RRP surgery. It will need to be determined whether there are enough patients to undergo robotic surgery to make it feasible, how many more patients would be drawn by the robot and for unrelated types of care, and whether or not the institution

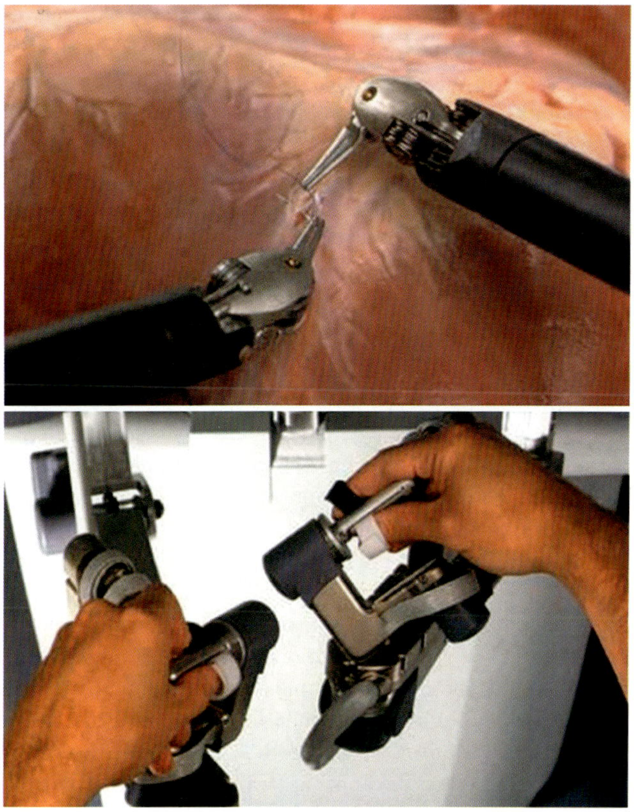

FIGURE 10–1 The Endowrist technology mimics the surgeon's natural hand and wrist movements.

will increase its market share by acquiring the robot. For example, in Nashville, Tennessee, there are already six robots at five institutions, and other institutions are considering acquisition, not to increase their market share, but rather to maintain case volumes and surgeons. These are important issues, but they are not always easy to answer or calculate. Evaluating the current referral base for the institution will give insight into the acceptance of new technology by referring physicians. Although some referring physicians may be excited to offer this opportunity to their patients, others may be concerned about losing their own patient base and the resultant impact on their own practices. Given that the advantages of robotic surgery are controversial, a tertiary center must consider how their community will respond to this advanced technology.

Another step in the market analysis is to determine which surgeons will be using the robot and for which procedures. The list of possible surgeries that can be performed using the robot has grown substantially (Box 10–1). This provides an initial basis on which to gauge surgical volume, operative times, and reimbursement data. It also provides an opportunity to assess buy-in by the participating surgeons and their commitment to the success of the overall program. Current volumes enable gross projections of case volumes following establishment of the robotic surgery program and will provide insight into the number of ORs and staff needed to cover these cases. Once the program is established, these data can be used as a benchmark to determine whether the program is growing and developing into a profitable entity.

Box 10–1

Surgical Procedures Performed with Robotic Assistance

Urologic
Prostatectomy
Pyeloplasty
Cystectomy
Nephrectomy
Sacrocolpopexy
Vasovasostomy
Pediatric urologic procedures (nephrectomy, partial nephrectomy, pyeloplasty, antireflux)
Adrenalectomy
Ureterolysis, ureteroureterostomy

Cardiothoracic
Internal mammary artery takedown
Left internal thoracic artery takedown
Coronary artery bypass graft
Totally endoscopic coronary artery bypass
Minimally invasive direct coronary artery bypass
Off-pump coronary artery bypass
Robotically sutured anastomosis via sternotomy
Mitral valve repair
Epicardial lead placement
Esophagectomy
Thymectomy

General surgery
Nissen fundoplication
Gastric bypass
Gastroplasty
Colon resection
Heller myotomy
Splenectomy
Cholecystectomy

CREDENTIALING

The surgeons who will use the robot need to be credentialed. A good credentialing system involves (1) board certification or board eligibility in the surgeon's appropriate surgical board, (2) privileges for both the open and laparoscopic surgery to be performed robotically, (3) completion of a specified robotic training course, (4) performance of robotic surgery in an animal model, (5) observation of expertly performed robotic surgery, (6) acting as bedside assistant for robotic surgery, (7) observation by a proctor of initial robotic surgical cases, and (8) ongoing monitoring of surgical outcomes of robotic surgical cases.[10] Our institution has a similar system in place and created a robotic surgery committee prior to system acquisition to establish credentialing, monitor safe implementation and ongoing use, and prepare in advance for the arrival of the new technology. This creates minimal downtime and prevents the financial loss of an unused robotic system.

FACILITY REQUIREMENTS

The OR and storage of the robotic system deserves careful consideration. The amount of space dedicated in the operative theater to the robot for the surgeon's console, robotic arm tower, and vision tower system is substantial. The layout of the room and amount of space required should be mapped out in advance (Figure 10–2). A room dedicated specifically to robotic surgery is beneficial. Appropriate numbers and types of electrical circuits, cables, and engineering input are required for the setup of the robot. The imaging monitors and the determination of which types (e.g., plasma screen, 3D) need to be well thought and mapped out, and the capability to upgrade them over time can be helpful. Determining which surgical services and surgeons require block time and access must be negotiated to allow for efficient, cost-effective utilization. We have constructed a specialized robotic surgical suite that can also be used for minimally invasive surgical and open procedures.

The ordering, stocking, and monitoring of the procedure-specific equipment and supplies necessary for the operative room are other important administrative issues. The robotic system uses a specialized, nonsterile, drapable camera, sterilizable 30- and 0-degree lens systems, and reusable robotic instruments (including cautery scissors, needle drivers, graspers, and special drapes). In addition, the different surgical teams may identify preferences for particular items. Often, as services increase volumes to include multiple patients and procedures in a single operative day, acquisition of a second lens systems and increasing duplication of equipment may be necessary to reduce turnover times.

TRAINING

Training of personnel can be the most time- and labor-intensive part of developing the robotic surgery program. However, a trained robotic team is the most important component of initiating a successful RALP program. A typical case may include the surgeon, one or two assistants, the scrub nurse, the circulating nurse, and the anesthesia team. The number of assistants and who serves as assistants may vary from institution to institution and from surgeon to surgeon. For example, having a fourth arm on the robot may eliminate the need for a second assistant or allow the scrub nurse to act as the second assistant. The first assistant may be another trained laparoscopic surgeon, surgical technician, physician's assistant, trained nurse, resident, or fellow. Regardless of who acts as first assistant, a certain comfort and facility with laparoscopy and the intended surgical procedures in addition to robotic

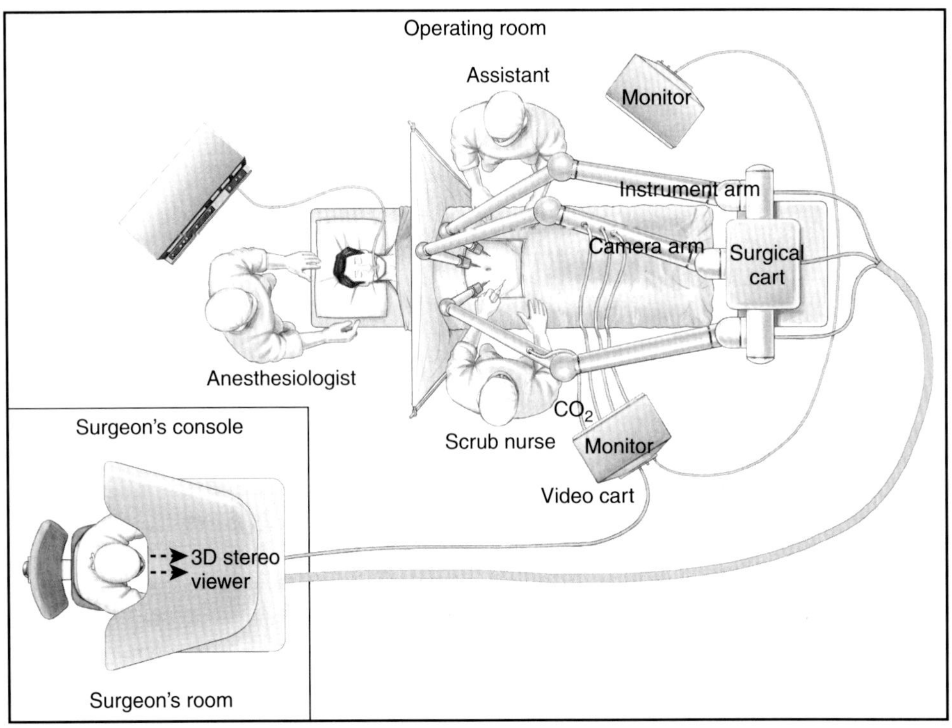

FIGURE 10–2 Schematic of the robotic operative suite including the operative staff required.

instrumentation training is necessary. At our institution, a highly experienced laparoscopic surgeon served as the table side surgeon for the first 40 to 50 cases by the open urologic oncologist. Residents, fellows, and a specialized, dedicated first assistant have been trained in case initiation, docking, assisting, and closure. We have found the decision to create a dedicated, first assistant position to be invaluable. This role provides for a highly specialized robotic laparoscopic first assistant who can train rotating residents and fellows and can be extremely valuable in providing consistent assistance and instruction.

Training in robotic surgery has been written about extensively. Robotic training courses and dedicated training centers are available throughout the United States. Several studies have evaluated a variety of instructional paradigms to become more adept at robotics prior to starting initial human cases. For example, Dasgupta et al.[11] described progressing from working in the robotic dry lab, to a cadaveric lab, to observing robotic surgery at another institution, to performing surgery while being mentored, and then finally performing the surgery themselves. Boehm et al.[12] described a similar method of training substituting increased animal lab procedural experience for the cadaveric lab. The cardiac surgeon authors introduced the robot clinically by performing one step robotically at a time and then doing the rest of the procedure in standard fashion through an open incision to become more facile with using the robot. Increasing portions of the cases incorporated the robot as their experience grew, and the size of their access to the chest was decreased over time.

Other published studies have evaluated robotic surgery training by comparing its learning curve to that of standard laparoscopy skills training. One study by Di Lorenzo et al.,[13] evaluating the robot for training, examined 20 experienced surgeons and 20 surgeons-in-training and evaluated their ability to use the robot for various tasks. They found that the experience of the surgeon affected results and found that the robot improved or simplified learning and perfecting surgical skills, and they theorized that it would therefore reduce the learning curve. Jourdan et al.[14] evaluated stereoscopic versus monoscopic vision use by eight laparoscopists for different surgical tasks and found that they performed tasks significantly better with stereoscopic vision. Hernandez et al.[15] also looked at the learning curve by evaluating 13 surgeons performing small bowel anastomoses and found a rapid learning curve using the robot. Ahlering et al.[9] evaluated the da Vinci for RALP and found that it took 12 cases to become proficient enough to perform the surgery in 4 hours or less for an open urologic oncologist. They also pointed out that this is significantly improved compared with that in the literature, where time for proficiency has classically been described as 80 to 100 cases for a laparoscopically naïve surgeon to perform laparoscopic prostatectomy and 40 to 60 cases for a skilled laparoscopic surgeon. Hubens et al.[16] came to a similar conclusion that the robot improves the learning curve compared with straight (manual) laparoscopic surgery by taking six medical students and comparing their learning curve with several tasks using both straight laparoscopy and the robot, with the learning curve being significantly shorter for the robot. Yohannes et al.[17] performed a similar study but involved eight novice and experienced laparoscopists who performed several different tasks and also found a shorter task learning curve when using the robot. In summary, the robot appears to substantially shorten the learning curve when compared with standard laparoscopy for a variety of task-oriented tests, as would be expected given the intuitive interface, albeit at a high financial cost. Although a variety of initial published studies in the urologic literature have commented on operative time as a measure of "learning curve" and proficiency, we would propose that the true learning curve for operations such as robotically assisted prostatectomy will be measured in terms of margin status combined with validated outcome measurements for continence and potency preservation.

OUTCOMES

Once the robotics program has been initiated, it is important to continually assess the key aspects of the program (Box 10–2). The financial impact is often the most important aspect to the hospital and includes the profit per case and the number of cases performed, as well as the marketing benefits realized. Continual assessment of per case instrumentation, personnel needs, and the reduction of operative times can reduce cost and potentially improve profit margins; however, the innate financial impact of the current one-vendor system limits cost reduction. To the patient and the surgeon, the case-specific outcomes are likely the most important aspect, which for RALP include margin status, continence, erectile function preservation, and complications.

Box 10–2

Important Outcome Measures for Robotic-Assisted Laparoscopic Prostatectomy (RALP)

Rate of conversion to open
Operating room time
Length of stay
Blood loss
Complications
Margin status
Continence
Potency

Although it is still too early in the robotic experience to make many definitive statements regarding the outcomes of robotic surgery in urology, initial experience has been encouraging, especially in the area of radical prostatectomy. Because of the lack of long-term outcomes based on prospective, randomized, multicenter studies, it is important to counsel patients appropriately. Patients must be informed that there are proven benefits to robotic prostate cancer surgery, including decreased blood loss. However, patients must also be informed that many benefits of RALP are potential and unproven, such as improved continence, erectile function, margin status, or even postoperative pain and length of stay at some institutions. At present, some institutions and studies have published data showing a marked advantage in their initial experience comparing robotic and open prostatectomy, although many of these studies' overall conclusions are limited by study design and the inherent lack of appropriate controls, randomization, and outcome measurements. In addition, the rapid and heavy penetration of robotic systems into many geographic areas combined with the competitive health care system environment and marketing may limit the unbiased assessment of outcomes. It is important that both the patient and the surgeon have realistic expectations. Surgeons must continually evaluate their own outcomes and resist the desire to quote results achieved in expert literature or at centers of excellence.

CONCLUSIONS

Establishing a robotic urologic surgery program for RALP requires careful forethought and planning, necessary financial expenditures, appropriate steps for establishing a dedicated OR and robotic team and for training personnel, and continual self-assessment. With the appropriate commitment, a robotic surgery program and urologic surgery robotics program can benefit the institution, the surgeons, and their patients. With ongoing study, we will continue to develop additional knowledge of this fascinating technology and the role it will assume in the armamentarium of urologic surgery.

REFERENCES

1. Steers WD, LeBeau S, Cardella J, et al: Establishing a robotics program. Urol Clin North Am 31:773–780, 2004.
2. Binder J, Kramer W: Robotically-assisted laparoscopic radical prostatectomy. BJU Int 87:408–410, 2001.
3. Eichel LAT, Clayman RV: Robotics in urologic surgery: risks and benefits. In: AUA Update Series, Vol 24, Lesson 13. Linthicum, MD, University of California, Irvine Medical Center, 2005, pp 106–111.
4. Nifong LW, Chitwood WR Jr: Building a surgical robotics program. Am J Surg 188(4A suppl):16S–18S, 2004.
5. Kaufman MR, Smith JA Jr, Baumgartner RG, et al: Positive influence of robotically assisted laparoscopic prostatectomy on the collaborative-care pathway for open radical prostatectomy. BJU Int 97:473–475, 2006.
6. Webster TM, Herrell SD, Chang SS, et al: Robotic assisted laparoscopic radical prostatectomy versus retropubic radical prostatectomy: a prospective assessment of postoperative pain. J Urol 174:912–914, 2005, discussion 914.
7. Patel YR, Donias HW, Boyd DW, et al: Are you ready to become a robo-surgeon? Am Surg 69:599–603, 2003.
8. Menon M, Shrivastava A, Tewari A, et al: Laparoscopic and robot assisted radical prostatectomy: establishment of a structured program and preliminary analysis of outcomes. J Urol 168:945–949, 2002.
9. Ahlering TE, Skarecky D, Lee D, et al: Successful transfer of open surgical skills to a laparoscopic environment using a robotic interface: initial experience with laparoscopic radical prostatectomy. J Urol 170:1738–1741, 2003.
10. Ballantyne GH, Kelley WE Jr: Granting clinical privileges for telerobotic surgery. Surg Laparosc Endosc Percutan Tech 12:17–25, 2002.
11. Dasgupta P, Hemal A, Rose K: Robotic urology in the UK: establishing a programme and emerging role. BJU Int 95:723–724, 2005.
12. Boehm DH, Arnold MB, Detter C, et al: Incorporating robotics into an open-heart program. Surg Clin North Am 83:1369–1380, 2003.
13. Di Lorenzo N, Coscarella G, Faraci L, et al: Robotic systems and surgical education. JSLS 9:3–12, 2005.
14. Jourdan IC, Dutson E, Garcia A, et al: Stereoscopic vision provides a significant advantage for precision robotic laparoscopy. Br J Surg 91:879–885, 2004.
15. Hernandez JD, Bann SD, Munz Y, et al: Qualitative and quantitative analysis of the learning curve of a simulated surgical task on the da Vinci system. Surg Endosc 18:372–378, 2004.
16. Hubens G, Coveliers H, Balliu L, et al: A performance study comparing manual and robotically assisted laparoscopic surgery using the da Vinci system. Surg Endosc 17:1595–1599, 2003.
17. Yohannes P, Rotariu P, Pinto P, et al: Comparison of robotic versus laparoscopic skills: is there a difference in the learning curve? Urology 60:39–45, 2002, discussion 45.

CHAPTER 11

Andreas Lunacek • Christian Schwentner • Wolfgang Horninger • Ashutosh Tewari • Georg Bartsch• Hannes Strasser

Anatomic Foundations of Nerve Sparing in Radical Prostatectomy

INTRODUCTION

During the past 10 years, the clinical course of prostate cancer has changed dramatically. Reasons for this change are better informed patients and improved screening methods. More patients then ever before are detected with localized prostate cancer, low prostate-specific antigen (PSA) values, and T_{1c} lesions.[1]

Radical retropubic prostatectomy is still the gold standard for effective treatment of organ-confined prostate cancer. Complete removal of the tumor is the main aim of surgery, but reduction of postoperative morbidity has also become very important to meet patients' expectations and to maintain a high quality of life after surgery.

To achieve an optimal postoperative outcome, good hemostasis of the dorsal vein complex and careful preservation of the pelvic plexus and the cavernous nerves are required. Excellent surgical experience as well as exact knowledge about topographic anatomy of the neurovascular bundles (NVBs) are prerequisites to reduce postoperative morbidity.

The main goals of the surgeon are cancer control, preservation of urinary control, and preservation of sexual function. After radical prostatectomy, urinary incontinence is usually secondary to intrinsic sphincter deficiency caused by injury during division of the dorsal vein complex or the urethra.[2] Therefore, meticulous apical dissection without destruction of the omega-shaped rhabdosphincter—the main structure of the urethral sphincter complex—and a precise mucosa-to-mucosa anastomosis are necessary to avoid this complication.[2–4]

Before the development of an anatomic approach to radical prostatectomy, virtually all patients were impotent, because the exact anatomic location of the autonomic branches from the pelvic plexus to the corpora cavernosa was unknown.[2] Walsh and Donker[5] described the anatomy of the cavernous nerves and recommended modifications in the surgical procedure that could preserve potency. The branches of the pelvic plexus that innervate the corpora cavernosa, the cavernous nerves, were shown to travel outside the prostatic capsule in the lateral pelvic fascia dorsolaterally between the rectum and the prostate. Although the nerves are microscopic in size, their location can be estimated intraoperatively by using the accompanying capsular prostatic vessels as a landmark.[2] The NVBs are located in the lateral pelvic fascia between the prostatic and levator ani fascia. At the level of the membranous urethra, they were shown to travel at the 3 and 9 o'clock positions.[5–10]

The fetal nerves are more prominent and relatively thicker than in adult specimens and can, therefore, be investigated more easily.[9,10] A histologic study was performed to investigate changes in the course of the cavernous nerves running in the NVBs during fetal development to provide morphologic data that could then be applied to improve the anatomic approach to radical prostatectomy.

MATERIALS AND METHODS

Fetal development of the pelvic plexus and the cavernous nerves was investigated in an extensive histologic study. Twenty-nine male fetal specimens were examined, and age of the fetuses ranged between 9 and 37 weeks' gestation. Crown-rump length was between 41 and 360 mm. The fetuses were all obtained after miscarriage and did not show any signs of maceration or macroscopic abnormalities.

The entire pelvic portion of the fetal trunk was dissected underneath the umbilicus. The plastination process started with preservation of the fetal specimens in 4% formaldehyde for about 12 weeks, followed by dehydration in acetone at −25° Celsius for about 6 weeks. Fat in the tissue was removed by embedding the specimens in methylene chloride at room temperature for 1 to 2 weeks. The specimens were then impregnated in a vacuum chamber with a mixture of the epoxy resin BiodurE12, hardener E1, and accelerator E600 for about 2 weeks. After polymerization, serial sections of the pelvic blocks were performed using the Well diamond wire-saw. Thickness of the serial sections ranged between 300 and 700 μm. The sections were polished before staining with azure II/methylene blue in alkaline solution and counterstaining with basic fuchsin. The sections were then used for examination and documentation. The individual sections of each block were investigated and photographed with a binocular microscope at a magnification of 4 to 400×.[11]

Then, the resulting morphologic data were used to modify dissection of the NVBs during nerve-sparing radical prostatectomy. All steps of the new operating technique were documented by photographs.

RESULTS

Fetal Anatomy of the Cavernous Nerves

The pelvic plexus presented as a prominent rectangular sagittal plate of densely packed nerve fibers between urinary bladder and rectum. This nerve plate and the other pelvic nerves could be demonstrated very clearly in fetal development as they were very thick compared with the surrounding tissue.

The fibers innervating the seminal vesicles, prostate, and the corpora cavernosa split off from this rectangular plate and passed caudally directly adjacent to the seminal vesicles, which were enclosed by the nerves (Figure 11–1). The pelvic plexus continued to remain in its original position as a rectangular plate between bladder and rectum throughout fetal development. Similarly, the cagelike embedding of the seminal vesicles with nerves was the same in all fetal stages. The pelvic plexus did not change its position during the entire period of fetal development.

The fibers of the cavernous nerves were shown to leave the caudal aspects of the pelvic plexus. The original course of the cavernous nerves could be demonstrated during the early stages of fetal development as the prostate did not start to develop before fetal week 13. Because of the absence of the prostate and the relatively thick nerves, the cavernous nerves were easy to identify as they ran downward lateral and dorsal to the prostatic and membranous urethra (Figure 11–2*A*). They were also situated dorsal and lateral to the omega-shaped rhabdosphincter, which covered the ventrolateral aspects of the prostatic and membranous urethra between the bulb of the penis and the bladder neck.

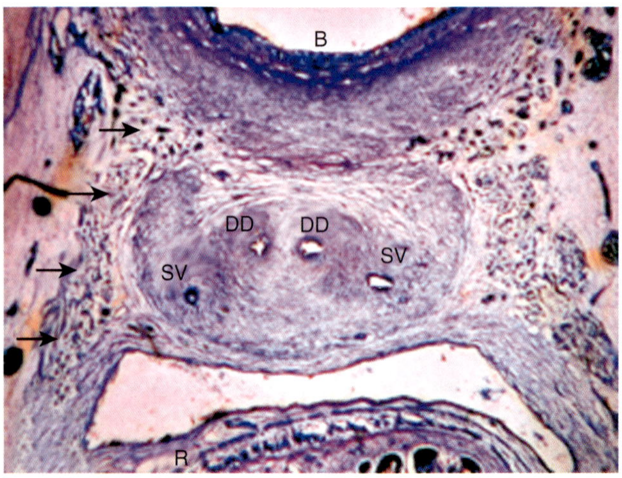

FIGURE 11–1 Fetal specimen, 12 weeks. The sagittally oriented pelvic plexus lateral to the pelvic organs is marked with arrows. B, bladder; DD, primordia of the deferential ducts; R, rectum; SV, primordia of the seminal vesicles.

After 13 weeks' gestation, the prostate began to develop. Because of growth and increasing volume of the prostate, the cavernous nerves were displaced further anteriorly, as the whole NVB fans out (Figure 11–2*B*). In this region the nerve fibers and the vessels were more and more fanned out along the convex surface of the prostatic capsule. Therefore, the cavernous nerves running in the NVB assumed a shape that can best be compared with the concave "steep turn of a bob run" or a concavely formed "curtain" covering both prostatic lobes (Figure 11–2*B* to *D*). At the apex of the prostate the nerve fibers of the NVBs converged again—like the exit of a steep turn of a bob run—and lay adjacent to the membranous urethra (Figure 11–2*C* and *D*).

Another striking finding of the present study was that the nerve fibers in the region of the prostatic and membranous urethra could be found all around the urethra between the 3 and the 9 o'clock positions and not only lateral to the urethra. The dorsal median raphe of the rhabdosphincter was the only area that was free of nerve fibers (Figure 11–3*A* and *B*). This finding could be demonstrated in all histologic specimens. The course of the cavernous nerves in the region of the rhabdosphincter and the membranous urethra was consistent in all specimens. The cavernous nerves passed caudally in both NVBs along the prostatic capsule and converged at the apex of the prostate to enclose the membranous urethra dorsolaterally.

Description of the Modified "Curtain Dissection" of the Neurovascular Bundles

According to the present anatomic findings, the surgical technique of radical retropubic prostatectomy has been modified. After incision of the ventral aspect of the membranous urethra and placement of the first four anastomotic sutures (Figure 11–4*A* to *C*) in the urethra without involvement of the cavernous nerves, the curtain dissection of both NVBs is performed (Figure 11–4*D*). Using magnifying lenses, dissection of the NVBs has to start very far anteriorly to preserve all the nerve fibers that are spread out concavely in a "bob run steep turn" or "curtain" shape along the surface of the lobes of the prostate (see Figure 11–2*C* and *D*). With this type of dissection, the majority of cavernous nerves forming the NVBs can be preserved.

After the NVBs have been spared, the urethra is cut at the apex of the prostate. Then, the dorsal aspect of the urethra is divided under direct vision (Figure 11–4*E*) and a traction suture is placed (Figure 11–4*E*), which is used to

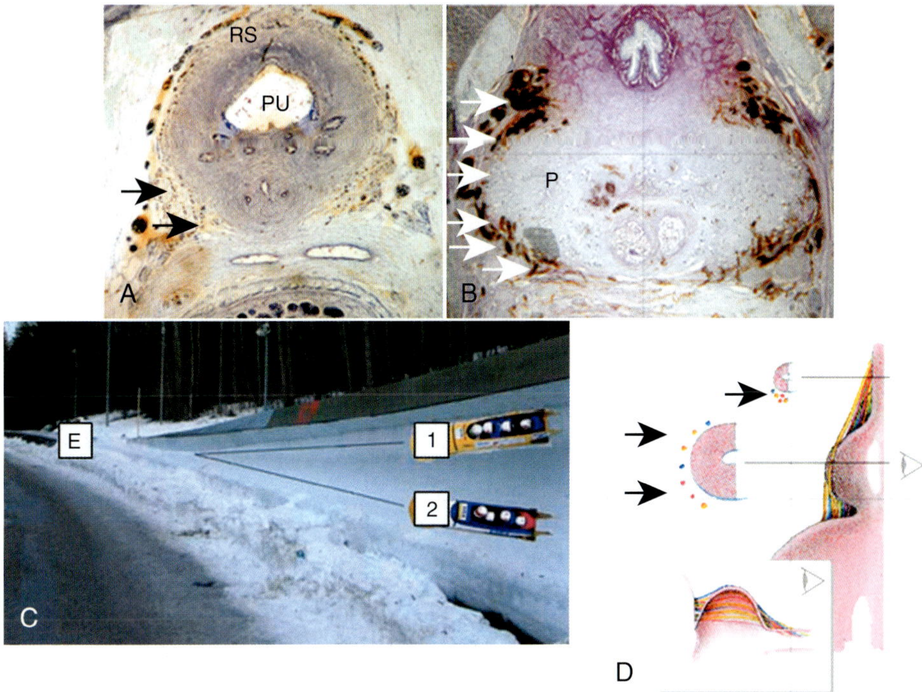

FIGURE 11–2 Change of course of the cavernous nerves after growth of the prostate. *A,* Before development of the prostate the cavernous nerves (marked with arrows) are situated lateral and dorsal to the prostatic (PU) and membranous urethra as well as the rhabdosphincter (RS). All around the urethra darkly stained blood vessels can be seen. *B,* Because of the growth of the prostate (P), the cavernous nerves and the blood vessels (darkly stained) running in the neurovascular bundle are more and more fanned out along the convex surface of the prostate. Therefore, they now assume a "bob run steep turn" or concave "curtain" shape (marked with arrows). Exit of a steep turn of the Olympic bob run in Igls/Innsbruck. Similar to the course of the faster bob sleigh (1) in the steep turn—compared with the slower bob sleigh (2)—dissection of the neurovascular bundle has to start more anteriorly to spare the majority of the cavernous nerves. The narrow exit (E) can be compared with the convergence of the neurovascular bundles in the region around the membranous urethra. *D,* Drawing of the "bob run steep turn" or concave curtain shape of the neurovascular bundle after development of the prostate. The two cross sections show the course of the neurovascular bundle along the surface of the prostate and along the dorsolateral aspect of the membranous urethra. The red line marks the anterior site of incision of the lateral pelvic fascia during the new curtain dissection of the neurovascular bundle. The blue line demonstrates the far more dorsally situated standard site of dissection of the neurovascular bundle. The green line marks the cavernous nerves that are situated dorsal and lateral to the membranous urethra. In the smaller drawing, the neurovascular bundle situated in the lateral pelvic fascia is shown after removal of the prostate. The course of the nerves can be compared with the steep turn of a bob run *(C).*

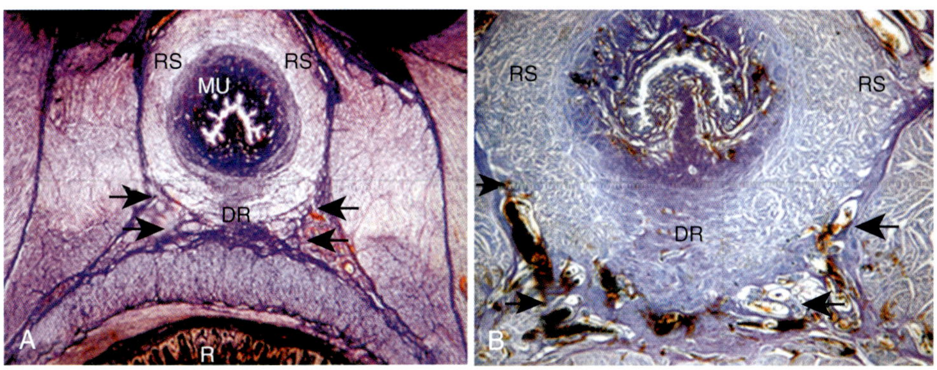

FIGURE 11–3 Membranous urethra of two fetal specimens after development of the prostate. The localization of both neurovascular bundles (marked by arrows) is not influenced by the growth of the prostate. The neurovascular bundles (marked with arrows) are situated dorsal and lateral to the membranous urethra (MU) and the rhabdosphincter (RS). DR, dorsal raphe of the rhabdosphincter; R, rectum. The dorsal median raphe (DR) of the rhabdosphincter (RS) does not contain nerve fibers (marked with arrows). Blood vessels are darkly stained.

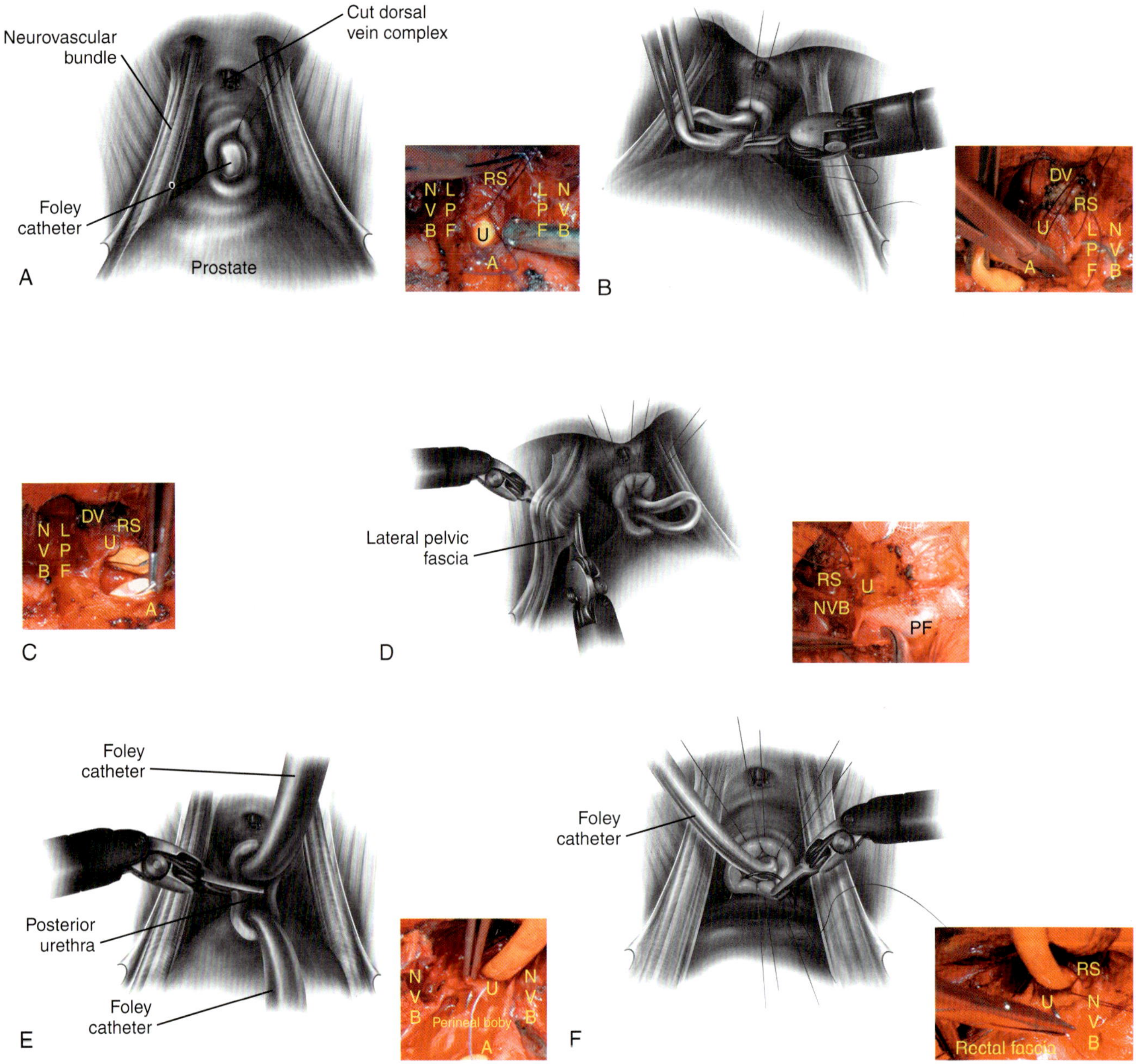

FIGURE 11–4 *A,* "Curtain dissection" of the neurovascular bundle and modified apical dissection. *B,* Placement of the second anastomotic suture (11 o'clock). *C,* The catheter is pulled up with a forceps (to the left side); placement of the third anastomotic suture (3:30 o'clock). *D,* The catheter is pulled up with a forceps (to the right side); placement of the fourth anastomotic suture (8:30 o'clock). *E,* Incision of the lateral pelvic fascia and curtain dissection of the neurovascular bundle has to start very far anteriorly to preserve all the nerve fibers that are spread out concavely in a "bob run steep turn" or "curtain" shape along the surface of the lateral lobe of the prostate (PF). The urethra is cut at the apex of the prostate; the urethra is not undermined with a clamp. Under direct vision the posterior part of the urethra and the perineal body are cut to the rectal fascia. *F,* A traction suture is placed at 6 o'clock. Pulling back the traction suture, the fifth anastomotic suture is placed (5 o'clock) medial to the neurovascular bundle. Then, the sixth anastomotic suture is placed as well on the other side. A, apex of the prostate; DV, dorsal vein complex; LPF, lateral pelvic fascia; NVB, neurovascular bundle; PF, prostatic fascia; RS, rhabdosphincter; U, urethra.

place the two dorsal anastomotic sutures in the urethral wall (Figure 11–4*F*).

Because the majority of the cavernous nerves are situated dorsolateral and dorsal to the membranous urethra, it is recommended not to use right angle clamps or other surgical instruments to dissect between the posterior urethra and the rectum (Figure 11–4*F*). Because the cavernous nerves are not only situated lateral to the urethra but are also running dorsal to the membranous urethra, except for the dorsal median raphe of the rhabdosphincter, minimal manipulation dorsal to the membranous urethra is critical for preservation of the erectile nerve fibers.

Another main finding of the present study is that the nerve fibers enclose the seminal vesicles very tightly. This fact supports earlier descriptions stating that dissection of the seminal vesicles has to be performed very accurately to avoid injury to the nerve fibers. No blunt dissection should be performed lateral to the seminal vesicles, because the nerve fibers are directly adjacent to the seminal vesicles. Therefore, the seminal vesicles have to be carefully dissected under direct vision. For control of bleedings small hemoclips are used, and electrocautery is avoided.

DISCUSSION

Based on anatomic studies, Walsh and Donker demonstrated that the cavernous nerves travel outside the prostatic capsule and Denonvilliers' fascia until they reach the region of the membranous urethra. As they exited the pelvic plexus, the cavernous nerves and the adjacent vessels were described to lie in the triangular space between prostate, levator ani muscle, and rectum, thereby forming the "neurovascular bundle," which is located between the prostatic and levator ani fascia.[2,5] At the apex of the prostate the nerves are only a few millimeters away from the urethral lumen. It has been thought that the cavernous nerves exit the pelvis lateral to the membranous urethra.[5–14]

The present study was performed to describe the exact course of the cavernous nerves. The goal was to provide an anatomic map to improve surgical technique. Preservation of potency during radical retropubic prostatectomy is possible,[15–17] if the surgeon has exact knowledge about the course of the cavernous nerves.

From the present anatomic data it has become clear that the growth of the prostate influences the course of the cavernous nerves running in the NVBs. As the prostate grows, the nerves become displaced anteriorly and fan out along the convex surface of the prostatic capsule. The NVBs assume a "steep turn of a bob run" or a concavely formed curtain shape covering both prostatic lobes (see Figure 11–2*B* to *D*). At the apex of the prostate, the nerve fibers of the NVBs converge again. The fibers are situated not only in the 3 and 9 o'clock positions but dorsal and lateral to the membranous urethra all along the 3 to 9 o'clock positions. Only in the area of the dorsal median raphe of the rhabdosphincter are nerve fibers absent.

The cavernous nerves are most prone to destruction during dissection of the NVBs along the prostate and during apical dissection. The modified curtain dissection described in the present article was introduced to improve preservation of the cavernous nerves running in the NVBs. Incision of the lateral pelvic fascia and dissection of the NVB has to be performed much more anteriorly than previously described to really spare the majority of cavernous nerves (see Figure 11–2*B* to *D*). It is also recommended not to use cauterization but to use small hemoclips to control bleedings from the NVBs during dissection and removal of the prostate.

In addition, apical dissection has to be performed very meticulously.[18–20] Any dissection of the tissue dorsal to the membranous urethra, including the caudal attachment of Denonvilliers' fascia to the perineal body, should be performed very carefully because the majority of nerves can be destroyed with any blunt surgical maneuver (see Figure 11–4*F*).

REFERENCES

1. Partin AW, Mangold LA, Lamm DM, et al: Contemporary update of prostate cancer staging nomograms (partin tables for the new millennium). Urology 58:843, 2001.
2. Walsh PC: Anatomic radical retropubic prostatectomy. In Walsh PC, Retik AB, Vaughan ED, et al (eds): Campbell's Urology, 8th ed. Philadelphia, WB Saunders Company, 2002.
3. Strasser H, Klima G, Poisel S, et al: Anatomy and innervation of the rhabdosphincter of the male urethra. Prostate 28:24, 1996.
4. Helweg G, Strasser H, Knapp R, et al: Transurethral sonomorphologic evaluation of the male external sphincter of the urethra. Eur Radiol 4:525, 1994.
5. Walsh PC, Donker PJ: Impotence following radical prostatectomy: insight into etiology and prevention. J Urol 128:492, 1982.
6. Lue TF, Zeineh SJ, Schmidt RA, et al: Neuroanatomy of penile erection: its relevance to iatrogenic impotence. J Urol 131:273, 1984.
7. Lepor H, Gregerman M, Crosby R, et al: Precise localization of the autonomic nerves from the pelvic plexus to the corpora cavernosa: a detailed anatomical study of the adult male pelvis. J Urol 133:207, 1985.
8. Walsh PC, Brendler CB, Chang T, et al: Preservation of sexual function in men during radical pelvic surgery. Md Med J 39:389, 1990.
9. Colleselli K, Strasser H, Moriggl B, et al: Anatomical approach in surgery on the membranous urethra. World J Urol 7:190, 1990.
10. Strasser H, Poisel S, Stenzl A, et al: Anatomy and innervation of the male urethra, the rhabdosphincter, and the corpora cavernosa. Part II, AUA update series, Lesson 16, Volume XX:122, 2001, American Urological Association Office of Education, Houston, TX.
11. Fritsch H, Hotzinger H: Topographical anatomy of the pelvic, visceral pelvic connective tissue and its components. Clin Anat 8:17, 1995.
12. Walsh PC, Lepor H, Eggleston JD: Radical prostatectomy with preservation of sexual function: anatomical and pathological considerations. Prostate 4:473, 1983.
13. Walsh PC, Marschke P, Ricker D, et al: Use of intraoperative video documentation to improve sexual function after radical retropubic prostatectomy. Urology 55:62, 2000.
14. Steiner MS: Anatomic basis for the continence-preserving radical retropubic prostatectomy. Semin Urol Oncol 18:9, 2000.

15. Quinlan DM, Epstein JI, Cartzer BS, et al: Sexual function following radical prostatectomy: influence of preservation of neurovascular bundles. J Urol 145:998, 1991.
16. Walsh PC: Patient-reported urinary continence and sexual function after anatomic radical prostatectomy. J Urol 164:242, 2000.
17. Walsh PC: Radical prostatectomy for localized prostate cancer provides durable cancer control with excellent quality of life: a structured debate. J Urol 163:1802, 2000.
18. Myers RP, Goellner JR, Cahill DR: Prostate shape, external striated urethral sphincter and radical prostatectomy: the apical dissection. J Urol 138:543, 1987.
19. Myers RP: Re: antegrade approach to radical retropubic prostatectomy in patients with difficult apical dissection. J Urol 148:1267, 1992.
20. Myers RP: Radical prostatectomy: making it a better operation in the new millennium. Int J Urol 8:9, 2001.

CHAPTER 12

Sagar R. Shah • Vipul R. Patel

Perioperative Outcomes of Robotic Radical Prostatectomy

INTRODUCTION

Prostate cancer accounts for 33% of all newly diagnosed cancers in men. It is estimated that in 2007 in the United States, the incidence of prostate cancer will be 218,890 cases, with approximately 27,050 deaths from the disease.[1] The current gold standard for surgical treatment is open radical retropubic prostatectomy (RRP), which has demonstrated a reduction in disease-specific mortality for patients with localized prostate cancer.[2] Approximately 77,000 radical prostatectomies are performed yearly for the treatment of prostate cancer. However, this treatment option is invasive and can potentially lead to significant perioperative morbidity, erectile dysfunction, incontinence, and reduced quality of life. As such, patients and surgeons alike have sought out less invasive surgical options with at least equivalent perioperative outcomes and possibly superior outcomes. One such alternative is robotic-assisted laparoscopic prostatectomy (RALP).

Initial reports of the use of telerobotic surgical systems to facilitate performance of laparoscopic radical prostatectomy (LRP) were presented in 2001 by Abbou et al.,[3] Pasticier et al.,[4] Binder and Kramer,[5] and Rassweiler et al.[6] Robotic assistance with the da Vinci Surgical System (Intuitive Surgical, Sunnyvale, CA) has been reported to aid in the performance of laparoscopic prostatectomy secondary to the following: (1) restoration of depth perception and improved vision as a result of the 10× magnification along with three-dimensional (3D) vision; (2) wristed miniature instrumentation with restoration of seven degrees of surgical freedom; (3) tremor filtering and scaling of movements, which aids in fine dissection and precise suturing; (4) intuitive finger-controlled movement; and (5) improved ergonomics and relaxed surgeon working position providing for reduced surgeon fatigue.[3–13] It has been reported that because of these advantages over conventional laparoscopy, robotic assistance has accelerated learning in the laparoscopically naïve surgeon and has reduced the learning curve to achieve 4-hour proficiency down to 12 to 18 cases without significant outcome variation.[13–16]

INDICATIONS AND CONTRAINDICATIONS

The indications for robotic-assisted laparoscopic prostatectomy via the transperitoneal approach have been described to be similar to those of open and laparoscopic prostatectomy. Patients should have localized prostate cancer, biologically significant disease, and life expectancy greater than 10 years.[7,17] It is often easier to perform RALP compared with conventional RRP in patients that have undergone prior laparoscopic inguinal herniorraphy.[17] Also, it is believed that robotic-assisted prostatectomies allow patients with increased comorbidities to undergo surgery, whereas otherwise they would have been considered poor candidates for the open surgical approach. Relative contraindication to RALP is weight greater than 300 pounds, body mass index (BMI) greater than 40, previously ruptured viscera, history of peritonitis, and prior pelvic radiation therapy.

OPERATIVE OUTCOMES

Operative Time

It is often difficult to compare operative times between various series because of variations in reporting of operative time to include setup and/or pelvic lymph node dissection. It must be noted that there is an initial learning curve not only for the surgeon with the procedure but also for the operating room staff with setup of the robot. The mean operative time for reported robotic series ranges from 141 to 540 minutes (Table 12–1).[1–10,14,16,18–32] In our experience, in a series of 200 cases, our operative time declined from a mean of 202 minutes for our first 50 cases to 141 minutes for the last 50 cases.[32] Our operative times have now declined further to the range of 90 minutes as our series has matured and advanced over 1000 cases. Ahlering et al.[14] have also reported a similar reduction in time with experience with a mean operative time of 184 minutes for their last 10 cases (in a series of 45) compared with the overall mean operative time of 207 minutes.

Table 12–1 Operative Characteristics and Outcomes of Robotic-Assisted Laparoscopic Prostatectomy (RALP)

	Mean Age in Years (range)	No. of Patients	Mean PSA in ng/mL (range)	Access	No. of Assistants	Mean Operative Time in Minutes (range)
Abbou et al.[3] (2001)	63 (NR)	1	7 (NR)	TP	1	420 (NR)
Pasticier et al.[4] (2001)	58 (55–63)	5	12.4 (6–23)	TP	1	222 (150–381)
Binder and Kramer[5] (2001)*	60.5 (57–69)	10	6.4 (0.5–22.4)	TP	1	540* (325–660)
Rassweiler et al.[5] (2001)*	47 (40–55)	6	9.7 (2.4–12)	TP	2	315* (242–480)
Samadi et al.[28] (2002)	67 (58–71)	11	8.9 (3.9-32)	TP	1	300 (200–420)
Menon et al.[16] (2002)	60.7 (NR)	40	5.7 (NR)	TP	2	274 (NR)
Menon et al.[8] (2003)	59.9 (42–76)	200	6.2 (0.6–41)	TP	2	160* (71–315)
Menon et al.[9] (2003)*	NR	100	NR	TP	2	165* 135 (NR)
Bentas et al.[31]	NR	40	NR	TP	NR	498 (NR)
Aherling et al.[14] (2003)	61.4 (46–71)	45	7.3 (1.1–24.0)	TP	1	207 (150–306)
Worlfram et al.[30] (2003)	63 (45–71)	81	8.96 (1.5–40)	TP	1	250 (150–390)
Aherling et al.[26] (2004)	62.9 (43–78)	60	8.1 (0.6–62)	TP	1	231 (160–340)
Cathelineau et al.[7] (2004)	NR	70 TP 35 EP	8 (4–24)	TP/EP	1	180 (120–190)
Patel et al.[32] (2005)	59.5 (40–78)	200	7.1 (1–90)	TP	1	141.2 (NR)

*Includes pelvic lymph node dissection.
EBL, estimated blood loss; EP, extraperitoneal; NR, not reported; TP, transperitoneal.

In a recent study, in patients undergoing RALP with BMI greater than 35, mean operative times (295.8 minutes) are significantly prolonged compared with those for patients with BMI less than 35 (236.1 minutes).[33] In series comparing RALP to RRP performed by the same surgeon or at the same institution, no significant difference has been observed between operative times in these studies.[11,26] Thus, it is safe to say that for experienced surgeons, RALP can be performed at least as fast as the other modalities and is showing a trend toward more rapid performance than LRP.

Blood Loss and Transfusion

As with any surgery, significant blood loss can occur with any form of prostatectomy and can be a source of significant morbidity from transfusion reactions, contraction of bloodborne infection from transfusion, and increased technical difficulty resulting from blood obscuring the operative field, preventing ideal operative outcome. It is known that transfusion rates do not always accurately represent blood loss associated with a procedure. A patient may have significant blood loss and still not require transfusion, which is dependent on surgeon variability with transfusion criteria. Decreased intraoperative blood loss has been reported to be a hallmark advantage of laparoscopic prostatectomy.[21,22,34–41] Because most intraoperative blood loss originates from the venous sinuses, the tamponade effect created by pneumoperitoneum helps diminish blood loss.[42] In addition, early identification and precise ligation of vessels facilitates the limitation of blood loss. The mean estimated blood loss in RALP series is 75 to 900 mL (see Table 12–1).[3–9,14,16,26,28,30–32] The transfusion rate after RALP has been reported to be 0% to 16.6%.[3–9,14,16,26,28,30–32] In many of the RALP series from the United States, there has been a 0% transfusion rate after RALP.[8,14,16,26,43] Menon et al.[17] report a 0% transfusion rate after 1100 RALPs. Tewari et al.[11] report a significantly higher rate of transfusion after RRP (67%) compared with RALP (0%) in their single-institution series comparing 100 RRPs performed by different surgeons and 200 RALPs performed by the same surgeon. Menon et al.[16] have also reported a higher rate of transfusion after LRP (2.5%) compared with RALP (0%). Thus, it appears that the currently available data show a trend for RALP to have at least equivalent if not superior outcome in regard to blood loss and transfusion rates when compared with RRP and LRP.

Mean EBL in mL (range)	Transfusion Rate in %	Mean Length of Stay in Days (range)	Mean Catheterization Time in Days (range)	% Intra-operative Complications	% Postoperative Complications	% Positive Margins
300 (NR)	0	4 (NR)	3 (NR)	0	0	0
800 (700–1600)	0	5.5 (4–7)	6.5 (5–9)	0	0	20
NR	10	NR	18 (5–23)	0	10	30
NR	16.6	NR	7.3 (5–14)	0	0	0
900 (400–1600)	NR	NR	NR (2–5)	0	0	36.4
256 (NR)	0	NR	NR	0	2.5	17.5
153 (NR)	0	1.2 (NR)	7 (NR)	0	4	6
150 (25–525)	NR	NR	4.2 (NR)	NR	NR	4
570 (NR)	NR	NR	NR	NR	NR	NR
134 (25–350)	0	1.5 (0.75–7)	7 (NR)	0	13	35.5
300 (100–1500)	12	NR	14 (6–28)	NR	NR	22.2
105 (25–400)	0	1.08 (0.75–4)	7 (NR)	0	6.7	16.7
500 (150–2000)	6	5.5 (3–13)	7 (NR)	0.9	6.7	22
75 (NR)	0	1.1 (1–3)	7.2 (5–15)	1	1	10.5

FUNCTIONAL OUTCOMES

Convalescence

One of the potential benefits of "minimally invasive" (i.e., laparoscopic) surgery has been shorter convalescence. Included in the definition of a shorter convalescence period is decreased postoperative pain, shorter length of hospital stay, and shorter catheter times.

Postoperative Pain

There is a perception of decreased postoperative pain with any type of laparoscopic surgery because of smaller incisions; however, there are very few studies comparing postoperative pain between groups of patients undergoing RALP and RRP from a single surgeon or institution. In the few published studies, there are conflicting reports on reduction in postoperative pain with RALP. In studies by Menon et al.[9,11] there was a statistically significant difference in visual analog pain score on postoperative day 1, with RALP having a mean score of 3 (1–7), compared with RRP, which had a mean score of 7 (4–10). In a study by Webster et al.,[44] the converse was reported with no statistical difference in pain on the day of surgery using the Likert pain scale, with RALP having a mean score of 2.52 compared with 2.88 in the RRP group. In the same study by Webster et al.,[44] mean pain scores were significantly lower, favoring the RRP group on postoperative day 1 (1.58 RRP versus 2.92 RALP), but at postoperative day 14, there was once again no difference between the two groups (2.81 RALP versus 2.10 RRP).

In our experience, pain after RALP is minimal. Our postoperative hospital orders do not contain any narcotics, but only Ketorolac 15 mg intravenously every 6 hours and the use of an ON-Q (I-flow corporation, Lake Forrest, CA) subcutaneously placed delivery system for 0.5% Marcaine are used. Further analysis in single-surgeon series with matched patient groups comparing postoperative pain with RRP and RALP with validated questionnaires is needed to confirm or refute the argument of decreased postoperative pain because of smaller incisions in LRP and RALP.

Length of Hospital Stay

Length of hospitalization is another component of convalescence after surgery and often considered a measure of well-being and marker of superior surgical outcome by patients undergoing treatment. The mean length of stay (LOS) in robotic series has been reported to be 1.08 to

5.5 days[3–10,14,16,26,27–32] (see Table 12–1). In more recent RALP series from the United States, the mean length of stay has been reported to be 1.08 to 1.5 days, declining with increasing experience.[8–10,12,14,16,26,30,32] It would be expected that patients after LRP and RALP would have similar LOS because RALP is no less invasive but simply uses robotic assistance for performance of LRP. Ahlering et al.[26] reported shorter LOS in patients after RALP compared with RRP (25.9 versus 52.8 hours) performed by the same surgeon. Menon et al.[10] reported similar findings, with the mean LOS for the RALP group being 1.2 days compared with 3.5 days for the RRP group. Thus, series comparing RALP to RRP from a single center or single surgeon have shown decreased LOS after RALP compared with RRP. In our experience, 95% of patients are discharged home on the first postoperative day.

Catheterization Time

Robotic assistance provides for improved vision with intuitive movements, lending to more facile performance of urethrovesical anastomosis. One could then infer that this would allow for a more watertight anastomosis and therefore earlier removal of catheter without fear of urinary retention. The mean catheterization time in reported RALP series ranges from 3 to 18 days (see Table 12–1).[3,4,7,8,14,26,32] When excluding the series with fewer than 40 patients, the majority of series report mean catheterization times ranging from 4.2 to 7.2 days. In a single-surgeon series by Ahlering et al.,[26] mean catheter time after RALP was 7 days compared with 9 days for RRP; however, this was not statistically significant. Tewari et al.[11] have reported duration of catheterization to be twice as long after RRP compared with RALP (15.8 versus 7 days) in their single-center study. Menon et al.[9] recently reported a reduction of catheter time following RALP to a mean of 4.2 days. Thus, there appears to be a trend for shorter time of catheterization with RALP in series comparing RALP to RRP outcomes for a single surgeon or center.

Erectile Function

Theoretically de novo erectile dysfunction after prostatectomy occurs because of injury of the neurovascular bundle. Damage to the neurovascular bundles can occur by direct incision, incorporation of the nerve into hemostatic suture or clips, and thermal or traction injury. Younger age, better preoperative potency, and extent of neurovascular bundle preservation are factors that have been shown to affect postoperative return of erectile function.[16,45,46]

Even after years of refinement of nerve-sparing technique in open surgery, the rate of erectile function recovery after RRP is not optimal and varies widely, depending on surgeon skill and definition of erectile dysfunction. In most instances, potency is defined as the ability to achieve erections and engage in intercourse with or without the use of oral medications, but it generally does not incorporate the measurement of erectile frequency or quality, which may be decreased from the preoperative state. Using this definition, overall potency rates after RRP are reported to be 62% to 68% at high-volume centers but as low as 10% to 30% in patient-reported surveys.[47–56] In series by Quinlan et al.,[46] potency rates are 90% for men younger than 50 years undergoing RRP with preservation of one or both neurovascular bundles, with a reduction in potency rate for men older than 50 years, especially if both neurovascular bundles are not preserved. Walsh et al.[57] have also reported an overall rate of potency defined by intercourse with or without the use of sildenafil to be 38% at 3 months, 54% at 6 months, 73% at 12 months, and 86% at 18 months.

It has been proposed that RALP may prevent damage to the neurovascular bundle because dissection occurs in an antegrade fashion, reducing traction on the nerve; because vision is improved as a result of magnification; and because the reduced blood in the surgical field allows more precise dissection, preventing inadvertent incision or incorporation into the suture or clip. In their initial comparative series from a single center, Bhandari et al.[15] reported a return to the preoperative baseline potency in 29.4% (5/17) of patients undergoing RALP at mean follow-up of 1.5 months compared with 25% (3/12) in the LRP group at a mean follow-up of 6.5 months. In their initial series, Ahlering et al.[14] only had two preoperatively potent (sexual health inventory in men [SHIM] >20) patients with adequate follow-up and reported a 50% rate of potency at 6 to 9 months, with the postoperatively impotent patient receiving only a unilateral nerve-spring procedure. In a recent series of 565 RALPs, Tewari et al.[11] report that 82% of preoperatively potent patients younger than 60 years had a return of some sexual activity and 64% had sexual intercourse at 6 months. In patients older than 60, 75% had some return of sexual activity and 38% had intercourse at 6 months postoperative. If potency is defined as ability to have intercourse, return of potency in men younger than 60 in Tewari's RALP series[11] compares favorably with Walsh's RRP series.[57] In an earlier series, Tewari et al.[11] also compared the outcomes of 200 RALP procedures to those of 100 RRPs performed over the same time period at a single institution; they reported a more rapid return of erection after RALP (50% return at a median follow-up of 180 days for RALP versus 440 days for RRP, $P < .05$) and a more rapid return to intercourse (50% at 340 days for RALP versus <50% at >700 days for RRP). Of note, both Menon and Ahlering have noticed improved potency rates after scissors and bipolar electrocautery became available for use with the da Vinci system in the posterior dissection.[8,14]

Recently, more series have presented outcomes based on validated questionnaires. One routinely used questionnaire is the International Index of Erectile Function (IIEF) and its abridged version, the IIEF-5. Rosen et al.[58] reported that an IIEF-5 score greater than 21 had a 98% negative predictive value for diagnosing erectile dysfunction. When using a cutoff of IIEF-5 less than 21 as defining erectile dysfunction, the percentage of men potent after RRP ranges from 10% to 74%.[59–61] In a recent LRP series, 17% of men attained IIEF-5 scores of more than 21 postoperatively.[60] In a recent study by Menon et al.[62] using their "veil of Aphrodite" technique, they report that 86% of men (mean age, 57.4) retained IIEF-5 scores of more than 21 postoperatively following RALP when they were preoperatively potent as defined by a score greater than 21.

No consensus exists on the ideal tools to document preoperative and postoperative potency in relation to any form of prostatectomy. There also appears to be great variation in the methodology used for describing potency outcomes among all available literature for RRP, LRP, and RALP.[19,35,36,39,63,64] However, it does appear that RALP has similar rates of postoperative potency compared with the best-reported rates after RRP and LRP and is showing a trend toward improved outcomes, especially when comparing data that have used validated questionnaires for evaluation of postoperative erectile function.

Continence

One of the primary surgical objectives when performing prostatectomy is maintenance of continence. This is often a significant area of concern for the patient when considering treatment options. Precise mucosa-to-mucosa approximation and optimal preparation of the urethral stump are important in preservation of continence and prevention of stricture.[12] Younger age, preservation of the neurovascular bundle, and absence of preoperative stricture have also been reported to increase the chance of retaining or regaining continence after surgery.[45]

In earlier series of RRP, the rates of incontinence based on patient-reported surveys were as high as 50%.[48–51] Walsh et al.[57] reported continence (no pad usage in past 4 weeks) to be 54% at 3 months, 80% at 6 months, 93% at 12 months, and 93% at 18 months. The pad-free rate after RRP at 3 months postoperative has been reported to be between 50% and 76%.[26,65,66] The majority of series report continence rates after RRP to be greater than 90% and up to 95% in one series at 12 months postoperative.[45,53–57,65,67,68]

It has been proposed that RALP can potentially result in better continence rates or earlier return of continence by improved preservation of urethral sphincter and urethral length. The theory is that superb visualization of the apex allows the surgeon to gently sweep away urethral sphincter muscular tissue from the anterior prostate and that improved hemostasis prevents blood from obscuring the apex, which leads to inadvertent injury to the sphincter.[42] Ahlering et al.[14] have reported continence rates of 33%, 63%, and 81% at 1 week, 1 month, and 3 months, respectively, after RALP. In a comparative study, Ahlering et al.[26] found no significant difference in overall continence rates after RALP (76%) compared with RRP (75%) when performed by the same surgeon. However, Tewari et al.[11] have shown return to continence to be quicker in the RALP group, with 50% being continent at 44 days compared with 160 days for RRP. In the landmark initial reports of RALP, Pasticier et al.[4] reported 80% of patients to be continent at 9 days postoperative, and Binder and Kramer[5] reported a 50% rate of continence at 1 month. Recently, Menon et al.[12] have reported a continence rate (no pads) of 96% at 3 months postoperative. In our study[32] of 200 patients, continence was described as the use of no pads daily and continence at 1, 3, 6, 9, and 12 months was 47%, 82%, 89%, 92%, and 98%, respectively. In a recent study using multivariate analysis, obesity (BMI > 30) was found to be a significant predictor ($P = .016$) of pad-free continence at 6 months postoperative following RALP, with 47% of patients with BMI greater than 30 having pad-free continence compared with 91% of patients with BMI less than 30 being continent ($P < .001$).[33]

Based on reported data, return of continence does appear to be earlier for RALP with a trend toward improved overall continence rates (98% for RALP versus 95% in RRP in best reported results) even when including cases in the learning curve.

Oncologic

The primary goal of any sort of operative intervention for prostate cancer is oncologic cure. Men with high tumor stage, large tumor volume, multiple positive biopsies, high biopsy grade, and high preoperative prostate-specific antigen (PSA) are more likely to have a positive margin after surgery.[69–71] Positive margin is a well-established independent risk factor for PSA recurrence.[43] As such, any modifications of the gold standard must provide for equivalent oncologic outcomes to be considered viable options of treatment. It is theorized that the lack of tactile feedback associated with LRP and RALP may prevent equivalent oncologic results because the surgeon is unable to palpate the tumor. Others have theorized that magnified 3D vision and minimal blood in the surgical field can improve vision, helping the dissection, and potentially lead to decreased positive surgical margins.

Most contemporary open RRP series report overall margin positive rates (MPR) of 12% to 25%.[68,71] In literature review, Weider et al.[70] reported positive margin rates after RRP to range from 0% to 77%, with an overall average of 28% in reviewed RRP series. In this review, they also report MPR for T_{2a} disease to be 0% to 38% with an average of 17%, 11% to 77% with an average of 36% for T_{2b} disease, and 25% to 59% with an average of 53% for T_3 disease.[70] Han et al.[72] have reported MPRs as low as 2.7% for T_2 disease after RRP. Eastham et al.[69] report significantly increased risk of positive margins with RRP when performed by surgeons with lower surgical volume.

Table 12–2 Positive Margin Rates

	No. of Patients	pT_1	pT_{2a}	pT_{2b}	pT_2
Abbou et al.[3] (2001)	1	—	—	—	—
Pasticier et al.[4] (2001)	5	—	0/2 (0%)	1/3 (33.3%)	1/5 (20%)
Binder and Kramer[5] (2001)	10	—	0/2 (0%)	0/4 (0%)	0/6 (0%)
Rassweiler et al.[6] (2001)	6	—	0/3 (0%)	0/2 (0%)	0/5 (0%)
Samadi et al.[28] (2002)	11	—	NR	NR	1/8 (12.5%)
Aherling et al.[14] (2003)	45	—	1/6 (16.7%)	3/21 (14.3%)	4/27 (14.8%)
Wolfram et al.[30] (2003)	81	—	NR	NR	7/55 (12.7%)
Aherling et al.[26] (2004)	60	—	NR	NR	2/44 (4.5%)
Cathelineau et al.[7] (2004)	105	—	NR	NR	9/75 (11.7%)
Patel et al.[77] (2006)	500	—	NR	NR	10/390 (2.5%)

NR, not reported.

In RALP, the surgeon is made devoid of tactile feedback because laparoscopic instruments are controlled by robotic arms without haptic feedback to the surgeon. With this, the fear of poorer oncologic outcomes was heightened initially, but it has subsided because most surgeons can overcome the lack of tactile feedback through the improved 3D vision and magnification. The reported MPR after RALP in reported series ranges from 0% to 36.4%.[3–9,14,16,26,28,30–32] When broken down by stage, MPR ranges from 0% to 16.7% for T_{2a} disease, 0% to 33.3% for T_{2b} disease, 0% to 20% for T_2 disease, 0% to 81.8% for T_{3a} disease, 20% to 50% for T_{3b} disease, 0% to 75% for combined T_3 disease, and 33.3% to 66.6% for T_4 disease (Table 12–2).[3–9,14,16,26,28,30–32] This appears to be similar to those outcomes for RRP. In a comparative series, Ahlering et al.,[26] in a single-surgeon series, reported a trend toward higher rates of positive surgical margins in the open RRP group (20%) compared with the RALP group (16.7%), even though it did not reach statistical significance because of low sample size. In this same series, they reported an MPR associated with T_2 disease of 4.5% for RALP, compared with 9.1% in RRP.[26] In our series of 500 patients, the MPR was 9.4% for the entire series (Patel VR[77]). The MPR was 13% (cases 1–100), 8% (cases 101–200), 13% (cases 201–300), 5% (cases 301–400), and 8% (cases 401–500). MPR was 2% for T_{2a} disease, 4% for T_{2b} disease, 2.5% for T_{2c} disease, 23% for T_{3a} disease, 46% for T_{3b} disease, and 53% for T_{4a} disease. For organ-confined disease (T_2), the MPR was 2.5%, and for non–organ-confined disease, the MPR was 31%. There were a total of 47 positive margins, 26 (56%) posterolateral, 4 (8.5%) apical, 4 (8.5%) bladder neck, 2 (4%) seminal vesicle, and 11 (23%) multifocally.

True oncologic outcome can only be evaluated based on long-term survival data. Because LRP and RALP are so new, these data are not available at this time. Short-term PSA data from the majority of series are promising. The variability in margin status reporting and pathologic specimen handling also makes cross-series analysis very difficult. This prevents definitive comparison of RALP, RPP, and LRP in regard to superiority of oncologic outcome until long-term biochemical recurrence and survival data are available.

COMPLICATIONS

Complications can occur with any operative intervention; however, our goal should be to perform the intervention and provide the best outcome while minimizing risk of complication. Complications must also be reported and critically analyzed so that appropriate adjustments can be made in operative technique to prevent future occurrences. Rates of intraoperative and postoperative complications after RALP are 0% to 1% and 0% to 13%, respectively (see Table 12–1).[3–9,14,16,26,28,30–32] In a series comparing rates of postoperative complications between obese patients (BMI > 30) and nonobese patients following RALP, obese patients have a significantly higher rate of postoperative complications (26.3%) compared with the nonobese patients (4.9%).[33]

Intraoperative

The major intraoperative complications associated with prostatectomy are rectal injury, ureteral injury, and nerve (obturator, femoral) injury. In recent open RRP series, rectal injury rates were reported to be 0.05% to 2.5%.[47,68,73,74] In LRP series, rectal injury has been reported to occur at a rate of 1.3% to 1.5%.[20,23,35,36] In RALP series, rectal injury is reported to occur at a rate of 0% to 1%.[4,6,7,11,17,28,32] Bowel injury other than the rectum has been reported to be 0.5% in one LRP series.[35] In RALP, rates of bowel injury have

pT_{3a}	pT_{3b}	pT_{3a+b}	pT_4	pT_{3+4}
0/1 (0%)	—	0/1 (0%)	—	0/1 (0%)
—	—	—	—	—
2/2 (100%)	1/2 (50%)	3/4 (75%)	—	3/4 (75%)
0/1 (0%)	NR	NR	—	0/1 (0%)
NR	NR	2/3 (66.6%)	—	2/3 (66.6%)
9/11 (81.8%)	1/5 (20%)	10/16 62.5%)	2/3 (66.7%)	12/19 (63.2%)
NR	NR	11/26 (42.3%)	—	11/26 (42.3%)
NR	NR	NR	NR	8/16 (50%)
NR	NR	13/30 (43%)	—	13/30 (43%)
14/58 (24%)	8/20 (40%)	22/78 (28%)	7/11 (63%)	12/44 (32.6%)

been reported to be 0% to 0.95%.[4,6,7,17,28] Ureteral injury rates during RRP are 0% to 1.6%.[47,68,73,74] For LRP, these rate have been reported to be 0.5% to 0.7%.[23,34] To date, no intraoperative ureteral injuries have been reported with RALP.[4,6–8,14,17,26,28,29,75] Open conversion rate secondary to intraoperative complication during LRP has been by Guillonneau et al.[35] to be 10% in their first 70 cases, but it decreased to 0% in the next 497. Rassweiler et al.[20] also reported a high conversion rate initially (8.1% of first 60 patients), with it declining to 1.7% in the next 60 patients. Open conversion rate during RALP has been reported to be 0% to 1% in recent series.[1,4,11,28,29]

Postoperative

Postoperatively, complications may occur that are specifically related to the surgery or that are medical complications that are a risk with any surgery. Rates of deep venous thrombosis (DVT) after open RRP have been reported to be 1.1% to 7.8%.[47,67,73,74] The rates of DVT after LRP have been lower with reported rates of 0.35% to 0.72%.[23,35] The rates of DVT after RALP are also lower than those with RRP and are reported to be 0% to 2.22%.[4,5,8,11,14,17,28,75] Rates of DVT in obese patients (BMI > 30) after RALP have been reported to be 5.55%.[33] A complication more specific to LRP is prolonged ileus, which occurs as a result of transperitoneal approach and manipulation of bowel. Ileus is reported to occur in 1.1% to 3.3% of patients after LRP.[20,23,33,35] After RALP, ileus occurs at a rate of 0% to 2.5%.[11,16,17,26,28] A common complication after RRP is anastomotic urinary leak, which is reported to occur at a rate of 0.1% to 21.7%.[73,76] After RALP, urinary leak rates are 0% to 4.44%.[4,5,7,14,26,28,33] Another significant complication after prostatectomy is bladder neck contracture, and rates after RRP are reported to be 0.5% to 9%, with one series reporting a rate of 17.5%.[50] Rassweiler et al.[20] reported a bladder neck contracture rate of 3.6% after LRP. Although there are limited data available because of short-term follow-up, bladder neck contracture after RALP has been reported to be 0.5% to 1.6%.[17,32] Specific complications to laparoscopic surgery include port site hernia and port site bleed. After RALP, port site hernias and delayed port site bleed are reported to occur at a frequency of 0% to 1.5% and 0% to 2.22% of patients, respectively.[4,6,8,11,14,17,26,28]

It appears that overall complication rate and rates of specific complications after RALP are at least equivalent to if not better than the alternatives of RRP and LRP. Further diligent reporting of complications is still needed as new centers begin to perform this procedure so that further refinements in technique can be performed to avoid these complications. Updates on complication rates for LRP and RRP are also needed so that accurate comparison can be made between current complication rates of these procedures and RALP since they have been refined.

CONCLUSIONS

Our review of the data for transperitoneal robotic-assisted laparoscopic radical prostatectomy shows a promising procedure in evolution. It is estimated that in 2008, the majority of radical prostatectomies in the United States will be performed robotically. Although there appears to be increasing adoption worldwide, it should be recognized that the procedure is still young and in evolution. The limitations of robotic technology, such as bulky instrumentation and lack of haptic feedback, seem to be outweighed by the advantages of improved visualization and miniature wristed instrumentation. The short-term data are growing quickly and are encouraging when compared with the current gold standard in terms of functional and oncologic outcomes as is demonstrated previously in this chapter. As robotic technology evolves and becomes more prevalent, we expect to see continued adoption, innovation, and improved surgical outcomes. If the long-term biochemical recurrence-free and survival rates with RALP are equivalent to or better than those of RRP and long-term functional outcome results with RALP continue with the current trend, RALP will prove to have a durable place in the treatment of localized prostate cancer.

REFERENCES

1. Ries LAG, Melbert D, Krapcho M, et al: SEER Cancer Statistics Review, 1975–2004. Bethesda, MD, National Cancer Institute, 2007.
2. Holmberg L, Bill-Axelson A, Helgesen F, et al: A randomized trial comparing radical prostatectomy with watchful waiting in early prostate cancer. N Engl J Med 347:781–789, 2002.
3. Abbou C-C, Hoznek A, Salomon L, et al: Laparoscopic radical prostatectomy with a remote controlled robot. J Urol 165:1964–1966, 2001.
4. Pasticier G, Rietbergen JBW, Guillonneau B, et al: Robotically assisted laparoscopic radical prostatectomy: feasibility study in men. Eur Urol 40:70–74, 2001.
5. Binder J, Kramer W: Robotically-assisted laparoscopic radical prostatectomy. BJU Int 87:408–410, 2001.
6. Rassweiler J, Frede T, Seemann O, et al: Telesurgical laparoscopic radical prostatectomy. Eur Urol 40:75–83, 2001.
7. Cathelineau X, Rozet F, Vallancien G: Robotic radical prostatectomy: the European experience. Urol Clin North Am 31:693–699, 2004.
8. Menon M, Tewari A, Vattikuti Institute Prostatectomy Team: Robotic radical prostatectomy and the Vattikuti Urology Institute technique: An interim analysis of results and technical points. Urology 61(suppl 4A):10–20, 2003.
9. Menon M, Tewari A, Peabody J, et al: Vattikuti Institute prostatectomy: technique. J Urol 169:2289–2292, 2003.
10. Menon M, Tewari A, Baise B, et al: Prospective comparison of radical retropubic prostatectomy and robot-assisted anatomic prostatectomy: the Vattikuti Urology Institute experience. Urology 60:864–868, 2002.
11. Tewari A, Srivasatava A, Menon M, et al: A prospective comparison of radical retropubic and robot-assisted prostatectomy: experience in one institution. BJU Int 92:205–210, 2003.
12. Menon M, Hemal AK, Tewari A, et al: The technique of apical dissection of the prostate and urethrovesical anastomosis in robotic radical prostatectomy. BJU Int 93:715–719, 2004.
13. Hemal AK, Menon M: Robotics in urology. Curr Opin Urol 12:89–93, 2004.
14. Ahlering TE, Skarecky D, Lee D, et al: Successful transfer of open surgical skills to a laparoscopic environment using a robotic interface: initial experience with laparoscopic radical prostatectomy. J Urol 170:1738–1741, 2003.
15. Bhandari A, Peabody JO, Tiwari A, et al: Does surgical robot assist in safe learning of laparoscopic radical prostatectomy? AUA Abstract, presented May 10, 2004.
16. Menon M, Shrivastava A, Tewari A, et al: Laparoscopic and robot assisted radical prostatectomy: establishment of a structured program and preliminary analysis of outcome. J Urol 168:945–949, 2002.
17. Menon M, Tewari A, Peabody JO, et al: Vattikuti Institute prostatectomy, a technique of robotic radical prostatectomy for management of localized carcinoma of the prostate: experience of over 1100 cases. Urol Clin North Am 31:701–717, 2004.
18. Scheusler WW, Schlaum PG, Clayman RV, et al: Laparoscopic radical prostatectomy: initial short term experience. Urology 50:854–857, 199.
19. Guillonneau B, Vallancien G: Laparoscopic radical prostatectomy: the Montsouris experience. J Urol 163:418–422, 2000.
20. Rassweiler J, Seemann O, Schulze M, et al: Laparoscopic versus open radical prostatectomy: Comparative study at a single institution. J Urol 169:1689–1693, 2003.
21. Rassweiler J, Sentker L, Seeman O, et al: Laparoscopic radical prostatectomy with the Heilbronn technique: an analysis of the first 180 cases. J Urol 166:2010–2108, 2001.
22. Turk I, Deger S, Winkelmann B, et al: Laparoscopic radical prostatectomy. Eur Urol 40:46–51, 2001.
23. Salomon L, Levrel O, Taille A, et al: Radical prostatectomy by the retropubic, perineal, and laparoscopic approach: 12 years of experience in one center. Eur Urol 42:104–111, 2002.
24. Eden CG, Chaill D, Vass JA, et al: Laparoscopic radical prostatectomy: the initial UK series. BJU 90:876–882, 2002.
25. Sulser T, Guillonneau B, Vallancien G, et al: Complication and initial experience with 1228 laparoscopic radical prostatectomies at 6 European centers. J Urol 165(suppl):150, 2001.
26. Ahlering TE, Woo D, Eichel L, et al: Robot-assisted versus open radical prostatectomy: a comparison of one surgeon's outcomes. Urology 63:820–822, 2004.
27. Abbou CC, Hoznek A, Olsson LE, et al: Telerobotic laparoscopic radical prostatectomy. AUA Abstract, presented May 27, 2002.
28. Samadi DB, Nadu A, Olsson E, Hoznek A, Salomon L, et al: Robot assisted laparoscopic radical prostatectomy: Initial experience in eleven patients. AUA Abstract, presented May 29, 2002.
29. Fumo M, Shrivastava A, DePeralta M, et al: Does routine preservation of the neurovascular bundle result in poor oncological outcomes in patients undergoing robotic radical prostatectomy? AUA Abstract, presented April 29, 2003.
30. Wolfram M, Brautigam R, Engl T, et al: Robotic-assisted laparoscopic radical prostatectomy: the Frankfurt technique. World J Urol 21:128–132, 2003.
31. Bentas W, Wolfram M, Jones J, et al: Robotic technology and the translation of open radical prostatectomy to laparoscopy: The early Frankfurt experience with robotic radical prostatectomy and one year follow up. Eur Urol, 44:175-181.
32. Patel VR, Tully AS, Linday J: Robotic radical prostatectomy in the community setting: the learning curve and beyond: initial 200 cases. J Urol 174:269–272, 2005.
33. Ahlering TE, Eichel L, Edwards R, et al: Impact of obesity on clinical outcomes in robotic prostatectomy. Urology 65:740–745, 2005.
34. Guillonneau B, Rozet F, Barrett E, et al: Laparoscopic radical prostatectomy: assessment after 240 procedures. Urol Clin North Am 28:189, 2001.
35. Guillonneau B, el-Fettouh H, Baumert H, et al: Laparoscopic radical prostatectomy: oncological evaluation after 1,000 cases at Montsouris Institute. J Urol 169:1261–1266, 2003.
36. Hoznek A, Salomon L, Olsson LE, et al: Laparoscopic radical prostatectomy: the Creteil experience. Eur Urol 40:38–45, 2001.
37. Gill IS, Zippe CD: Laparoscopic radical prostatectomy: technique. Urol Clin North Am 28:423–436, 2001.
38. Dahl D, L'esperance JO, Trainer AF, et al: Laparoscopic radical prostatectomy: initial 70 cases at a U.S. university medical center. Urology 58:570–572, 2001.
39. Turk I, Deger S, Winkelmann B, et al: Laparoscopic radical prostatectomy: technical aspects and experience with 125 cases. Eur Urol 40:46–52, 2001.

40. Anastasiadis AG, Salomon L, Katz R, et al: Radical retropubic versus laparoscopic prostatectomy: a prospective comparison of functional outcome. Urology 62:292–297, 2003.
41. Fabrizio MD, Tuerk I, Schellhammer PF: Laparoscopic radical prostatectomy: decreasing the learning curve using a mentor initiated approach. J Urol 169:2063–2065, 2003.
42. Smith JA Jr: Robotically assisted laparoscopic prostatectomy: an assessment of its contemporary role in the surgical management of localized prostate cancer. Am J Surg 188:63S–67S, 2004.
43. Ahlering TE, Eichel L, Edwards RA, et al: Robotic radical prostatectomy: a technique to reduce pT2 positive margins. Urology 64:1224–1228, 2004.
44. Webster TM, Herrell SD, Baumgartner RG, et al: Robotic assisted laparoscopic prostatectomy versus radical retropubic prostatectomy: assessment of perioperative pain. AUA Abstract, presented May 8, 2004.
45. Eastham J, Scardino P: Radical prostatectomy. In: Campbell's urology, 4th ed. Philadelphia, WB Saunders, 2002, pp 3080–3106.
46. Quinlan DM, Epstein GI, Carter BS, et al: Sexual function following radical prostatectomy: influence of preservation of neurovascular bundles. J Urol 145:998–1002, 1991.
47. Catalona WJ, Carvalhal GF, Mager DE, et al: Potency, continence, and complication rates in 1870 consecutive radical retropubic prostatectomies. J Urol 162:433–438, 1999.
48. Fowler FJ Jr, Barry MJ, Lu-Yao G, et al: Patient-reported complications and follow up treatment after radical prostatectomy. Urology 42:622–629, 1993.
49. Geary ES, Dendinger TE, Frieha FS, et al: Nerve sparing radical prostatectomy: a different view. J Urol 154:145–149, 1995.
50. Geary ES, Dendinger TE, Frieha FS, et al: Incontinence and vesical neck strictures following radical retropubic prostatectomy. Urology 45:1000–1006, 1995.
51. Talcott JA, Ricker P, Propert KJ, et al: Patient reported impotence and incontinence after nerve sparing radical prostatectomy. J NCI 89:1117–1123, 1997.
52. Moul JW, Mooneyhan RN, Kao TC, et al: Preoperative and operative factors to predict incontinence, impotence, and stricture after radical prostatectomy. Prostate Cancer Prostatic Dis 5:242–249, 1998.
53. Walsh PC, Partin AW, Epstein JI: Cancer control and quality of life following anatomical radical retropubic prostatectomy: results at 10 years. J Urol 152:1831–1836, 1994.
54. Catalona WJ, Basler JW: Return of erections and urinary continence following nerve sparing radical retropubic prostatectomy. J Urol 150:905–907, 1993.
55. Eastham JA, Kattan MW, Roger SE, et al: Risk factors for urinary incontinence after radical prostatectomy. J Urol 156:1707–1713, 1996.
56. Palapattu JS, Stapelton AM, Seale-Hawkins CK, et al: A change in technique in radical retropubic prostatectomy markedly improves post-operative potency. J Urol 155:647a, 1996.
57. Walsh PA, Marschke P, Ricker D, et al: Patient-reported urinary continence and sexual function after anatomic radical prostatectomy. Urology 55:58–61, 2000.
58. Rosen RC, Cappelleri JC, Smith MD, et al: Development and evaluation of an abridged, 5-item version of the International Index of Erectile Function (IIEF-5) as a diagnostic tool for erectile dysfunction. Int J Impot Res 11:319, 2002.
59. Schover LR, Fouladi RT, Warneke CL, et al: Defining sexual outcomes after treatment of localized prostate carcinoma. Cancer 95:1773, 2002.
60. Hara I, Kawabata G, Miyake H, et al: Comparison of quality of life after laparoscopic and open prostatectomy for prostate cancer. J Urol 169:2045, 2003.
61. Parsons JK, Marshke P, Maples P, et al: Effect of methylprednisolone on return of sexual function after nerve sparing radical retropubic prostatectomy. Urology 64:987, 2004.
62. Menon M, Kaul S, Bhandari A, et al: Potency following robotic radical prostatectomy: a questionnaire based analysis of outcomes after conventional nerve sparing and prostatic fascia sparing techniques. J Urol 174:2291–2296, 2005.
63. Rassweiler J, Sentker L, Seemann O, et al: Laparoscopic radical prostatectomy: technique and first experiences. Akt Urol 31:238–247, 2000.
64. Bollens R, Vanden Bossche M, Roumeguere T, et al: Extraperitoneal laparoscopic radical prostatectomy: results after 50 cases. Eur Urol 40:65–69, 2001.
65. Walsh PC: Patient-reported urinary continence and sexual function after anatomic radical prostatectomy. J Urol 164:242, 2000.
66. Lepor H, Nieder AM, Fraiman MC: Early removal of urinary catheter after radical retropubic prostatectomy is both feasible and desirable. Urology 58:425, 2001.
67. Lepor H, Nieder AM, Ferrandino MN: Intraoperative and postoperative complications of radical retropubic prostatectomies in a consecutive series of 1,000 cases. J Urol 166:1729, 2001.
68. Zincke H, Bergstralh EJ, Blute ML, et al: Radical prostatectomy for clinically localized prostate cancer: long-term results of 1,143 patients from a single institution. J Clin Oncol, 12:2254–2263, 1994.
69. Eastham JA, Kattan MW, Riedel E, et al: Variations among individual surgeons in the rate of positive surgical margins in radical prostatectomy specimens. J Urol 170:2292–2295, 2003.
70. Weider JA, Soloway MS: Incidence, etiology, location, prevention and treatment of positive surgical margins after radical prostatectomy for prostate cancer. J Urol 160:299–315, 1998.
71. Hull GW, Rabbani F, Abbas F, et al: Cancer control with radical prostatectomy alone in 1,000 consecutive patients. J Urol 167:528–534, 2002.
72. Han M, Chan DY, Partin AW: An evaluation of the decreasing incidence of positive surgical margins in a large radical retropubic prostatectomy series. J Urol 169(suppl):448, 2003.
73. Gheiler EL, Lovisolo JA, Tiguert R, et al: Results of clinical care pathway for radical prostatectomy patients in an open hospital-multiphysician system. Eur Urol 35:210, 1999.
74. Hammerer P, Hubner D, Gonnermann D, et al: Perioperative and postoperative complications of pelvic lymphadenectomy and radical prostatectomy in 320 consecutive patients. Urologe A 34:334–342, 1995.
75. Guillonneau B, Cathelineau X, Doublet JD, et al: Prospective assessment of functional results after laparoscopic radical prostatectomy. AUA Abstract, presented June 4, 2001.
76. Shekarriz B, Upadhyay J, Wood DP: Radical prostatectomy: intraoperative, perioperative, and long-term complications of radical prostatectomy. Urol Clin North Am 28:639–653, 2001.
77. Patel VR, Shah SR, Arend D: Histopathologic outcomes of robotic radical prostatectomy. Sci World J 6:2566–2572, 2006.

CHAPTER 13

Thomas E. Ahlering • James F. Borin • Douglas W. Skarecky

Oncologic Outcomes of Robotic Radical Prostatectomy

The annual incidence of prostate cancer is increasing; it has risen 2.3% per year since 1996 while mortality has continued to decline.[1] Although some of this may be attributed to stage migration and screening with prostate-specific antigen (PSA), a recent study comparing radical prostatectomy with watchful waiting demonstrated the benefit of surgery in reducing the risk of progression, metastases, cancer-specific mortality, and overall mortality based during a median follow-up of 8.2 years.[2] Although the comparative success of other treatments is debatable because mature, randomized clinical trials are lacking, radical prostatectomy offers the advantage of precise staging and grading and ease of detection of disease eradication or recurrence via PSA nadir or PSA rise.[3] Because of a significant reduction in perioperative morbidity and long-term complications, in the year 2000, 36% to 41% of men with prostate cancer chose to undergo radical prostatectomy. With the advent of minimally invasive techniques to rival the minimal perioperative morbidity of brachytherapy and external beam radiation, that number is most likely rising.

The key principle of radical prostatectomy, whether retropubic, perineal, laparoscopic, or robotic, is oncologic control, that is, eradication of all local disease present. Disease recurrence has been linked to a number of parameters, including pretreatment PSA; primary and secondary Gleason grade; tumor, nodes and metastases (TNM) stage (clinical and pathologic); and margin status.[4] However, ultimately only two factors will lead to eventual biochemical recurrence: subclinical micrometastases present at the time of surgery or lapse in technique. Improved oncologic outcomes, then, can be achieved only through careful patient selection and superior technique as evidenced by a low rate of positive margins.[5]

POSITIVE MARGINS

The impact of a positive margin on biochemical recurrence and cancer-specific survival is controversial, especially in pT_2 disease. However, most authors believe that a positive margin is a poor prognostic sign and will ultimately result in a higher rate of biochemical recurrence and decreased survival.[6] A positive surgical margin (PSM) is defined as tumor present at the inked margin of a specimen. The 5-year risk of biochemical failure for PSM is reported between 42% and 64%, which is significantly higher than that for patients with negative surgical margins (NSMs).[7] Swindle and colleagues[5] looked at 1389 consecutive patients who underwent radical retropubic prostatectomy, performed by two surgeons, from 1983 to 2000 for clinical T_1 to T_3 prostate cancer. The overall rate of PSM was 12.9%, with 6.8% for T_2 and 23% for T_3. At a median follow-up of 50 months, the probability of being free of PSA progression was 58% versus 81% ($P < .00005$) for PSM and NSM, respectively, which translated into a relative risk of failure of 1.2 to 2.7. The authors concluded that a PSM is associated with an increased risk of recurrence even after adjusting for concurrent risk factors such as pretreatment PSA, Gleason grade, and clinical and pathologic stage. A similar study of more than 2500 patients by Blute et al.[8] supports these findings.

ROBOTIC PROSTATECTOMY: ADVANTAGES AND DISADVANTAGES

Minimally invasive approaches to urologic disease have been shown to reduce length of hospital stay and convalescence. Robotic-assisted surgery is merely an extension of laparoscopy and would be expected to confer all of its advantages as well. In addition, robotic surgery allows for a shorter learning curve than pure laparoscopy, with more ready transfer of open skills in a laparoscopically naïve surgeon as well as features such as tremor filtering, motion scaling, three-dimensional visualization, and wristed instruments with six degrees of freedom and supraphysiologic 540-degree rotation.[9] Disadvantages of robotic surgery include a lack of significant haptic feedback and higher cost, even in the setting of a reduced hospital stay. One study estimated the cost differential compared with open prostatectomy at $1726 and laparoscopy at $1239.[10] This is primarily because of the costs associated with the purchase and maintenance of the robot, $857 per case, which the authors amortized over 7 years, as well as the limited-life reusable robotic instruments. In this study, theoretical cost equivalence could be achieved only if all major associated costs—purchase price, annual service contract, and disposable robotic instruments—were decreased by approximately 67%.

TECHNIQUE TO REDUCE MARGIN POSITIVITY

During radical prostatectomy, meticulous apical dissection is critical in preserving the fibers of paraurethral skeletal muscle, which contribute to the external urethral sphincter. In addition, the prostatourethral junction must be well identified to preserve urethral length without risking a positive margin. We previously described a technique using the da Vinci robotic system that enhances one's ability to more precisely dissect the apex and reduce surgical margins.[11] The PSM rate in our initial 50 patients was 36%, and after altering our apical technique, this rate was reduced to 18%. In our initial 50 cases, we used two sutures to control the dorsal venous complex (DVC), one proximally and distally. The prostate was freed, and, finally, the DVC and urethra were divided. However, a bundle of fat obscured the apex, leading to positive apical margins. To more precisely visually define the apex, we developed the following method (Figure 13–1). First, all fat overlying the DVC and prostate is removed. Second, the levator fibers are fully dissected off of the prostatic apex and then the puboprostatic ligaments are cut to increase the DVC length. Finally, the DVC is stapled and divided. For the next 200 consecutive cases, the overall margin rate was 18% and 7.2% for pT_2 (Table 13–1).

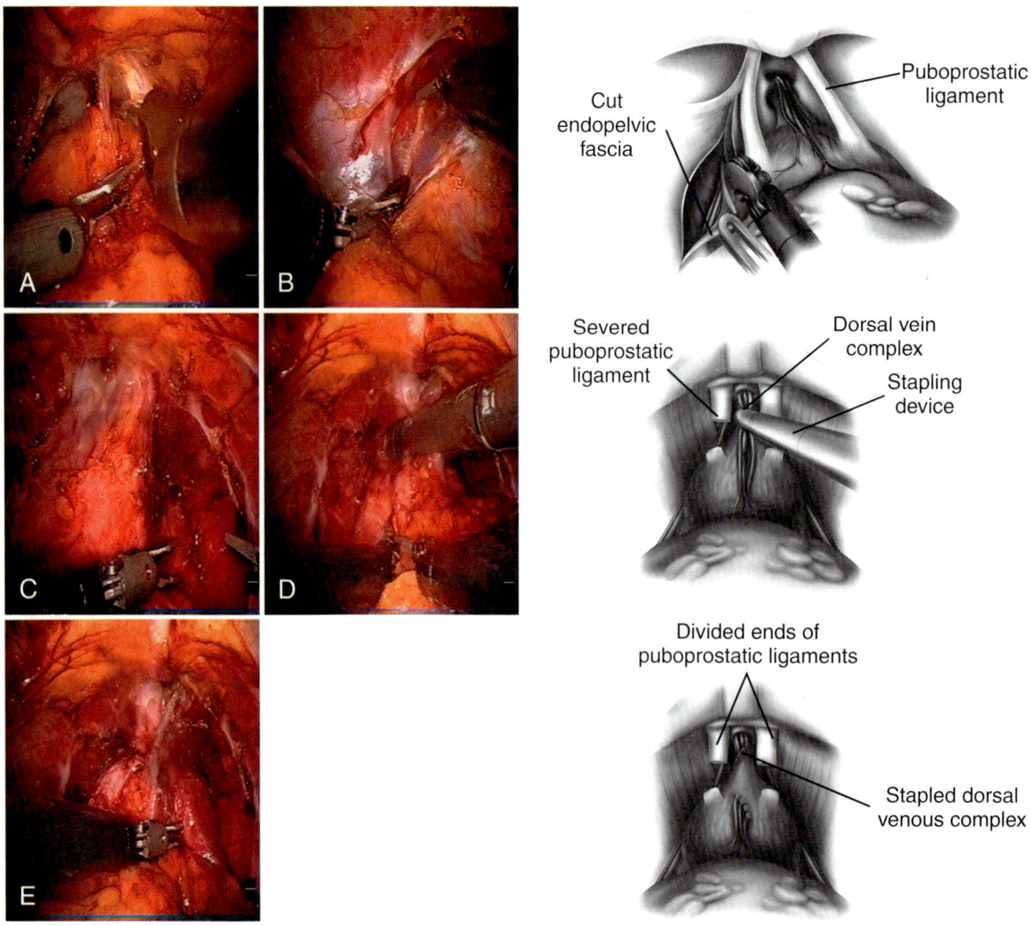

FIGURE 13–1 Technique to reduce positive margins. *A*, All fat overlying the prostate is removed from the dorsal venous complex (DVC) and puboprostatic ligaments to the level of the bladder neck. *B* and *C*, Endopelvic fascia is incised, the levator fibers are fully dissected off of the prostatic apex, and then the puboprostatic ligaments are cut to increase the DVC length. *D*, The DVC is stapled and divided with an EndoGia stapler such that the apex and prostatourethral junction can be readily identified *(E)*.

After careful clinical and pathologic review of this group, we further altered the technique (Figure 13–2). During the apical dissection, we had always endeavored to preserve urethral length so as not to compromise continence. However, an interim analysis of these 200 robotic-assisted laparoscopic radical prostatectomies (RALRPs) demonstrated no effect of intraoperative urethral stump length on time of return to continence or overall continence (Figure 13–3). Patients were assessed prospectively by validated questionnaires at 1, 3, 6, and 12 months. Continence was defined as requiring no pads. Urethral stump length was assessed intraoperatively: (0) the stump is retracted below the distal urethral sphincter (urogenital diaphragm) and requires perineal pressure to perform the urethrovesical anastomosis, (1) the stump is at the level of the sphincter, and (2) there is at least 1 cm of urethral stump above the level of the distal sphincter. Pathologic data were collected prospectively from our last 270 consecutive cases. All specimens were inked and sectioned according to standard protocol as described previously.[11] Briefly, the apex was transected perpendicular to the axis of the urethra and sliced radially, generating five to eight segments. The remainder of the prostate and seminal vesicles were serially sectioned in the transverse plane at 3- to 5-mm intervals. A PSM was defined by the presence of tumor cells at the resection margin (i.e., cancer cells with ink on them). We noted that the majority (75%) of positive margins were focal and located at the apex. Therefore, in our last 70 patients, a more aggressive apical dissection has been performed, resulting in a statistically significant decrease in overall positive margin rate from 18% to 5.7% (P = .01). Positive margin rates for pT_2 and $pT_{3/4}$ improved from 7.2% to 3.3% and 52% to 22%, respectively (both P = NS) (see Table 13–1).

Table 13–1 Comparison of Positive Margin Rates for Patients Undergoing Robotic-Assisted Radical Prostatectomy Prior and Subsequent to an Interim Analysis and Change in Technique

	Before Interim Analysis (N = 200)		After Interim Analysis (N = 70)		
Stage	SM+	SM+ at Apex	SM+	SM+ at Apex	P Value*
pT_2	11/152 (7.2%)	73%	2/61 (3.3%)	50%	0.36
$pT_{3/4}$	25/48 (52%)	74%	2/9 (22%)	100%	0.15
Overall	18%	74%	5.7%	75%	0.01

*Two-sided Fisher's exact test.
SM+, positive surgical margin.

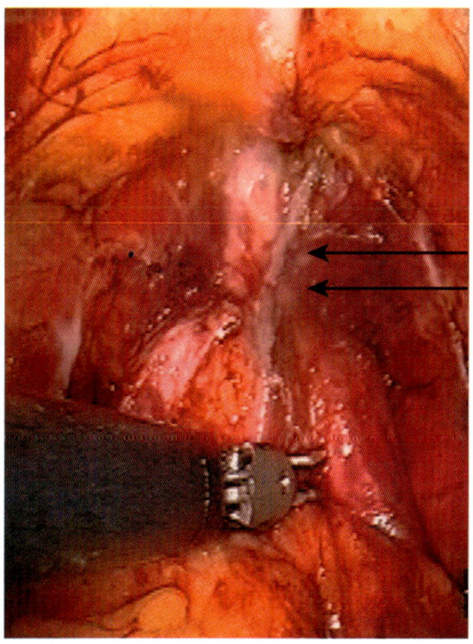

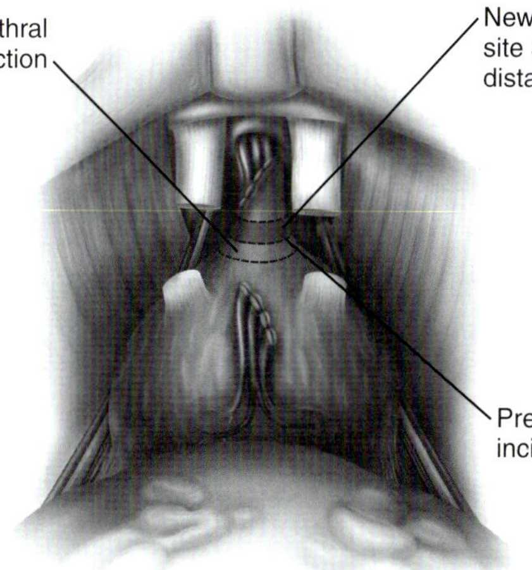

FIGURE 13–2 Change in technique of urethral transection. Old incision at prostatourethral junction resulted in 18% rate of positive margins, with 74% at the apex. By incising 3 to 7 mm distally (new), positive margin rate decreased to 5.7% without any compromise in continence. In the left figure, the upper arrow demonstrates the new incision site and the lower arrow, the previous site.

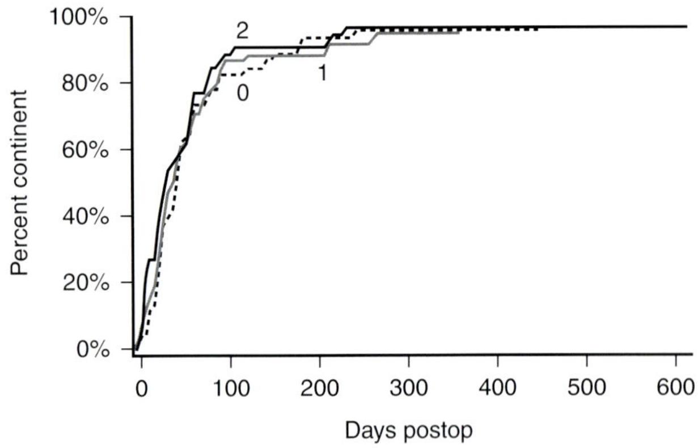

FIGURE 13–3 Percentage of men achieving pad-free continence determined by membranous urethra length evaluated by analysis of variance (ANOVA). Urethral stump position was defined as follows: 0, the stump is below the urogenital (UG) diaphragm and requires perineal pressure to perform the urethrovesical anastomosis; 1, the stump is at the level of the UG diaphragm; and 2, there is at least 1 cm of urethral stump lying well above the UG diaphragm. There was no statistically significant difference in % continence between groups at 1, 3, 6, 9, or 12 months.

EXCISION OF THE NEUROVASCULAR BUNDLE

Radical prostatectomy, first and foremost, is a cancer operation and must remain so, despite any technologic advancements. Excision of the neurovascular bundle (NVB) may be required to achieve adequate control and to ensure negative margins. Intraoperative prostate examination has been proposed to help determine when a wide excision is necessary. One study looked at 403 patients who underwent open radical prostatectomy at the University of Chicago from 1997 to 2004.[12] All patients had intraoperative prostate examination with a palpable abnormality at the NVB in 12%. All of these patients had a wide excision of the NVB, and 37% were found to have extraprostatic extension at the site of the palpable abnormality with only one PSM. A total of 354 patients had a normal intraoperative prostatic examination and thus a nerve-sparing procedure. Among these patients, there was an 8.5% incidence of extraprostatic extension at the NVB with 23% PSM. In this series, intraoperative prostate examination had a positive predictive value of 37% for extraprostatic extension and a negative predictive value of 92%. The authors conclude that intraoperative examination is an important part of radical prostatectomy and advocate its use to guide clinical decision making regarding excision of the NVB. However, as the authors acknowledge, the very low positive predictive value of this technique translates into a substantial number of unnecessary NVB excisions.

Another approach has been suggested by Lepor's group, who created a nerve-sparing algorithm based on analysis of 535 patients who underwent radical retropubic prostatectomy.[13] A total of 263 patients were evaluated preoperatively, and the ipsilateral NVB was excised for tumors with a Gleason score of 6 or less with 50% or more tumor volume in the biopsy specimen and perineural invasion, for tumors with a Gleason score of 7 with 30% or more tumor volume or perineural invasion, and for tumors with a Gleason score of 8 to 10 when there was 10% or greater tumor volume or perineural invasion. Compared with a cohort of 272 prostatectomies that did not have prospectively defined criteria governing excision of the NVB, the study group had fewer PSM (8% versus 14%, $P = .027$) while significantly more NVBs were preserved. The sensitivity, specificity, positive and negative predictive values, and accuracy of the algorithm were 18%, 93%, 28%, 89%, and 84%, respectively. In cases of extraprostatic extension, ipsilateral wide excision of the NVB was associated with positive margins in 33% versus 22% when the NVB was preserved ($P = .42$).

We favor Lepor's approach and will determine whether NVBs will be excised based on the following criteria. First, the patient must be a candidate for a nerve-sparing procedure. This requires a score of more than 21 (of 25) on the sexual health inventory of men (SHIM), a validated, multidimensional questionnaire of erectile function. If the patient has T_{1c} disease and is a candidate for nerve sparing, we will elect to widely excise the ipsilateral NVBs if the biopsy demonstrates more than two cores with Gleason scores of $\geq 4 + 3$ in more than 30%. If the patient has palpable disease ($\geq T_{2a}$), the threshold for wide excision is lowered.

RESULTS

There are few published studies with long-term follow-up after RALRP. Table 13–2 compares results from recent large series of radical retropubic and perineal prostatectomy with current laparoscopic and robotic series. The rate of positive margins ranged from 9% to 26%. The largest series, from Johns Hopkins, had 9035 radical retropubic prostatectomies with 14.7% positive margins.[14] The selected laparoscopic series represent more than 1750 patients with 18.6% to 26% positive margins. The series of RALRP, which are among the largest reported series in the literature, represent 1300 patients with 9% to 14.8% positive margins, which is commensurate with the reported series of open prostatectomy.

Margin positivity is generally assessed as described previously, by inking the margins of the specimen. Of note, some authors will obtain frozen section biopsies from the periurethral tissues anterior and posterior to the prostatic apex, the prostatovesical junction and from tissues anterior to the NVBs and use these results to determine margin status.[24] Lepor and Kaci[25] recommend routine biopsy of the apical soft tissue margin because this intervention led to a

Table 13–2 Comparison of Results from Contemporary Large Series of Radical Prostatectomy: Retropubic, Perineal, Laparoscopic, and Robotic

Institution	Technique	*N*	Positive Margins (%)	Mean Follow-up (mo)	PSA Progression-Free (%)
Johns Hopkins[14]	Retropubic	9035	14.7		
NYU[15]	Retropubic	1000	19.9		
Mayo Clinic[16]	Retropubic	3170	24	60	52 at 10 yr
Baylor[17]	Retropubic	1000	12.8	53	75
Duke[18]	Perineal	1242	23	60	Organ confined 92 Specimen confined 65 Positive margin 35
Heilbronn[19]	Laparoscopic	450	18.6	23	91
Henri Mondor[20]	Laparoscopic	330	26		
Monstouris[21]	Laparoscopic	1000	19.2	12	90.5
Vattikuti Institute[22]	Robotic	530	9	6	92
Alabama[23]	Robotic	500	9.4	9.7	95
UC Irvine (unpublished)	Robotic	270	14.8	7.6	93

reduction in their apical positive margins by 3.8%. However, they note that there was a 98% negative predictive value of the surgical specimen to predict apical soft tissue positivity. We do not routinely biopsy the apical soft tissue and favor reporting margin status based on inked margins of the entire specimen.

PROGRESSION

PSA recurrence, although simple and convenient, has not clearly demonstrated its value to predict progression to bone metastasis or cancer-specific death. However, in those patients who develop biochemical recurrence, PSA doubling time (PSADT) is emerging as potentially the best predictor of disease progression. For example, Stoergel et al.[26] studied 121 patients with PSA recurrence after radical prostatectomy and found that 60% of those with a PSADT of less than 6 months eventually developed metastatic disease, versus 0% of those with a doubling time greater than 12 months. Ahlering and Skarecky[27] evaluated 204 patients who underwent radical prostatectomy from 1984 to 1994. As expected, these patients had more disease at prostatectomy than would be found in the current era. PSA recurrence occurred in 44%, and 17% of these patients died of prostate cancer at a mean of 7.6 years, versus 27% who died of other causes. Of those with recurrence, 40% required no intervention or hormone therapy at 10 years. Once again, PSADT was the best predictor of progression. In this cohort, a PSADT greater than 18 months was most consistent with a successful course of observation. In patients who develop biochemical recurrence as evidenced by a PSA greater than 0.2 ng/ml, it is our current practice to offer hormonal therapy for those with a PSADT less than 12 months. Patients whose PSADT is greater than 12 months are actively monitored for signs of clinical progression.

CONCLUSIONS

RALRP has emerged as a viable alternative for the treatment of organ-confined prostate cancer. The magnified view and pneumoperitoneum provide for superior visualization with little blood loss. With meticulous technique, positive margin rates can remain very low. Although the data are short term, RALRP appears to offer excellent oncologic control, at least equivalent to its open and pure laparoscopic counterparts.

REFERENCES

1. Weir HK, Thun MJ, Hankey BF, et al: Annual report to the nation on the status of prostate cancer, 1975-2000, featuring the uses of surveillance data for cancer prevention and control. J Natl Cancer Inst 95:1276–1299, 2003.
2. Bill-Axelson A, Holmberg L, Ruutu M, et al: Radical prostatectomy versus watchful waiting in early prostate cancer. N Engl J Med 352:1977–1984, 2005.
3. Bianco FJ Jr, Scardino PT, Eastham JA: Radical prostatectomy: long-term cancer control and recovery of sexual and urinary function ("trifecta"). Urology 66:83–94, 2005.
4. Stephenson AJ, Scardino PT, Eastham JA, et al: Postoperative nomogram predicting the 10-year probability of prostate cancer recurrence after radical prostatectomy. J Clin Oncol 23:7005–7012, 2005.
5. Swindle P, Eastham JA, Ohori M, et al: Do margins matter? The prognostic significance of positive surgical margins in radical prostatectomy specimens. J Urol 174:903–907, 2005.
6. Wieder JA, Soloway MS: Incidence, etiology, location, prevention and treatment of positive surgical margins after radical prostatectomy for prostate cancer. J Urol 160:299–315, 1998.
7. Ohori M, Scardino PT: Localized prostate cancer. Curr Probl Surg 39:833–957, 2002.
8. Blute ML, Bergstralh EJ, Iocca A, et al: Use of Gleason score, prostate specific antigen, seminal vesicle and margin status to predict biochemical failure after radical prostatectomy. J Urol 165:119–125, 2001.
9. Basillote JE, Ahlering TE, Skarecky DW, et al: Laparoscopic radical prostatectomy: review and assessment of an emerging technique. Surg Endosc 18:1694–1711, 2004.
10. Lotan Y, Cadeddu JA, Gettman MT: The new economics of radical prostatectomy: cost comparison of open, laparoscopic and robot assisted techniques. J Urol 172:1431–1435, 2004.
11. Ahlering TE, Eichel L, Edwards RA, et al: Robotic radical prostatectomy: a technique to reduce pT2 positive margins. Urology 64:1224–1228, 2004.
12. Rapp DE, Orvieto MA, Lucioni A, et al: Intra-operative prostate examination: predictive value and effect on margin status. BJU Int 96:1005–1008, 2005.
13. Shah O, Robbins DA, Melamed J, et al: The New York University nerve sparing algorithm decreases the rate of positive surgical margins following radical retropubic prostatectomy. J Urol 169:2147–2152, 2003.
14. Han M, Partin AW, Chan DY, et al: An evaluation of the decreasing incidence of positive surgical margins in a large retropubic prostatectomy series. J Urol 171:23–26, 2004.
15. Lepor H, Nieder AM, Ferrandino MN: Intraoperative and postoperative complications of radical retropubic prostatectomy in a consecutive series of 1,000 cases. J Urol 166:1729–1733, 2001.
16. Zincke H, Oesterling JE, Blute ML, et al: Long-term (15 years) results after radical prostatectomy for clinically localized (stage T2c or lower) prostate cancer. J Urol 152:1850–1857, 1994.
17. Hull GW, Rabbani F, Abbas F, et al: Cancer control with radical prostatectomy alone in 1,000 consecutive patients. J Urol 167:528–534, 2002.
18. Iselin CE, Robertson JE, Paulson DF: Radical perineal prostatectomy: oncological outcome during a 20-year period. J Urol 161:163–168, 1999.
19. Rassweiler J, Seemann O, Hatzinger M, et al: Technical evolution of laparoscopic radical prostatectomy after 450 cases. J Endourol 17:143–154, 2003.
20. Ruiz L, Salomon L, Hoznek A, et al: Comparison of early oncologic results of laparoscopic radical prostatectomy by extraperitoneal versus transperitoneal approach. Eur Urol 46:50–54, 2004.
21. Guillonneau B, El-Fettouh H, Baumert H, et al: Laparoscopic radical prostatectomy: oncological evaluation after 1,000 cases at Montsouris Institute. J Urol 169:1261–1266, 2003.
22. Tewari A, Kaul S, Menon M: Robotic radical prostatectomy: a minimally invasive therapy for prostate cancer. Curr Urol Rep 6:45–48, 2005.
23. Patel V, Tully S: Robotic radical prostatectomy: outcomes of 500 cases. J Endourol 19:A133, 2005 [Abstract].
24. Menon M, Tewari A, Peabody J: Vattikuti Institute prostatectomy: technique. J Urol 169:2289–2292, 2003.
25. Lepor H, Kaci L: Role of intraoperative biopsies during radical retropubic prostatectomy. Urology 63:499–502, 2004.
26. Soergel TM, Koch MO, Foster RS, et al: Accuracy of predicting long-term prostate specific antigen outcome based on early prostate specific antigen recurrence results after radical prostatectomy. J Urol 166:2198–2201, 2001.
27. Ahlering TE, Skarecky DW: Long-term outcome of detectable PSA levels after radical prostatectomy. Prostate Cancer Prostatic Dis 8:163–166, 2005.

CHAPTER 14

Justin Harmon • François Rozet • Xavier Cathelineau • Eric Barret • Guy Vallancien

Robotic versus Standard Laparoscopic Prostatectomy

INTRODUCTION: FROM LAPAROSCOPY TO ROBOTICS

The urologic profession has openly embraced the growing trend for minimally invasive surgery. The radical prostatectomy itself has perhaps experienced more of this evolution than any other genitourinary oncologic procedure. Historically, Schuessler and colleagues[1] attempted the first laparoscopic radical prostatectomy (LRP) in 1992. They eventually published their series of nine prostatectomies, concluding that the procedure offered no advantage to standard open prostatectomy.[1] In the same year, Raboy and colleagues[2] performed the first extraperitoneal LRP. In 1998, Vallancien and Guillonneau began performing their first LRPs at Montsouris.[3,4] After refining the technique of LRP, patients began to experience the documented benefits of diminished postoperative pain and convalescence as well as lower blood losses and the suggestion of better functional outcomes because of the improved visualization acquired with the laparoscope.[5–7]

In May 2000, Binder performed the first robotic-assisted laparoscopic prostatectomy (RALP) in Frankfurt, Germany. Shortly thereafter, Vallancien performed an RALP in Detroit, Michigan, along with Menon, who would later go on to develop the technique.[8]

Our current series at Montsouris consists of more than 2500 LRPs, of which more than 130 have been performed using the robotic technique. In this chapter, we review the key technical points for both procedures based on our experience and a review of the literature. We also discuss the relative advantages and disadvantages of each approach.

INDICATIONS

The standard indications for LRP or RALP do not differ from those of open radical retropubic prostatectomy. There are no particular patient characteristics that lend to one approach or the other. However, as with open surgery, the adequate selection of patients who are candidates for a surgical treatment will affect the results obtained with either approach.

As in open surgery, LRP can be performed in selected $T_3N_0M_0$ stages without neurovascular bundle preservation. In such cases, the patient must always be cautioned on the risk of residual disease and the possible requirement of complementary therapy. Also, salvage LRP after radiotherapy or brachytherapy has been reported[9]; however, it is important to keep in mind that this surgery by either open or laparoscopic approach involves a higher risk of damage to the rectum. Such series do not exist for the RALP at this time.

CONTRAINDICATIONS

As with open radical prostatectomy, there are no anatomic contraindications for LRP or RALP. However, there are preoperatively identified factors considered as potentially challenging that have been described in the literature. These include a large-volume prostate of more than 100 g,[10,11] neoadjuvant hormone therapy,[12] previous prostatic surgery (transurethral resection of the prostate [TURP] or simple prostatectomy),[13] a history of prostatitis, radiotherapy, brachytherapy,[9] or previous major abdominal or pelvic surgery because of the formation of adhesions.[14] Finally, the history of a previous hernia repair with mesh is associated with dense scarring in the space of Retzius, making the extraperitoneal dissection difficult; thus, care must be taken when taking this approach.[15]

It is important for surgeons at the beginning of their learning curve to remember these ideas and to carefully select their patients until their skill level matures.

PATIENT POSITIONING

Laparoscopic Radical Prostatectomy

LRP, by the transperitoneal or extraperitoneal approach, is performed under general anesthesia, with the patient placed in a dorsal supine position. During the transperitoneal technique an exaggerated Trendelenburg position is preferred compared with a moderate position in the extraperitoneal approach. The lower limbs are abducted for intraoperative access to the rectum. The upper limbs are positioned alongside the body to avoid the risk of stretch injuries to the brachial plexus. Two security belts are placed across the thorax in an "X" pattern to ensure that there is no movement during surgery and to avoid pressure injuries.

The surgeon stands on the left side of the patient with the scrub nurse and instrument table, and the assistant stands on the right side of the operating table. The video tower is placed between the legs of the patient.

Robotic-Assisted Laparoscopic Radical Prostatectomy

Prior to the patient entering the room, the robotic system is started and a self-testing procedure is performed, during which it recognizes spatial positioning and components. The cameras are black and white balanced and calibrated. The patient positioning is the same as LRP except for a slight flexion of the lower limbs to allow close entry of the robot. A metal tray, locked to the operating room (OR) table, is positioned over the patient's face to serve as protection and a stand for instruments during installation. The surgeon remains at the console for the entire procedure, and a scrub nurse and assistant remain on the left side of the patient.

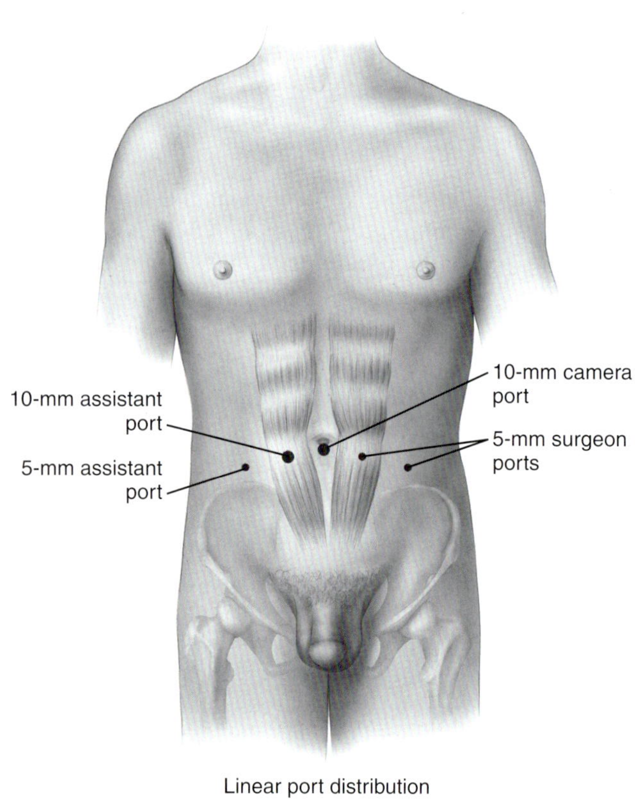

FIGURE 14–1 Linear port distribution.

TROCAR PLACEMENT

Laparoscopic Radical Prostatectomy

At Montsouris, five trocars are used for both the extraperitoneal and transperitoneal approaches. Extraperitoneal trocars are placed slightly more caudad when compared with those in the transperitoneal approach. Depending on surgeon preference, they may be positioned in either a linear or triangular distribution.

In the *linear distribution,* a 10-mm trocar is introduced at the umbilicus for the camera. The surgeon's working ports consist of two 5-mm trocars that are introduced to the left of midline; one roughly one fingerbreadth above and medial to the iliac spine and another lower and lateral to the umbilical port. The assistant ports consist of a 5-mm trocar placed above and medial to the right iliac spine and a second 10-mm trocar between the umbilical and lateral ports on the right (Figure 14–1).

In the *triangular distribution,* the surgeon's working ports are altered such that one 5-mm port on the left side is placed between the umbilical port and the left iliac spine and the other is placed two-thirds of the distance between the umbilical port and the suprapubic rim along the midline (Figure 14–2).

Additional variations have been described. The Hielbron technique[16] uses a six-trocar W-shaped configuration: a 12-mm umbilical port, 10-mm trocars in the medial and inferior position bilaterally, two 5-mm trocars positioned more cephalad and lateral, and a 5-mm trocar in the right suprapubic region. The Erasme technique[17] uses a five-trocar extraperitoneal approach: a 12-mm camera port, two 10-mm ports just medial to the anterior iliac spine, and two 5-mm ports (one 5 cm above the pubic arch and the other cephalad to the right-sided 10-mm port).

Robotic-Assisted Laparoscopic Radical Prostatectomy

At Montsouris, a three-armed robot is used, and trocar placement does not differ for the extraperitoneal or transperitoneal approach. A 12-mm trocar is introduced at the umbilicus for the camera, and two 8-mm trocars for the robotic arms are placed on both sides five fingerbreadths lateral to the optic port and slightly lower. For the assistant, a 5-mm trocar is introduced above and medial to the left iliac spine, and a 10-mm trocar for suture introduction is placed slightly higher between the optic and right robotic trocar (Figure 14–3). The primary port placement for the RALP described here is based on the description given by Menon and Hemal.[18] Here, the authors also describe the placement of a

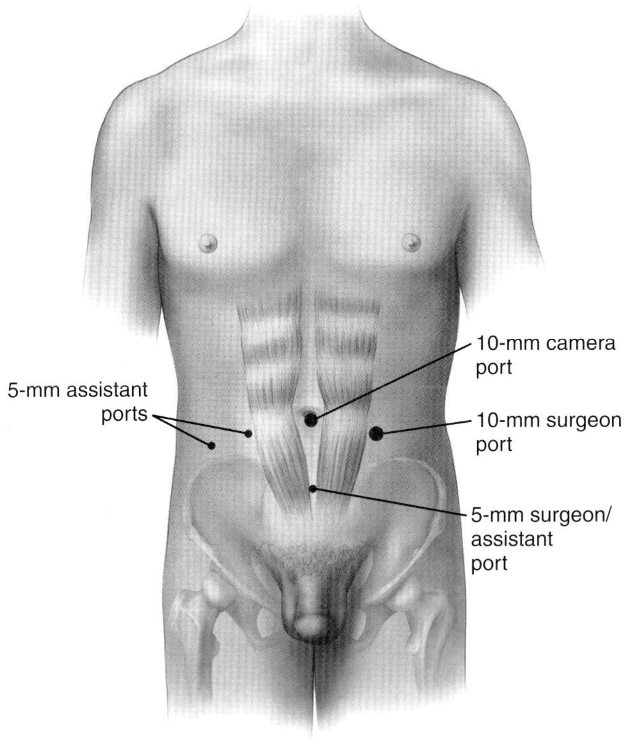

FIGURE 14–2 Triangular port distribution.

sixth port depending on exposure. There have been several other subtle variations described,[19,20] and some authors have used the fourth arm for stable retraction.[21]

LRP OPERATIVE TECHNIQUES

Transperitoneal Approach

This approach was the first to be described for LRP,[4] and it has been divided into six critical steps:

1. Incision of the posterior vesical peritoneum with dissection of the vasa deferentia and seminal vesicles. Denonvilliers' fascia is also incised.
2. Dissection of the space of Retzius. The endopelvic fascia is incised with selective suture ligation of Santorini's plexus.
3. The bladder neck is then identified and dissected and the seminal vesicles delivered.
4. The lateral surfaces of the prostate are dissected in the intrafascial plane to preserve the neurovascular bundles (when indicated).
5. Selective dissection of the urethra with the aid of a metal Béniqué dilator.
6. A vesicourethral anastomosis is performed with interrupted or running Vicryl sutures. Finally, the prostate is extracted using a laparoscopic bag.

Variations have been described in the literature regarding this technique. Hoznek et al.[22] prefer to divide Santorini's plexus after having opened the bladder neck, which is identified by palpation with scissors to distinguish a mobile bladder wall from the solid prostatic substance. Another difference is that the urethrovesical anastomosis is performed with two hemi-circumferential running sutures.

Rassweiler et al.[16] begins the procedure first with an "ascending part," by immediately accessing the space of Retzius, incising the endopelvic fascia, transecting the puboprostatic ligaments, and then ligating and dividing the dorsal venous complex to gain access to the urethra at the level of the apex. The "descending part" of the surgery begins with traction of the prostate ventrally for the dissection of the bladder neck to gain access to the seminal vesicle by a retrovesical approach. Finally, the anastomosis is done with interrupted sutures.

These and other modifications demonstrate that the steps of the LRP can be performed according to the surgeon's preferences and that a continuous evolution is necessary to reach optimal oncologic and functional results.

Extraperitoneal Approach

This approach has been previously described in the literature and can be divided into steps similarly[23,24]:

1. The space of Retzius is dissected by blunt dissection with the laparoscope or by the use of a balloon.
2. The endopelvic fascia is opened.
3. The bladder neck is dissected and reveals the initial plane of dissection of the seminal vesicles and Denonvilliers' fascia.
4. The lateral surfaces of the prostate are dissected in the intrafascial plane to preserve the neurovascular bundles (when indicated).
5. The dorsal venous complex is suture ligated, and the prostatic apex is dissected and mobilized for a selective section of the urethra.
6. A vesicourethral anastomosis is performed with interrupted or running Vicryl sutures, and the prostate is extracted with a laparoscopic bag.

The retropubic, or extraperitoneal, approach, described after the experience gained with the transperitoneal prostatectomy, has experienced a lot of interest because it is argued that the anatomy is more comparable to that of the open technique and that by avoiding the peritoneum, the danger of gastrointestinal damage is diminished.[23] What has been learned from experience is that it also allows

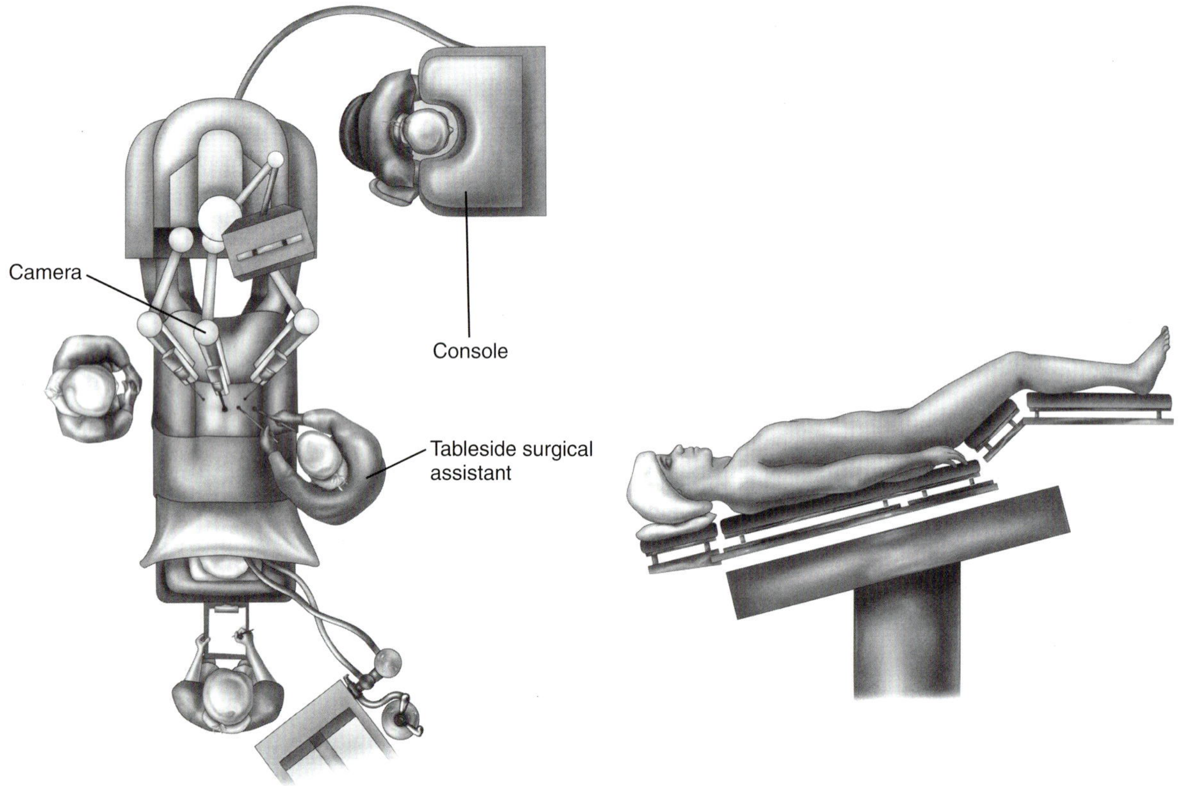

FIGURE 14–3 Telerobotic system.

a better identification of the epigastric vessels, which is very helpful during the placement of the lateral ports. Finally, an anastomotic leak can be better managed by maintaining an intact peritoneum to exclude bowel contact with urine.[23]

RALP OPERATIVE TECHNIQUES

The da Vinci system (Intuitive Surgical, Sunnyvale, CA) is a master-slave surgical robot, consisting of a slave (or work) unit and a master (or control unit), which are connected by a computer-based system. The slave unit will move the camera and two to three instrument arms. The master unit, located in the remote console, will transmit movements that the surgeon performs. The role of the assistant is limited to exposing the operative field, aiding in hemostasis by suction and irrigation and applying clips.[25] Once the robot is assembled and trocars are inserted, the prostatectomy proceeds as previously described for the standard LRP. Both transperitoneal[8,20] and extraperitoneal[26,27] approaches have been described.

LRP VERSUS RALP

The benefits of LRP when compared with open radical retropubic prostatectomy have been well documented.[5] These benefits occur without sacrificing the oncologic standards established by the open approach.[28] With the advent of the RALP, patients and surgeons have witnessed similar improvements over the open technique.[29–31]

The robot offers several advantages and disadvantages to the surgeon when compared with standard laparoscopy. Perhaps no benefit has been more recognized than the reduction of the learning curve. Historically, the mastery of LRP required a steep learning curve with even experienced laparoscopists requiring nearly 60 cases to obtain proficiency.[32] Now that the techniques for LRP have been well developed and refined, the learning curve for the laparoscopically naïve surgeon may be shorter than once reported.[33,34] Significantly shorter learning curves have been reported with the RALP. Ahlering et al.[19] described the successful transfer of skills from a laparoscopically naïve surgeon to proficiency in RALP in 12 cases. When comparing the operative times of LRP to RALP, Menon et al.[35] observed a progressive decrease in the time of RALP with surgeon experience that was not seen in the LRP group. This trend has been reported in most early series of RALP.[19,20] A patient side assistant with intermediate to advanced laparoscopic skill is required, however, to achieve this outcome with RALP.[19,35,36] Setup of the robot also may require more time during the learning curve, but this can be easily overcome.[19]

Technical factors that may be attributed to shortening the learning process of RALP include visualization in three-dimensions,[37] as opposed to two with standard laparoscopy. The surgeon also enjoys six degrees of freedom from the instrument tips of the robot compared with only four with standard laparoscopy. Further advantages of the robot include the ability to filter hand tremor with motion scaling of 1:5 and an ergonomic surgeon console to limit fatigue.

A drawback to both RALP and LRP is the lack of tactile feedback. The robot requires the surgeon to use visual cues to determine suture tension or tissue consistency. This is enhanced, however, with its three-dimensional imagery. Standard laparoscopy also does not allow the direct tactile feedback of open surgery, but additional information can be obtained by "instrument palpation."

Cost analyses have also been performed comparing RALP and LRP.[38–40] An initial purchasing cost of $1.2 million is required for the da Vinci, followed by a $100,000 per year maintenance fee.[38] Lotan et al.[38] reported a cost advantage of $1239 in favor of LRP compared with RALP. Menon et al.[41] estimated that an institution must perform 75 cases per year with an average operating time of 3 hours per case to be cost-effective in the United States.

With regard to patient outcomes, the literature for these minimally invasive approaches is not fully mature. A second generation of series, however, is now emerging (Table 14–1) related to LRP that present data from beyond the initial learning curve of an institution.[5,17,42–49] A better comparison between LRP and RALP is therefore possible because the biggest advantage to the surgeon with RALP is removed (learning curve) and the patient-related outcomes can more equally be analyzed. The first series of LRP described by Schuessler et al.[1] has been included in Table 14–1 to demonstrate this progression. Table 14–2 shows the most recent series of RALP.[19,20,27,50,51]

Similar to the single institution comparison data that are available for open surgery versus LRP,[5,28,52] RALP and LRP comparisons have been published.[35,41,53] The RALP and LRP comparison series are seen in Table 14–3[35,41,53] along with outcomes from the first 2208 LRPs performed at Montsouris compared with the first 105 RALPs performed.

OPERATIVE TIME

The operative times for the LRP and RALP series are given in Tables 14–1 and 14–2. The average time across series for LRP is 234 minutes, with a range of 151 minutes to 453 minutes. This is a dramatic reduction compared with the time of 564 minutes observed with Schuessler et al.'s[1] original description.[1] At Montsouris, the operative time has also decreased from 200 minutes in the earlier series[54] to 173 in the most recent series.[43] Two authors have noted significantly shorter times for the extraperitoneal approach compared with the transperitoneal approach for LRP, stating that this approach is similar to the retropubic open procedure and therefore familiar to the surgeon.[45,46] This trend has not been observed, however, with all comparative studies.[44,55] Operative times for RALP (see Table 14–2) range from 141 to 250 minutes, with a mean time across series of 182 minutes. At Montsouris, a time of 180 minutes for the LRP group was compared with 155 minutes for the RALP group (see Table 14–3), and no statistically significant difference was observed. This finding is true for other single institution studies.[35,41,53]

ESTIMATED BLOOD LOSS

Estimated blood loss for LRP ranges from 185 to 850 mL, with an average across series of 482 mL (see Table 14–1). At Montsouris, this statistic has not changed when comparing our earlier and later series.[43,54] As with operative time and LRP, authors have noticed significant differences in blood loss when comparing the extraperitoneal to the transperitoneal approach; however, no unanimity can be reached with regard to the superiority of one or the other.[45,46] Estimated blood loss for the RALP averages 234 mL, with a range of 75 to 500 mL (see Table 14–2). Table 14–3 shows each series having significantly different blood loss between approaches. Menon et al.[41] and Joseph et al.[53] each report less blood loss with the RALP (391 mL for LRP versus 256 mL for RALP in Menon et al. and 299 mL for LRP versus 206 mL for RALP in Joseph et al.). At Montsouris, the contrary was found. Mean estimated blood loss for the LRP series was 360 mL, whereas an estimated blood loss of 500 mL was observed in the RALP group. The rate of transfusion differed significantly in our series from 3% in the LRP to 9.8% in the RALP group. The other series did not report this observation.[41,53] In summary, differences in blood loss vary by institution, and although a trend toward less blood loss can be seen in the RALP series, definitive conclusions cannot be made at this time.

COMPLICATIONS

The reporting and description of complications varies greatly between authors. Table 14–1 shows a range of overall complication rates from 4% to 34% in the LRP series. Table 14–2 shows a range of 1% to 8.8% in the RALP series. Because of the large discrepancy between these series, important information is gained by looking at the single-institution studies in Table 14–3. At Montsouris, we observed a 7.3% complication rate with the LRP and a 7% rate with the RALP. The other authors in Table 14–3 agree that no significant differences are seen between each approach.[35,41,53]

As institutional experience increases, conversion rates tend to decrease. Table 14–3 shows that it is relatively rare to convert to open surgery (2.5% in the Menon et al. series of LRP) and that conversion from RALP to LRP (two patients in the Montsouris RALP series) and from extraperitoneal to transperitoneal laparoscopy (two patients in the Joseph et al. series) are more common based on surgeon

Table 14–1 Laparoscopic Radical Prostatectomy

Series	*N*	Approach	OR Time (min)	EBL (mL)	Transfusion %	Conversion (%)
Stolzenburg et al.[1]	700	Extraperitoneal	151	220	0.9	0
Rozet et al.[5]	599	Extraperitoneal	173	380	1.2	0
Brown et al.[17]	122	Transperitoneal	197	n.r.	3.27	1
	34	Extraperitoneal	191	n.r.	0	5.8 to transperitoneal
Eden et al.[42]	100	Transperitoneal	238.9*	310.5*	2	1
	100	Extraperitoneal	190.6*	201.5*	0	0
Ruiz et al.[43]	165	Transperitoneal	248.5*	678*	1.2	n.r.
	165	Extraperitoneal	220*	803*	5.4	n.r.
Roumeguere et al.[44]	85	Extraperitoneal	288	400	n.r.	2.3
Rassweiler et al.[45]	438	Transperitoneal	218 (last 219)	800 (last 219)	9.6	0.5
Gregori et al.[46]	80	Transperitoneal	218	376	53 auto/6	0
Hara et al.[47]	26	Transperitoneal	453	850	3.8	0
Turk et al.[48]	125	Transperitoneal	265	185	2	0
Schuessler et al.[49]†	9	Transperitoneal	564	583	n.r.	0

*$P < .05$.
†Reference series.
auto, autotransfusion; b/l sp, bilateral nerve sparing; EBL, estimated blood loss; n.r., not reported; OR, operating room.

Table 14–2 Robotic-Assisted Radical Prostatectomy

Series	*N*	Approach	OR Time (min)	EBL (mL)	Transfusion %
Patel et al.[19]	200	Transperitoneal	141	75	0
Cathelineau et al.[20]	105	Transperitoneal/extraperitoneal	155	500	6
Menon et al.[27]	250	Transperitoneal	160	153	0
Ahlering et al.[50]	45	Transperitoneal	207	145	n.r.
Wolfram et al.[51]	81	Transperitoneal	250	300	12

EBL, estimated blood loss; LRP, laparoscopic radical prostatectomy; n.r., not reported; OR, operating room.

Table 14–3 Single-Institution Series

Series	Approach	Year	*N*	Approach	OR Time (min)
IMM	LRP	2005	2208	Transperitoneal/extraperitoneal	180
	RALP		105	Transperitoneal/extraperitoneal	155
VIP[35,41]	LRP	2002	40	Transperitoneal	258
	RALP		40	Transperitoneal	274
U. Rochester, NY[53]	LRP	2005	50	Extraperitoneal	264
	RALP		50	Extraperitoneal	277

*$P < .05$.
EBL, estimated blood loss; LRP, laparoscopic radical prostatectomy; n.r., not reported; OR, operating room; RALP, robotic-assisted laparoscopic prostatectomy.

Complications (%)	Hospital Stay (days)	Positive Margin (%)	Continence (%)	Potency (%)
2 major, 9.7 minor	n.r.	10.8 pT_2, 31.2 pT_3	92	47.1 b/l sp.
2.3 major, 9.2 minor	6.3	17.7	84	64
11	2.1	24	87	55
12	1.6	21	75	25
8	3.8*	16	56	61
4	2.6*	16	80	82
9,1	6.7	23	n.r.	n.r.
6,1	6.3	29.7	n.r.	n.r.
5 major, 24.6 minor	6	7.8 pT_2	80.7	65
10	12	23.7	95.8	n.r.
23	4.5	31.25	n.r.	n.r.
19	n.r.	n.r.	100	71
34	7.5	26.4	92	59
33	7.3	11	66	50

Conversion (%)	Complications (%)	Hospital Stay (days)	Positive Margin (%)	Continence (%)	Potency (%)
0	1	1	10.5	98	n.r
2 to LRP	7	5.5	22	70	79
n.r.	4	1.2	6	96	82 (<60 yr)
n.r.	8.8	1.5	35.5	81	n.r.
n.r.	n.r.	n.r.	22.2	n.r.	n.r.

EBL (mL)	Transfusion %	Conversion (%)	Complications (%)	Hospital Stay (days)	Positive Margin (%)
360*	3*	0	7.3	4	15.8
500*	9.8*	2 to LRP	7	5.5	22
391*	n.r.	2.5 to open	10	n.r.	25
256*	n.r.	0	5	1	17.5
299*	0	2 to transperitoneal	4	2	14
206*	0	0	8	2	12

experience and comfort level.[35,41,53] Overall, there is no difference in conversion when comparing LRP with RALP.

HOSPITAL STAY

Hospital stay is another factor that is difficult to standardize based on varying international hospital practice policies for discharge. Table 14–1 shows a range of 1.6 to 12 days in the LRP group, whereas a range of 1 day to 5.5 days is reported for RALP in Table 14–2. In the combined series (see Table 14–3), there is no significant difference between the number of days spent in the hospital between the LRP and RALP groups.

ONCOLOGIC OUTCOMES

Long-term outcomes data on PSA progression are not yet available for LRP or RALP because of their relatively short existence, but encouraging short-term data are becoming available for LRP.[56] In several large series comparing LRP with radical retropubic prostatectomy, no difference was observed in rates of positive surgical margins.[5,28,52] A mean positive surgical margin rate of 20.6% is observed across recent series of LRP (see Table 14–1), with a range of 11% to 29.7%. Similarly, a range of 10.5% to 35.5% (mean, 19.24%) is seen in Table 14–2 for RALP. At Montsouris, a 15.8% rate of overall positive surgical margins was seen in the LRP group, compared with 22% in the RALP group ($P > .05$). When comparing other single-institution series, there is no statistically significant difference between the LRP and RALP groups in terms of overall positive surgical margins (see Table 14–3).[35,41,53]

FUNCTIONAL OUTCOMES

Continence outcomes for LRP can be seen in Table 14–1 and range from 56% to 100%. The definition of continence by pad number varies from series to series, making adequate comparison difficult. Similar problems exist with regard to erectile dysfunction. Table 14–1 shows a range of 25% to 82% depending on the type of preservation performed and the use of medications. Data for continence and potency are currently not mature enough for RALP to form adequate conclusions when comparing with LRP. Therefore, longer follow-up with standardized reporting is vital for true comparisons to be made.

CONCLUSIONS

Compared with LRP, RALP appears to offer a significant benefit to the laparoscopically naïve surgeon with respect to learning curve. This, however, comes at an increased cost. Intraoperative and postoperative outcomes appear to be comparable between the two approaches, and longer follow-up data are necessary to compare oncologic and functional outcomes.

REFERENCES

1. Schuessler WW, Schulam PG, Clayman RV, et al: Laparoscopic radical prostatectomy: initial short-term experience. Urology 50:854–857, 1997.
2. Raboy A, Ferzli G, Albert P: Initial experience with extraperitoneal endoscopic radical retropubic prostatectomy. Urology 50:849–853, 1997.
3. Guillonneau B, Cathelineau X, Barret E, et al: Laparoscopic radical prostatectomy: technical and early oncological assessment of 40 operations. Eur Urol 36:14–20, 1999.
4. Guillonneau B, Vallancien G: Laparoscopic radical prostatectomy: the Montsouris technique. J Urol 163:1643–1649, 2000.
5. Rassweiler J, Seemann O, Schulze M, et al: Laparoscopic versus open radical prostatectomy: a comparative study at a single institution. J Urol 169:1689–1693, 2003.
6. Salomon L, Sebe P, De la Taille A, et al: Open versus laparoscopic radical prostatectomy: part I. BJU Int 94:238–243, 2004.
7. Bhayani SB, Pavlovich CP, Hsu TS, et al: Prospective comparison of short-term convalescence: laparoscopic radical prostatectomy versus open radical retropubic prostatectomy. Urology 61:612–616, 2003.
8. Menon M, Tewari A, Peabody J: Vattikuti Institute prostatectomy: technique. J Urol 169:2289–2292, 2003.
9. Vallancien G, Gupta R, Cathelineau X, et al: Initial results of salvage laparoscopic radical prostatectomy after radiation failure. J Urol 170:1838–1840, 2003.
10. Sarle R, Tewari A, Hemal AK, et al: Robotic-assisted anatomic radical prostatectomy: technical difficulties due to a large median lobe. Urol Int 74:92–94, 2005.
11. Chang CM, Moon D, Gianduzzo TR, et al: The impact of prostate size in laparoscopic radical prostatectomy. Eur Urol 48:285–290, 2005.
12. Brown JA, Garlitz C, Strup SE, et al: Laparoscopic radical prostatectomy after neoadjuvant hormonal therapy: an apparently safe and effective procedure. J Laparoendosc Adv Surg Tech A 14:335–338, 2004.
13. Guillonneau B, el-Fettouh H, Baumert H, et al: Laparoscopic radical prostatectomy: oncological evaluation after 1,000 cases a Montsouris Institute. J Urol 169:1261–1266, 2003.
14. Parsons JK, Jarrett TJ, Chow GK, et al: The effect of previous abdominal surgery on urological laparoscopy. J Urol 168:2387–2390, 2002.
15. Stolzenburg JU, Anderson C, Rabenalt R, et al: Endoscopic extraperitoneal radical prostatectomy in patients with prostate cancer and previous laparoscopic inguinal mesh placement for hernia repair. World J Urol 23:295–299, 2005.
16. Rassweiler J, Sentker L, Seemann O, et al: Laparoscopic radical prostatectomy with the Heilbronn technique: an analysis of the first 180 cases. J Urol 166:2101–2108, 2001.
17. Roumeguere T, Bollens R, Vanden Bossche M, et al: Radical prostatectomy: a prospective comparison of oncological and functional results between open and laparoscopic approaches. World J Urol 20:360–366, 2003.
18. Menon M, Hemal AK: Vattikuti Institute prostatectomy: a technique of robotic radical prostatectomy: experience in more than 1000 cases. J Endourol 18:611–619, 2004; discussion 619.
19. Ahlering TE, Skarecky D, Lee D, et al: Successful transfer of open surgical skills to a laparoscopic environment using a robotic interface: initial experience with laparoscopic radical prostatectomy. J Urol 170:1738–1741, 2003.

20. Patel VR, Tully AS, Holmes R, et al: Robotic radical prostatectomy in the community setting—the learning curve and beyond: initial 200 cases. J Urol 174:269–272, 2005.
21. Smith JA Jr, Herrell SD: Robotic-assisted laparoscopic prostatectomy: do minimally invasive approaches offer significant advantages? J Clin Oncol 23:8170–8175, 2005.
22. Hoznek A, Salomon L, Olsson LE, et al: Laparoscopic radical prostatectomy. The Creteil experience. Eur Urol 40:38–45, 2001.
23. Bollens R, Vanden Bossche M, Roumeguere T, et al: Extraperitoneal laparoscopic radical prostatectomy. Results after 50 cases. Eur Urol 40:65–69, 2001.
24. Rozet F, Arroyo C, Cathelineau X, et al: Extraperitoneal standard laparo scopic radical prostatectomy. J Endourol 18:605–609m 2004. discussion 609–610.
25. Abbou CC, Hoznek A, Salomon L, et al: Laparoscopic radical prostatectomy with a remote controlled robot. J Urol 165(6 pt 1):1964–1966, 2001.
26. Gettman MT, Hoznek A, Salomon L, et al: Laparoscopic radical prostatectomy: description of the extraperitoneal approach using the da Vinci robotic system. J Urol 170(2 pt 1):416–419, 2003.
27. Cathelineau X, Rozet F, Vallancien G: Robotic radical prostatectomy: the European experience. Urol Clin North Am 31:693–699, viii, 2004.
28. Salomon L, Levrel O, de la Taille A, et al: Radical prostatectomy by the retropubic, perineal and laparoscopic approach: 12 years of experience in one center. Eur Urol 42:104–110; discussion 110–101, 2002.
29. Webster TM, Herrell SD, Chang SS, et al: Robotic assisted laparoscopic radical prostatectomy versus retropubic radical prostatectomy: a prospective assessment of postoperative pain. J Urol 174:912–914, 2005. discussion 914.
30. Menon M, Tewari A, Baize B, et al: Prospective comparison of radical retropubic prostatectomy and robot-assisted anatomic prostatectomy: the Vattikuti Urology Institute experience. Urology 60:864–868, 2002.
31. Tewari A, Srivasatava A, Menon M: A prospective comparison of radical retropubic and robot-assisted prostatectomy: experience in one institution. BJU Int 92:205–210, 2003.
32. Guillonneau B, Rozet F, Barret E, et al: Laparoscopic radical prostatectomy: assessment after 240 procedures. Urol Clin North Am 28:189–202, 2001.
33. Martina GR, Giumelli P, Scuzzarella S, et al: Laparoscopic extraperitoneal radical prostatectomy—learning curve of a laparoscopy-naive urologist in a community hospital. Urology 65:959–963, 2005.
34. Poulakis V, Dillenburg W, Moeckel M, et al: Laparoscopic radical prostatectomy: prospective evaluation of the learning curve. Eur Urol 47:167–175, 2005.
35. Menon M, Shrivastava A, Tewari A, et al: Laparoscopic and robot assisted radical prostatectomy: establishment of a structured program and preliminary analysis of outcomes. J Urol 168:945–949, 2002.
36. Lee DI, Eichel L, Skarecky DW, Ahlering TE: Robotic laparoscopic radical prostatectomy with a single assistant. Urology 63:1172–1175, 2004.
37. Tewari A, Peabody JO, Fischer M, et al: An operative and anatomic study to help in nerve sparing during laparoscopic and robotic radical prostatectomy. Eur Urol 43:444–454, 2003.
38. Lotan Y, Cadeddu JA, Gettman MT: The new economics of radical prostatectomy: cost comparison of open, laparoscopic and robot assisted techniques. J Urol 172(4 pt 1):1431–1435, 2004.
39. Scales CD Jr, Jones PJ, Eisenstein EL, et al: Local cost structures and the economics of robot assisted radical prostatectomy. J Urol 174:2323–2329, 2005.
40. Steers WD, LeBeau S, Cardella J, Fulmer B: Establishing a robotics program. Urol Clin North Am 31:773–780, x, 2004, review.
41. Menon M, Shrivastava A, Tewari A: Laparoscopic radical prostatectomy: conventional and robotic. Urology 66(5 suppl):101–104, 2005.
42. Stolzenburg JU, Rabenalt R, Do M, et al: Endoscopic extraperitoneal radical prostatectomy: oncological and functional results after 700 procedures. J Urol 174(4 pt 1):1271–1275; discussion 1275, 2005.
43. Rozet F, Galiano M, Cathelineau X, et al: Extraperitoneal laparoscopic radical prostatectomy: a prospective evaluation of 600 cases. J Urol 174:908–911, 2005.
44. Brown JA, Rodin D, Lee B, et al: Transperitoneal versus extraperitoneal approach to laparoscopic radical prostatectomy: an assessment of 156 cases. Urology 65:320–324, 2005.
45. Ruiz L, Salomon L, Hoznek A, et al: Comparison of early oncologic results of laparoscopic radical prostatectomy by extraperitoneal versus transperitoneal approach. Eur Urol 46:50–54; discussion 54–56, 2004.
46. Eden CG, King D, Kooiman GG, et al: Transperitoneal or extraperitoneal laparoscopic radical prostatectomy: does the approach matter? J Urol 172(6 pt 1):2218–2223, 2004.
47. Gregori A, Simonato A, Lissiani A, et al: Laparoscopic radical prostatectomy: perioperative complications in an initial and consecutive series of 80 cases. Eur Urol 44:190–194, 2003. discussion 194.
48. Hara I, Kawabata G, Miyake H, et al: Feasibility and usefulness of laparoscopic radical prostatectomy: Kobe University experience. Int J Urol 9:635–640, 2002.
49. Turk I, Deger S, Winkelmann B, et al: Laparoscopic radical prostatectomy. Technical aspects and experience with 125 cases. Eur Urol 40:46–52, 2001. discussion 53.
50. Menon M, Tewari A: Robotic radical prostatectomy and the Vattikuti Urology Institute technique: an interim analysis of results and technical points. Urology 61(4 suppl 1):15–20, 2003.
51. Wolfram M, Brautigam R, Engl T, et al: Robotic-assisted laparoscopic radical prostatectomy: the Frankfurt technique. World J Urol 21:128–132, 2003.
52. Remzi M, Klingler HC, Tinzl MV, et al: Morbidity of laparoscopic extraperitoneal versus transperitoneal radical prostatectomy verus open retropubic radical prostatectomy. Eur Urol 48:83–89, 2005. discussion 89.
53. Joseph JV, Vicente I, Madeb R, et al: Robot-assisted vs pure laparoscopic radical prostatectomy: are there any differences? BJU Int 96:39–42, 2005.
54. Guillonneau B, Cathelineau X, Doublet JD, et al: Laparoscopic radical prostatectomy: assessment after 550 procedures. Crit Rev Oncol Hematol 43:123–133, 2002.
55. Cathelineau X, Cahill D, Widmer H, et al: Transperitoneal or extraperitoneal approach for laparoscopic radical prostatectomy: a false debate over a real challenge. J Urol 171(2 pt 1):714–716, 2004.
56. Trabulsi EJ, Guillonneau B: Laparoscopic radical prostatectomy. J Urol 173:1072–1079, 2005.

CHAPTER 15

Michael J. Fumo • Ketan K. Badani • Mani Menon

Robotic Radical Cystectomy

INTRODUCTION

"As to diseases, make a habit of two things—to help, or at least to do no harm."

— Hippocrates, Epidemics, Book I, Section XI

With this quote, Hippocrates commands physicians to search out the means by which to cure with the least morbidity possible. This goal has remained constant; however, as technology and our self-understanding have increased, the methods have changed greatly. Recently, minimally invasive procedures have not only gained acceptance but have become an extremely popular standard of care. Radical cystectomy, an operation fraught with potential complications,[1] can now been reevaluated in the light of robotic technology. Robotics minimizes the morbidity of not only the extirpative but also the reconstructive aspects of radical cystectomy. This chapter seeks to discuss the methods of robotic radical cystectomy and the available data regarding outcomes after this procedure.

INDICATIONS

The major indication for cystectomy is carcinoma of the bladder. This includes patients with superficial tumors in whom endoscopic control has failed despite adjuvant intravesical therapy, those with high-risk factors for recurrence, and patients with locally infiltrating tumors. Radical resection includes removal of the bladder, associated peritoneum, perivesical fat, distal ureters, and, in men, the prostate, vasa, and seminal vesicles. In women, preservation of the uterus and vagina is feasible so that an anterior exenteration may or may not also be included.[2]

ALTERNATIVE THERAPIES

There are numerous protocols involving radiation, systemic chemotherapy, or a combination of both for the treatment of muscle-invasive malignancy of the bladder. These options are usually chosen for patients who are poor surgical candidates or who refuse surgery. Radical cystectomy is considered the standard of care.

PREPARATION

In anticipation of surgery, the patient is started on a clear liquid diet the day before surgery, along with a bowel preparation of the surgeon's choice. On the morning of surgery, the patient receives a broad-spectrum antibiotic along with deep venous thrombosis prophylaxis, including bilateral compression stockings and 5000 U of subcutaneous heparin. With the patient under general anesthesia, a nasogastric tube is placed and the patient is positioned in exaggerated Trendelenburg position with the arms adducted and tucked at the sides; adequate padding for all pressure points should be used. Foam padding is crisscrossed as a thoracic wrap to secure the patient in position. After sterile preparation and draping, a urethral catheter is placed as well.

PORT PLACEMENT

Pneumoperitoneum has been created at our institution using a Veress needle in more than 2000 cases without complication. Using either a Veress needle or Hassan technique, the surgeon insufflates the peritoneum to 15 mm Hg and places the initial 12-mm camera port at the umbilicus; peritoneoscopy is then performed with a 30-degree laparoscope. The remainder of the ports are placed under direct vision. Each of the two 8-mm robot trocars is placed just lateral to the rectus muscle on their respective side along a line 2 to 4 cm below the umbilicus.[3] This line may be moved cephalad depending on the height of the patient. A second 12-mm port is placed above the right iliac fossa approximately 3 cm above the iliac crest along the midaxillary line. Last, two 5-mm ports are placed: the first equidistant between the camera and right robotic port and the second in the mirror image of the right 12-mm port above the left iliac fossa (Figure 15–1).

EQUIPMENT

After port placement, the robot is brought into position at the patient's feet and docked with the robotic trocars. The standard robotic instruments include the da Vinci monopolar hook, triangular bipolar grasper, articulating scissors, and 8-mm needle drivers. The majority of the case can be performed with the robotic bipolar graspers and monopolar hook or articulating scissors. The assistant's instruments include a laparoscopic grasper, long suction-irrigator, and laparoscopic scissors needed for retraction and exposure.

DISSECTION

Posterior

Dissection should begin with the camera in the 30-degree down position; the peritoneum is then opened in a horizontal "U" with the base at the cul-de-sac and each arm following the course of the ureter if seen to the level of the bifurcation of the iliac vessels. The dissection is started posteriorly to take advantage of the bladder's natural adhesions anteriorly, thus supporting the bladder in space so that minimal extra retraction is required while dissection of the posterior surface of the bladder is performed. After the peritoneum is opened in men, the anterior sheath of Denonvilliers' fascia is encountered and excised in the midline such that a plane may be extended between the rectum and bladder distally as far as is easily possible to visualize. This space should be broadened laterally as much as possible. The ureterovesical junctions will be encountered in broadening this posterior space, and the ureter should be able to be seen extending from where it crosses the iliac vessels down to the bladder on each side. The seminal vesicles and vasa will act as landmarks; the vasa cross medially with the ureterovesical junction just lateral and posterior to the crossing vasa. The inferior vesical pedicle will be encountered in this area and must be controlled and divided (Figure 15–2). Once the ureters are fully dissected free, they can be clipped and divided and a biopsy of the distal end performed to ensure margins free of tumor. In men, the seminal vesicles can now be carefully dissected free as the neurovascular bundles course along the tips of the seminal vesicles. Once they are free, the posterior sheath of Denonvilliers' fascia is now encountered and divided so that dissection can be continued posteriorly to the apex of the prostate.

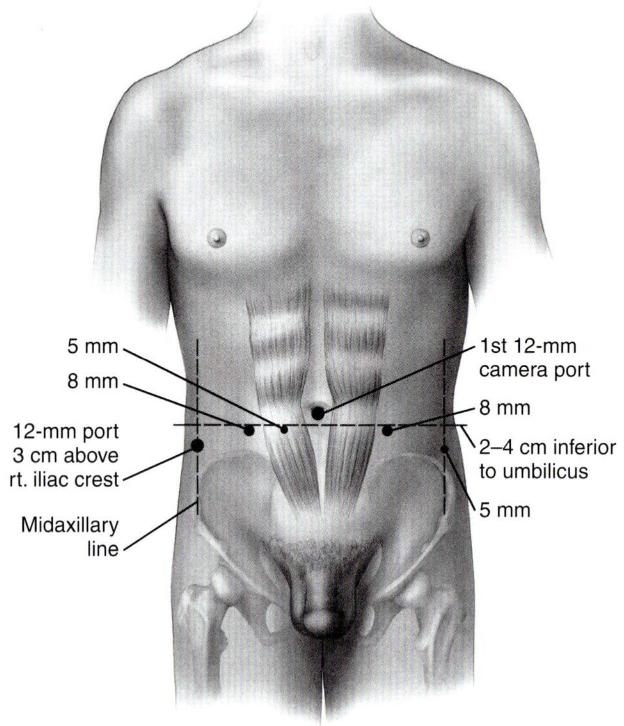

FIGURE 15–1 Anatomic positioning of port placement.

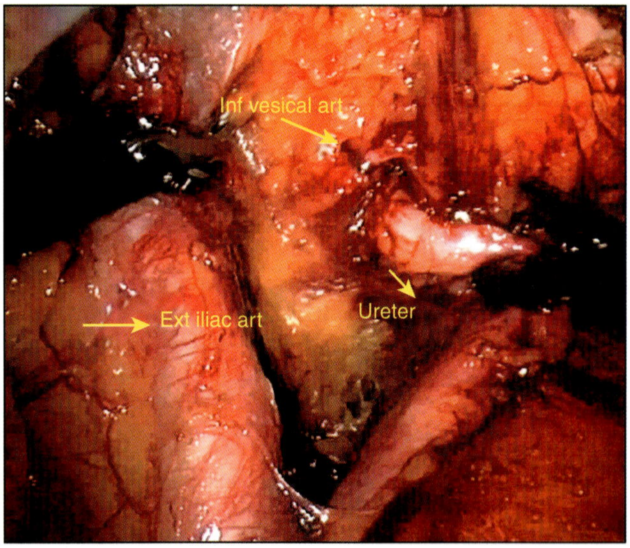

FIGURE 15–2 Posterolateral view of the ureterovesical junction. Note that the inferior vesical pedicle lies just above this and can be ligated after the ureter is transected.

Lateral Pedicle Control and Anterior Dissection

With the posterior dissection complete for the entire width of the bladder, attention is next turned to mobilizing the bladder laterally, performing the lymphadenectomy, and controlling the vascular pedicles. The dissection should start as far lateral as possible to remove the lymph nodes en bloc with the bladder before the pedicles are transected. The full description of the lymph node dissection is described later in this section. The camera can now be changed to be a 30-degree lens, looking upward, for the best visualization. The peritoneum is now incised just laterally to the median umbilical ligaments down to the vasa that are once again encountered as they exit from the inguinal ring. The vasa should be ligated and divided, which allows the dissection to progress such as to connect the lateral dissection posteriorly. Laterally, the dissection is carried along the bladder, encountering the superior vesicle pedicle that is controlled and divided, along with any other vessels that arise from the iliac vessels. Any lymphoid tissue is taken en bloc with the bladder because the dissection should extend as far laterally as possible and should skeletonize the iliac vessels. At this point the bladder is completely free down to the level of the endopelvic fascia, now opened to expose the lateral prostatic dissection. A dorsal venous suture may be placed to secure the venous complex prior to dissection of the prostate in males, as described in the robotic prostatectomy chapter of this book. Anteriorly, the peritoneum is incised, thus exposing the urachus and median umbilical ligaments that need to be divided and giving access to the space of Retzius (Figure 15–3).

Apex

In an attempt to maximize potency postoperatively, we spare the lateral prostatic fascia and the nerves that course through it. Thus, the lateral prostatic fascia is reflected off of the prostate controlling the vascular pedicle and dividing it. The dissection continues around the posterior surface of the prostate to completely free the gland posteriorly and laterally to the apex. The camera should be changed to a 0-degree lens for best visualization. At this point, attention is directed anteriorly to the puboprostatic ligaments that are divided along with the dorsal venous complex. Finally, the striated sphincter is freed from the rectourethralis muscle posteriorly before it is sharply divided while preserving as much urethra as possible (Figure 15–4). The

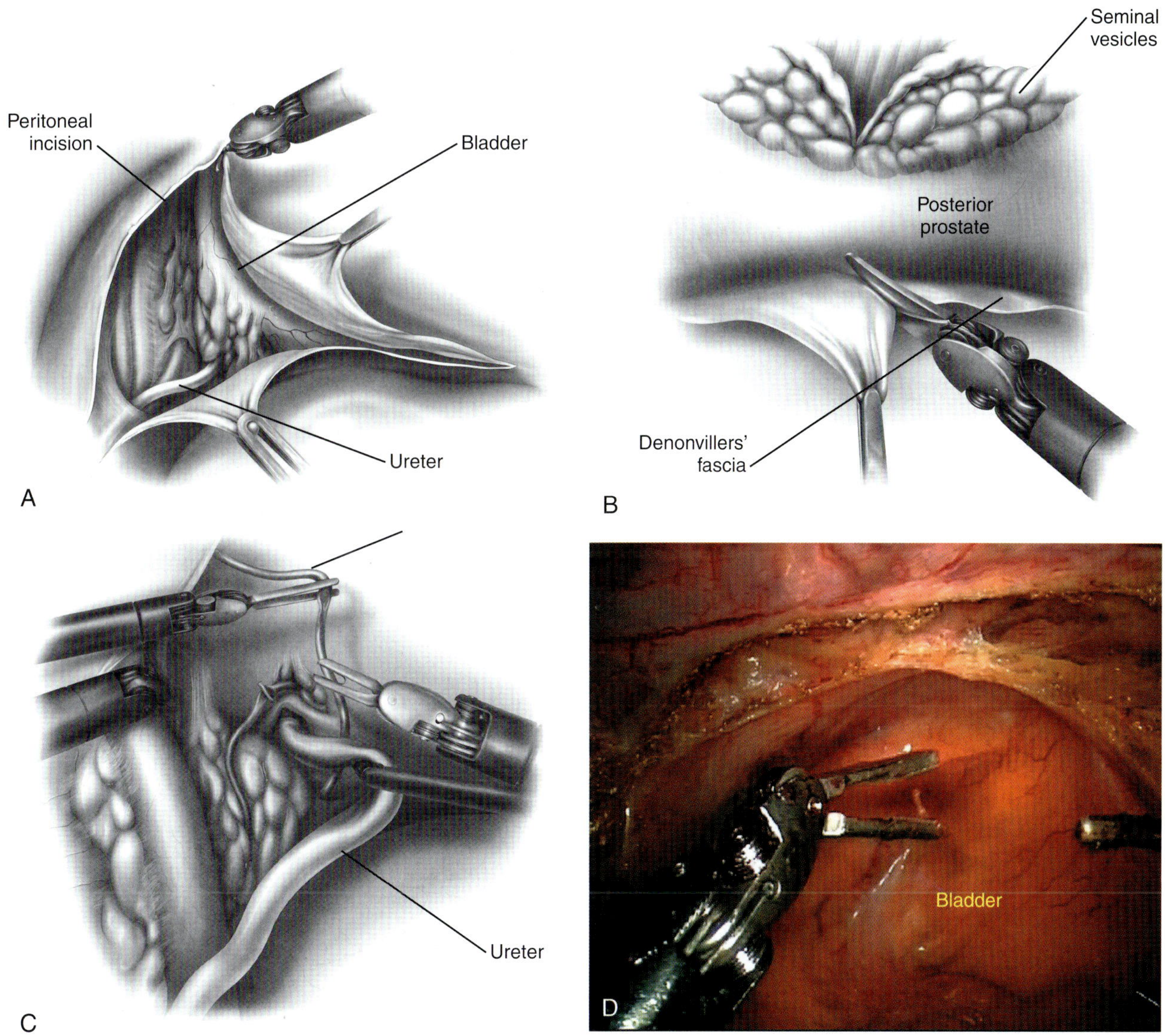

FIGURE 15–3 *A*, Left posterolateral dissection. *B*, Posterior dissection of prostate up to the apex. *C*, Division of the vas deferens and dissection of the left ureter en block with lymphoid tissue. *D*, Inverted "U" incision through peritoneum exposing urachus and median umbilical ligaments as bladder is not dropped off of the abdominal wall.

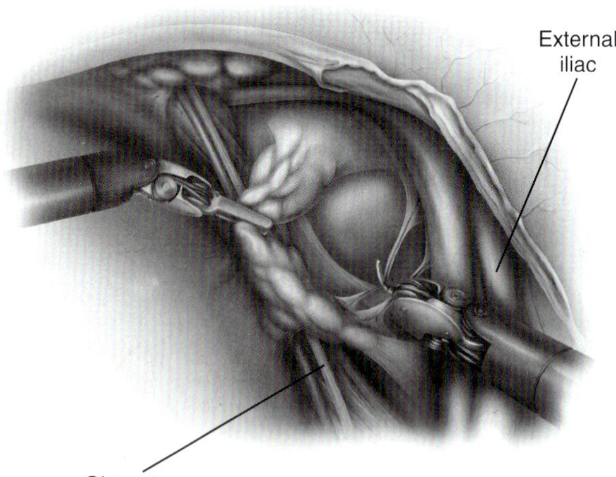

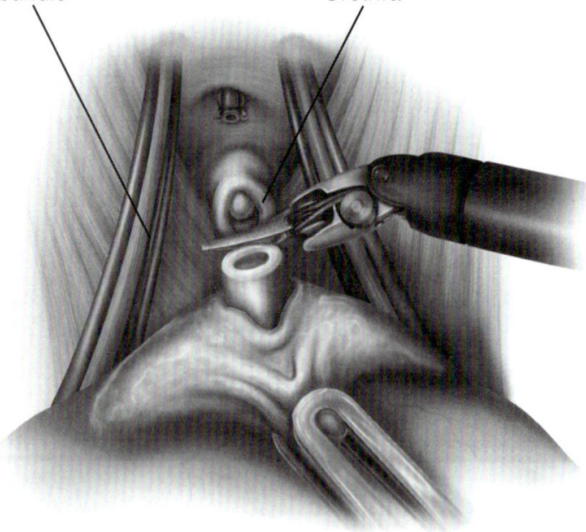

FIGURE 15–4 Apical dissection in the male. Urethra is preserved and biopsied for planned orthotopic bladder substitution. Note the extended preservation of the neurovascular bundles.

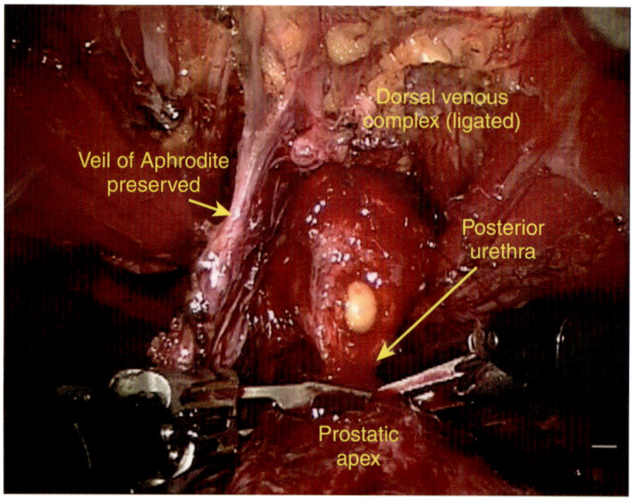

FIGURE 15–5 Lymphadenectomy along external iliac vessels.

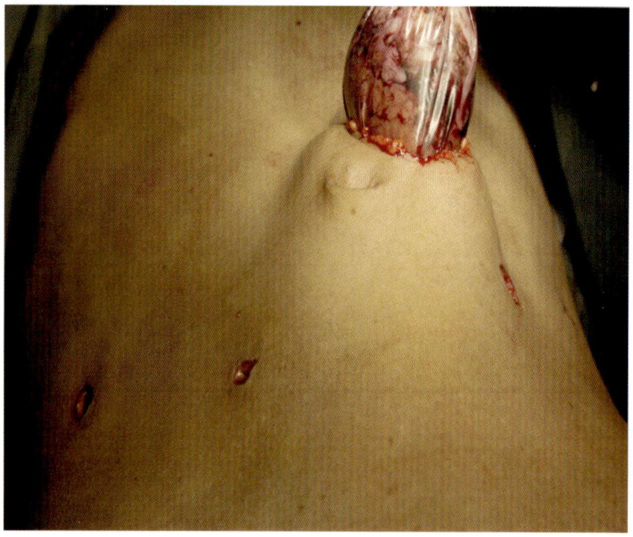

FIGURE 15–6 Removal of specimen in EndoCatch bag through minimal midline incision.

specimen can now be placed into a large EndoCatch (US Surgical) bag until final removal.

LYMPHADENECTOMY

Lymphadenectomy is often part of radical cystectomy because many nodes can be removed intact with the bladder (Figure 15–5). Once the bladder is removed, it is possible to further visualize any remaining nodes using the 30-degree lens directed downward. Using this lens is essential for adequate visualization of the common iliac lymph nodes. All nodal tissue is cleared from the genitofemoral nerve laterally, to the bladder wall medially, and from the distal common iliac artery superiorly, to the lateral circumflex iliac vein and the node of Cloquet inferiorly. The obturator fossa is cleared of nodal tissue, preserving the obturator nerve but sacrificing the obturator vessels if necessary. The nodal tissue seems to form two natural packages: one attached to the bladder wall and one lateral to it. Lymphadenectomy can be the most difficult part of the operation because of multiple small blood vessels that must be meticulously coagulated. If this is not done, the vessels retract into the tissues and give rise to hemodynamically insignificant but visually annoying oozing that impairs visibility. Leaving perivesical fat and nodal tissue attached to the bladder may decrease the oozing and allows a more anatomic operation.

URINARY DIVERSION AND URETHRONEOVESICOSTOMY

The specimen can now be retrieved through a 5-cm incision made midway between the umbilicus and pubic symphysis (Figure 15–6). This incision is planned so that next, a segment of ileum is extracted, isolated, detubularized, and

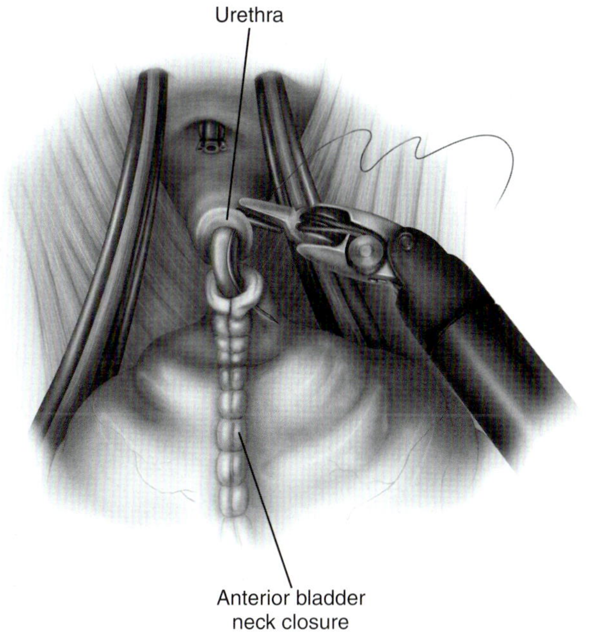

FIGURE 15–7 Watertight urethroneovesicostomy performed robotically after the neobladder is replaced into the abdomen and pneumoperitoneum reestablished.

reconfigured extracorporeally into the orthotopic diversion of choice. This small incision may also be used for any urinary diversion of choice. Once complete, the neobladder is replaced into the pelvis and a Foley catheter is passed per urethra into its neck, inflated, and then pulled down to the urethra. The abdominal incision is closed, and the robot is redocked. Two 5-inch sutures of 3-0 polydioxane, one dyed and one undyed, are tied together and each arm used to perform a continuous running (clockwise and counterclockwise) watertight urethroneovesicostomy (Figure 15–7).

DISCUSSION

As advances in technology have allowed for increasingly sophisticated procedures to be performed with greater ease, interest in laparoscopic radical cystectomy has advanced. Currently, patients and physicians alike are demanding that advances in technology be used to improve efficacy while decreasing morbidity. Initially, stapling devices were understood to significantly reduce blood loss in open cystectomy.[4] Recently, surgical series have been published highlighting the benefits of laparoscopic versus open cystectomy. Basillote et al.[5] highlighted equal operative time, blood loss, and complication rates between open and laparoscopic approaches but noted decreased postoperative pain and hospitalization after laparoscopic surgery. Laparoscopic series have reported less bowel fluid loss, less blood loss, lower incidence and duration of ileus, shorter pain duration, and shorter hospital stay. Robotic technology now improves on laparoscopy in that it facilitates the sophisticated, precise movements necessary in this complex procedure to preserve normal function while curing disease.

Parra et al. performed the first reported laparoscopic cystectomy for pyocystis in a retained bladder. Less than a year later, Sanchez de Badajoz et al. performed and reported the first radical cystectomy with extracorporeally constructed ileal conduit. Gill et al.[6,7] further raised the bar by reporting two cystectomy case series, first with a completely intracorporeal conduit diversion and later with an intracorporeal orthotopic neobladder creation. From this point on, the case series of laparoscopic cystectomy and urinary diversion fall into two categories: where the diversion was done either extracorporeally or intracorporeally with a conduit or continent diversion.

Menon et al.[2,8] successfully blended robotic assistance with extracorporeal diversion creation. This was done to maximize the benefit of the robotic dissection while using a needed incision for specimen extraction to efficiently create an extracorporeal orthotopic neobladder. Robotics can facilitates suturing as shown by Balaji et al.[9] who reported an ileal conduit that was created intracorporeally. Although compared with laparoscopy, robotics facilitates suturing intracorporeally, complete intracorporeal diversion creation is still technically difficult.

Currently, multiple centers are advancing laparoscopic or robotic cystectomy programs as longer-term follow-up becomes available. Cathelineau et al.[10] recently published a large series of intermediate follow-up after laparoscopic cystectomy. They reported decreased pain and blood loss with comparable oncologic outcomes but caution that long-term follow-up is needed. Overall, the majority of cases in the series have had negative oncologic margins and good short-term data. Furthermore, the operating time with the extracorporeal ileal conduit and neobladder diversion has ranged, respectively, from 4 to 9 hours and 5 to 12 hours. The times for completely intracorporeal ileal conduit and neobladder diversion have ranged from 10 to 11.5 hours and 7.4 to 12 hours, respectively. The blood loss has ranged from 300 to 1200 mL (Table 15–1). It appears that laparoscopic and robotic procedures at the very least minimize pain and hospitalization but probably minimize blood loss and ileus as well depending on technique and experience. The major advantage of a completely intracorporeal procedure is further minimizing the small abdominal incision, but it comes at the cost of the patient being under anesthesia for an additional 2 to 3 hours.

Although intracorporeal diversion creation is technically feasible, it seems to waste the opportunity for efficiency that the specimen retrieval incision offers. It can be done, but does it need to be? Should more efficient automatic suturing devices come about, a completely intracorporeal technique may make sense, but until then, robotic cystectomy with extracorporeal diversion creation offers decreased morbidity with faster recovery and, to date, equal short-term oncologic follow-up.

Table 15–1 Selected Series of Laparoscopic and Robotic Radical Cystectomy

Author	Operation	Diversion	Specimen Retrieval	Blood Loss (mL)	Operation Time (hr) (Cystectomy/ Diversion)	Hospital Stay
Parra	Laparoscopic simple cystectomy	—	—	—	2.2 cystectomy alone	5
Badajoz	LRC	Extracorporeal ileal conduit	Enlarged port site	—	—	—
Gill[6,7]	LRC	Intracorporeal ileal conduit and ONB	Abdominal incision	1000, 200– 400	10–11.5 conduit 8.5–10.5 ONB	6–12
Turk	LRC	Intracorporeal rectal sigmoid pouch	None	245	7.4 (total)	10
Simonato	LRC	Intracorporeal sigmoid ureterostomy, extra-corporeal ONB	Abdominal incision	310	2.7/7 ONB 2.7/5.7 sigmoid ureter-ostomy	7–9
Basillote[5]	LRC	Extracorporeal ONB	Abdominal incision	1000	7–9 (total)	5.1
Cathelineau[10]	LRC	Extracorporeal ileal conduit and ONB	Abdominal incision	550	4.3 (total)	12
Menon[2,8]	RRC	Extracorporeal ileal conduit and ONB	Suprapubic incision	100–300	1.8–2.8/2 conduit 3 ONB	—
Yohannes	RRC	Intracorporeal ileal conduit	Abdominal incision	435, 1800	10–12 (total)	6
Beecken	RRC	Intracorporeal ONB	Abdominal incision	200	8.5	—
Balaji[9] RRC	Intracorporeal ileal conduit	Abdominal incision	250	11.5 (total)	7.5	

LRC, laparoscopic radical cystectomy; ONB, orthotopic neobladder; RRC, robotic radical cystectomy. Parra RO, Andrus CH, Jones JP: Laparoscopic cystectomy: initial report on a new treatment for retained bladder. J Urol 148:1140–1144, 1992; Sanchez de Badajoz E, Gallego Perales JL, et al: Laparoscopic cystectomy and ileal conduit: case report. J Endourol 9:59–62, 1995; Turk I, Deger S, Winkelmann B, et al: Laparoscopic radical cystectomy with continent urinary diversion (rectal sigmoid pouch) performed completely intracorporeally: the initial 5 cases. J Urol 165:1863–1866, 2001; Simonato A, Gregori A, Lissiani A, et al: Laparoscopic radical cystoprostatectomy: our experience in a consecutive series of 10 patients with a 3 years follow-up. Eur Urol 47:785–790, 2005; Yohannes P, Puri V, Yi B, et al: Laparoscopy-assisted robotic radical cystoprostatectomy with ileal conduit urinary diversion for muscle-invasive bladder cancer: initial two cases. J Endourol 17:729–732, 2003; Beecken WD, Wolfram M, Engl T, et al: Robotic-assisted laparoscopic radical cystectomy and intra-abdominal formation of an orthotopic ileal neobladder. Eur Urol 44:337–379, 2003.

REFERENCES

1. Skinner DG, Crawford ED, Kaufman JJ: Complications of radical cystectomy for carcinoma of the bladder. J Urol 123:640–643, 1980.
2. Menon M, Hemal AK, Tewari A, et al: Robot-assisted radical cystectomy and urinary diversion in female patients: Technique with preservation of the uterus and vagina. J Am Coll Surg 198:386–393, 2004.
3. Hemal AK, Eun D, Tewari A, et al: Nuances in the optimal placement of ports in pelvic and upper urinary tract surgery using the da Vinci robot. Urol Clin North Am 31:683–692, 2004.
4. Chang SS, Smith JA Jr, Cookson MS: Decreasing blood loss in patients treated with radical cystectomy: a prospective randomized trial using a new stapling device. J Urol 169:951–954, 2003.
5. Basillote JB, Abdelshehid C, Ahlering TE, et al: Laparoscopic assisted radical cystectomy with ileal neobladder: a comparison with the open approach. J Urol 172:489–493, 2004.
6. Gill IS, Fergany A, Klein AE, et al: Laparoscopic radical cystoprostatectomy with ileal conduit performed completely intracorporeally: the initial 2 cases. Urology 56:29–30, 2000.

7. Gill IS, Kaouk JH, Meraney AM, et al: Laparoscopic radical cystectomy and continent orthotopic ileal neobladder performed completely intracorporeally: the initial experience. J Urol 168:13–18, 2002.
8. Menon M, Hemal AK, Tewari A, et al: Nerve-sparing robot-assisted radical cystoprostatectomy and urinary diversion. BJU Int 92:232–236, 2003.
9. Balaji KC, Yohannes P, McBride CL, et al: Feasibility of robot-assisted totally intracorporeal laparoscopic ileal conduit urinary diversion: initial results of a single institutional pilot study. Urology 63:51–55, 2004.
10. Cathelineau X, Arroyo C, Rozet F, et al: Laparoscopic assisted radical cystectomy: the Montsouris experience after 84 cases. Eur Urol 47:780–784, 2005.

CHAPTER 16A

Justin M. Albani • David I. Lee • Ralph V. Clayman

Robotic Renal Surgery: Pyeloplasty

INTRODUCTION

In 1993, laparoscopic pyeloplasty was initiated by Schuessler and colleagues in an effort to duplicate the technique and success rates of open pyeloplasty while offering the advantages of minimally invasive surgery.[1,2] Contemporary series have now confirmed that these success rates are equivalent to those reported for open ureteropelvic junction obstruction (UPJO) repair.[3,4] However, because of the technically demanding nature of the procedure, laparoscopic pyeloplasty still is largely limited to certain clinical centers of laparoscopic excellence.

Sung and Gill[5] initially demonstrated the feasibility and efficacy of performing completely robotic-assisted laparoscopic pyeloplasties in an acute porcine model. Two robotic surgical systems using master-slave manipulators were initially available: Zeus (formerly Computer Motion, Goleta, CA) and da Vinci (now, both of Intuitive Surgical, Sunnyvale, CA); the da Vinci system, with its three-dimensional viewing system, articulating instruments, and intuitive platform, proved superior. Following the initial clinical reports of robotic-assisted pyeloplasty (RAP) using the da Vinci surgical system in 2001, these procedures are increasing in prevalence.[6,7]

INDICATIONS AND PREOPERATIVE EVALUATION

RAP can be offered as first-line treatment for primary or secondary UPJ obstruction. However, in general, the widely accepted indications for selecting pyeloplasty over endopyelotomy are presence of anterior crossing vessels, grade 3-4 hydronephrosis, or percent function of the affected kidney in the 15% to 25% range. Also, for those patients in whom primary endopyelotomy has failed, RAP can still be offered.

Preoperatively for patients with a primary UPJO, standard imaging with intravenous urography (IVU) demonstrating a delay in function associated with a dilated pelvicaliceal system and a narrowed ureteropelvic junction (UPJ) and normal ureter is often sufficient for the initial diagnosis. However, our preference is also to obtain nuclear imaging with technetium ^{99m}Tc-diethylenetriamenepentacetic acid (^{99m}Tc-DTPA) with and without furosemide washout to quantify the degree of obstruction and to determine split function. Rarely, invasive pressure perfusion studies using the Whitaker test are used in cases in which the clinical significance of a dilated system remains in question despite prior radiographic evaluation.[8] We also routinely obtain a spiral computed tomography (CT) angiogram with three-dimensional reconstruction to delineate the presence or absence of crossing vessels. We believe this test is indispensable in the management of secondary UPJ obstruction because it can detect the presence of stones and determine the position of a scarred UPJ in relation to the medial surface of the kidney, as well as detect any crossing vessels that may be present. Retrograde pyelography is usually not performed until the time of surgery.

As with all surgical patients, a preoperative evaluation must confirm the presence of normal coagulation studies, sterile urine, and a thorough medical evaluation before intervention is planned.

SURGICAL TECHNIQUE

With use of the da Vinci robotic surgical system, traditional open techniques of the Anderson-Hynes dismembered pyeloplasty and nondismembered Foley Y-V plasty and Fengerplasty have been successfully performed and are listed in Table 16A–1.[9–21] In many centers, conventional laparoscopy is performed until the UPJ is exposed and the robotic surgical system is docked for the dismemberment and reconstruction of the UPJ. In other centers, the entire procedure is performed with the robot. In either case, a standard set of laparoscopic instruments should be available for the assistant during the surgery (5-mm suction device, needle drivers, electrosurgical scissors, a fenestrated bowel grasper, and other instruments [± harmonic shears, hook electrode, soft tip dissectors]). Finally, we typically use the following robotic instruments at our two institutions: monopolar cautery scissors, Maryland bipolar cautery graspers, Potts scissors, and two needle drivers.

Table 16A–1 Published Experience with Robotic-Assisted Laparoscopic Pyeloplasty

Author	Year	No. of Cases	Technique	Success Rate (%)	Mean FU (mo)	Mean OR Time (min)	EBL (mL)	Mean Stent Removal (wk)
Graham et al.[6]	2001	1	TP	—	—	—	—	—
Guillonneau et al.[7]	2001	1	TP	100	—	—	—	1.5
Gettman et al.[9]	2002	6	TP	100	3	140	<50	3–6
Gettman et al.[10]	2002	9	TP	88.9	4.1	138.8	<50	6
Yohannes and Burjonrappa[18]	2003	1	TP	100	1.5	300	150	6
Hubert[12]	2003	12	TP	—	—	153	—	—
Bentas et al.[13]	2003	11	TP	100	21	197	—	5–6
Munver et al.[14]	2003	10	TP	90	3	168	—	—
Peschel et al.[11]	2004	41	TP	100	7.4	124	<50	6
Luke et al.[21]*	2004	5	TP	80	3	225	68	3–6
Mendez-Torres et al.[15]	2005	32	TP	89	8.6	300	50	6
Siddiq et al.[16]	2005	26	TP	95	6	245	69	4–6
Palese et al.[17]	2005	35	TP	94	7.9	216.4	73.9	4–6
Rubinstein et al.[19]	2005	5	RP	100	6	145	36	—
Patel[20]	2005	50	TP	96	11.7	122	40	2.5

*Zeus robotic platform.

EBL, estimated blood loss; FU, follow-up; OR, operating room; RP, retroperitoneal; TP, transperitoneal.

TRANSPERITONEAL APPROACH

By far the most common laparoscopic approach to the kidney, the transperitoneal approach provides a familiar operative field for the urologist and the greatest amount of working space for performing reconstructive surgery.

PATIENT POSITIONING AND OPERATING ROOM CONFIGURATION

Informed consent is obtained. A standard bowel preparation is not routinely performed. In an unproven effort to decompress the bowels, half a bottle of magnesium citrate can be administered the night before surgery. One gram of cefazolin is administered preoperatively. Obese patients are routinely given 5000 U of heparin subcutaneously 2 hours before the procedure. Generally, we do not place a stent preoperatively and will place it antegrade at the time of the procedure. If the patient had a stent placed preoperatively, we simply use that stent for the repair of the UPJ. Alternatively, a retrograde ureterogram can be performed at the outset of the procedure and an external ureteral stent (e.g., 7-French, 11.5-mm occlusion balloon catheter) can be positioned. Inflation of the balloon allows the catheter to be snugged down at the UPJ, facilitating the subsequent dissection. At the end of the procedure, the external stent is exchanged for an indwelling stent.

General anesthesia is induced. Pneumatic compression stockings are placed on the lower extremities. After placement of the Foley catheter and orogastric tube, the patient is secured in the lateral decubitus position using Stulberg Hip Positioners (Innomed, Savannah, GA) placed at the hip and shoulder along the posterior aspect of the patient. We prefer these positioners because they attach directly to the operating room table using existing table adapters and consist of upright pads of semidense foam that directly pad pressure points. We prefer this to a bulky bean bag that may interfere with the surgery. The bean bag is also very hard and may contribute to postoperative neurologic complications. If so inclined, the entire table can be padded with a gel pad, which we prefer to the use of foam eggcrates. We gently flex the bed to open the space between the iliac crest and costal margin and either do not use the kidney rest or elevate it only during the initial brief part of the procedure when the pneumoperitoneum is being obtained. Although many surgeons place the patient in a modified 45-degree lateral decubitus position, we prefer to position our patients in 70-degree flank position. This facilitates movement of the bowel out of the surgical field.

The operating room configuration is important because the robot, surgical cart, console, and tower are large pieces of equipment. Proper preoperative planning allows for all members of the operative team to have sufficient room to work and view the monitors, for all appropriate cords to reach the proper connections, and for the surgical cart to have ample room to move to and away from the patient. The table side assistant is placed opposite the lowermost midline 5-mm port (Figure 16A–1). This provides the assistant with the optimal approach to the UPJ. The scrub nurse is present adjacent to but behind the assistant, and the video tower is adjacent to the surgical cart in the direct line of sight of the assistant.

Access and Port Placement

After sterile preparation and draping the patient appropriately, a 12-mm curvilinear incision around the umbilicus on the side the surgery is made with a scalpel. The underlying

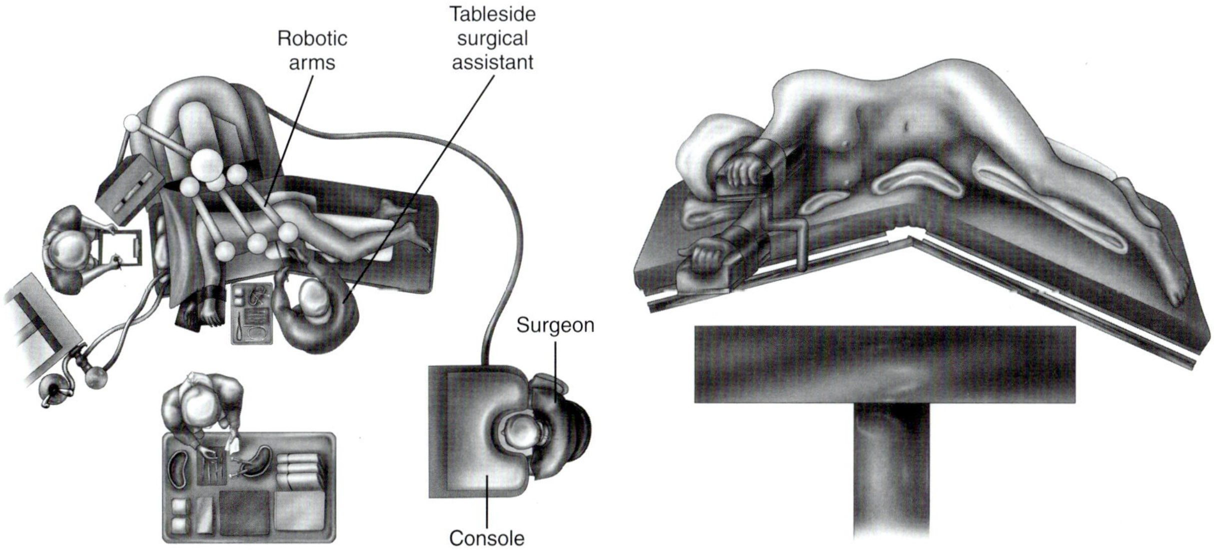

FIGURE 16A–1 Operating room configuration for left-sided robotic-assisted (da Vinci) dismembered pyeloplasty.

dermis and subcutaneous adipose tissue is transected using cautery until the underlying fascia is reached. After pneumoperitoneum is established with a Veress needle at this site, the ports are placed as in Figure 16A–2, beginning with the periumbilical trocar as described by Peschel et al.[11] We prefer to use the Ethicon 12-mm dilating trocar (Ethicon Endo-Surgery, Cincinnati, OH) for the camera port. This port is placed under direct vision with the 0-degree lens inside the clear plastic port; it is important to incise the periumbilical fascia to 10 mm to ease passage of this port into the abdomen. The two 8-mm working ports (Intuitive Surgical, Sunnyvale, CA) for the robotic arms are placed under laparoscopic control in a triangular fashion such that one is placed in the upper midline near the xiphoid process and the other is placed at the lateral border of the rectus inferior to the umbilicus. These ports are optimally placed by ensuring at least 8 cm exists between the camera port and each working port to avoid robotic arm collisions during the surgery (see Figure 16A–2). Many variations exist for the assistant port, but we have found that placement of a 5-mm port infraumbilically along the midline provides excellent

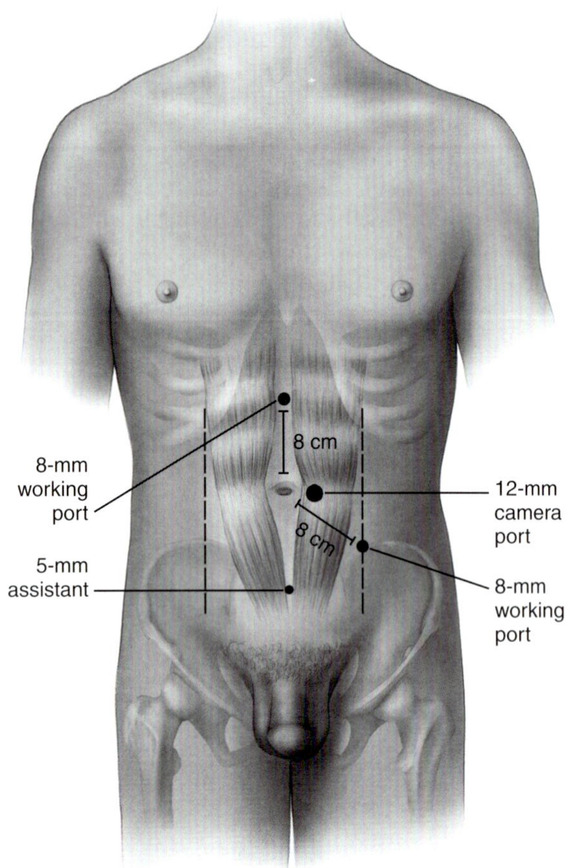

FIGURE 16A–2 Port placement for left-sided robotic-assisted (da Vinci) transperitoneal pyeloplasty. Mirror image is used for the right-sided procedure.

mobility for the assistant. Likewise, this port should be at least 8 cm away from the camera port. Sutures can easily be passed in and out of the 8-mm robotic instrument port, obviating the need for a second 12-mm cannula. In the obese patient, this port placement moves laterally such that the initial 12-mm port is placed in the pararectus line at a level with or just above the umbilicus; the other ports are likewise moved laterally in a similar manner. In general, it is most helpful to have the camera port on a direct line with the UPJ; on occasion, this may necessitate placing all three robotic ports in the midline with the 12-mm port midway between the umbilicus (8-mm port) and the xiphoid (another 8-mm port would be placed in the midline below the xiphoid). Again, all robotic ports need to be 8 cm apart.

Exposure of the Obstructed Ureteropelvic Junction

Citing greater comfort with standard laparoscopic dissection for renal surgery, many authors (including RVC) report obtaining exposure of the UPJ without robotic assistance.[9,15–18] Others (JA, DL) prefer to complete the entire laparoscopic procedure with the robot.

For patients with a left-sided UPJO, the line of Toldt is incised and the descending colon is mobilized medially to expose Gerota's fascia. For a UPJ that is laterally placed, it may be necessary to mobilize only the colon and its splenic flexure away from the spleen. For a more medially placed UPJ, complete mobilization of the spleen may be necessary to adequately visualize the pelvis and ureter; this may include incision of the splenophrenic attachments as well as the splenic flexure and rarely the splenorenal ligament. The gonadal vein can also be used as a guide to the ureter itself if the area is approached from a more distal location as the gonadal vein reliably crosses anterior to the ureter usually at the level of the lower pole of the kidney. Extensive dissection of the renal hilum is usually not necessary.

For patients with a right-sided UPJO, the ascending colon can usually be mobilized medially by incising the colon's peritoneal reflection on the anteriormedial aspect of the kidney, allowing for prompt recognition of Gerota's fascia. A Kocher maneuver may be performed on the duodenum to fully expose the distended renal pelvis. An incision into Gerota's fascia is performed, and the perirenal fat at the lower pole of the kidney is mobilized to expose the obstructed UPJ and the surface of the renal pelvis. If done robotically, these maneuvers are performed with a monopolar scissors and Maryland bipolar grasper. Extensive dissection of the proximal ureter is avoided to maintain the vascular supply to the ureter and UPJ; as such, usually only 3 to 4 cm of the proximal ureter are dissected.

On either side, as the dissection of the UPJ is carried from the ureter toward the UPJ, it is important to be aware of the crossing vessels that may exist in this area. Gentle dissection can be aided by gentle grasping of the renal pelvis. When done laparoscopically, this entails use of 5-mm Kittner dissectors and an atraumatic grasper (e.g., bowel forceps or Atrac grasper [Applied Medical, Rancho Santa Marguerita, CA]). Certainly, any manipulation of the ureter must be kept to a minimum, especially when using the robotic platform where one cannot "feel" how hard one is squeezing tissue.

Alternatively, to maintain optimal exposure of the UPJ, a single 3-0 absorbable braided (polyglactin-910) suture on an SH needle can be placed through the uppermost area of the dissected renal pelvis and secured to the abdominal side wall or, if this part of the procedure is being done laparoscopically, brought through one of the port sites prior to transection of the UPJ. In the latter case, the suture is delivered onto the abdominal surface and the port is removed and replaced, thereby exteriorizing the suture from the port. This provides the surgeon with excellent orientation to the UPJ throughout the remainder of the procedure. If necessary, a vessel loop can be placed directly through the skin with a Carter-Thomason device and brought under the ureter and out the same needle tract to provide constant upward traction on the ureter during mobilization.

Pyeloplasty/Stent Insertion

We prefer performing the Anderson-Hynes dismembered pyeloplasty for the treatment of UPJO because it allows complete excision of an anatomically or functionally abnormal UPJ with transposition of crossing vessels, if necessary. The UPJO is partially transected using the monopolar cautery scissors. It is very important at this point to identify and keep track of the orientation of the ureter to spatulate the ureter in the proper direction, thus preventing overrotation or spiraling of the ureter during the anastomosis. If a stent is indwelling, great care must be taken to not transect the stent during the cutting of the ureter. The ureter can be opened anteriorly and the stent gently grasped and pulled anteriorly. The remainder of the ureter can then be completely transected. If anterior crossing vessels exist, then the pelvis can be pulled cranially before transection of the UPJ. A key maneuver is to completely mobilize the pelvis away from its anterior attachments of the crossing vessels and its posterior attachments to the retroperitoneum; additional attention should be paid to also separating the lateral aspect of the UPJ from the medial aspect of the kidney. This allows easy transposition of the UPJ before the anastomosis.

Of note, if the robot is to be docked after a standard laparoscopic dissection, it is helpful to bring the robot into position such that it is in line with the laparoscope as it is directed at the UPJ. This provides additional room between the robotic arms and appears to work better than a direct perpendicular attachment of the robot to the umbilical port.

The dismembering incision is begun on the pelvis, thereby opening the pelvis so that the UPJ can be directly visualized. The goal is to incise the pelvis in such a way that the lateral, inferior portion of the incision remains dependent. At this point, any redundant renal pelvis can be excised. Alternatively, if only a small opening has been made in the pelvis, it can be spatulated medially and cephalad to facilitate the subsequent anastomosis of the ureter.

The proximal ureter is spatulated laterally for 1 cm, and the obstructing stenotic segment is excised or can be left in place to serve as a "handle" to facilitate the subsequent anastomosis, thereby limiting handling of the "good" part of the ureter that is being anastomosed to the renal pelvis. Once the spatulation is completed, the incision in the UPJ is then completed, thereby dismembering it from the renal pelvis.

Prior to beginning the UPJ anastomosis, the pneumoperitoneum pressure is lowered to 5 mm Hg and excellent hemostasis is obtained. Next, the ureteropelvic anastomosis is performed using either of two methods: an adaptation of the Van Velthoven technique described for performing a laparoscopic vesicourethral anastomosis or three separate sutures.[22] The van Velthoven technique incorporates two 5-inch lengths of 4-0 absorbable monofilament (poliglecaprone 25, e.g., Monocryl) sutures on an SH needle tied together at the loose ends and thus allows for a one-knot pyeloplasty to be performed as described previously.[23] One length is dyed, and the other length is clear to aid in distinguishing the anterior from the posterior suture. Assigning the lateral spatulation of the ureter the 3 o'clock position, the first two sutures are placed at the 2:30 and 3:30 position from outside to inside through the renal pelvis, then inside to outside through their corresponding positions on the lateral wall of the proximal ureter. When both sutures are drawn up, the ureter is pulled along a broad arc of 30 degrees, which then firmly secures the site of spatulation to the renal pelvis. The single knot joining the two sutures functions as a buttress to pull the pelvis down to the ureter and prevents subsequent shortening of the suture arms or potential "sawing" from occurring. After completion of the posterior wall with the left arm of the suture, if an external stent was not placed at the outset of the procedure, then an indwelling stent can be placed now. To do this, an 8 French/10 French Amplatz dilator/sheath system (Cook Urological Inc., Spencer, IN) is introduced via the assistant port or via the uppermost 8-mm robotic port; the latter is in a more direct line with the ureteral lumen; however, the robotic arm must be undocked to gain access to this port. The 8-French catheter is replaced with a 5-French Kumpe ureteral access catheter (Cook Urological Inc., Spencer, IN), which is advanced until the tip of the catheter rests in the proximal ureter. A 0.035-inch nitinol guide wire is then advanced until it is felt to coil in the bladder. The Kumpe catheter is removed and a 7-French double J indwelling ureteral stent is advanced through the 10-French Amplatz sheath over the guidewire and into the ureter. The stent is selected such that it will likely be "too long"; hence in most patients shorter than 5 feet 10 inches, a 28-cm stent is used, whereas in those taller than 5 feet 10 inches, a 30-cm stent is selected. The stent is then advanced with a pusher until the proximal black marker is seen exiting the 10-French Amplatz sheath. The Amplatz sheath is withdrawn followed by the guidewire. The proximal coil of the stent is then advanced into the renal pelvis. Indigo carmine–stained saline solution is then inserted into the bladder through the Foley catheter; if the distal coil of the stent is properly located within the bladder, the blue stained saline should reflux up the stent and into the surgical field around the open renal pelvis. The anterior wall of the UPJ anastomosis is then sutured using the right arm of the suture. A transition stitch is then performed with the left arm of the suture by passing the suture outside-in from the proximal ureter to inside-out on the renal pelvis to allow the knot to cross the anastomosis and thus provide optimal tissue coaptation and strength.

If the pelvis requires no further closing, the anastomosis is completed and the needles are removed, with the resulting knot lying on the outside of the pelvis. If the renal pelvis does require further suturing, the stitches are continued cephalad in a shoelace-type fashion until the entire pelvis is closed. This technique is demonstrated in Figure 16A–3.

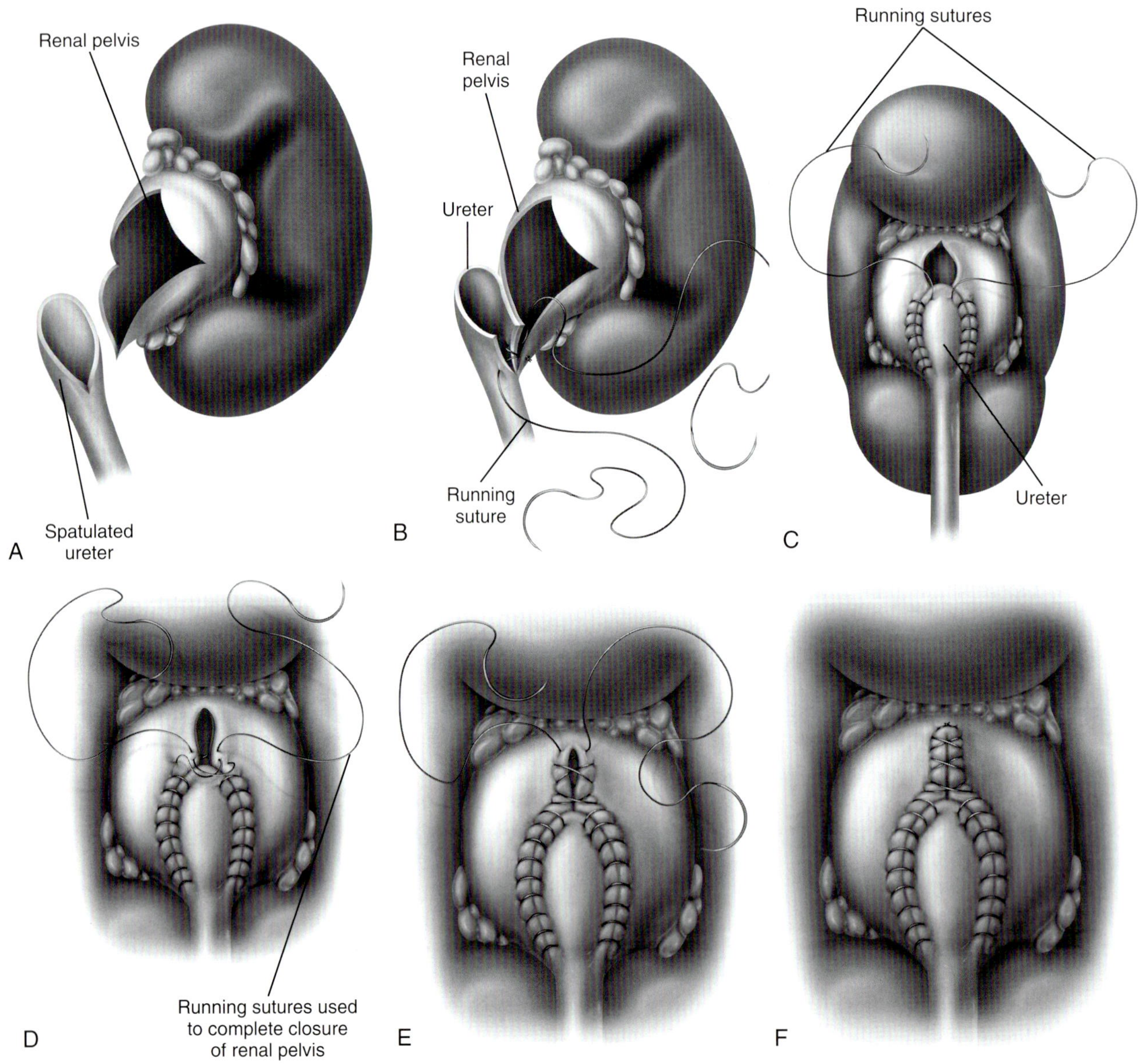

FIGURE 16A–3 Suturing technique of one-knot pyeloplasty. *A*, Diamond-shaped defect in renal pelvis and spatulated ureter. *B*, Each arm of double-armed suture is passed outside-in on the renal pelvis and then inside-out on the ureter. *C*, Suture is run up each side of anastomosis in a continuous manner. *D* and *E*, At the top of the ureter, one side of double-armed suture is reversed in direction as a transition stitch such that it is passed from the inside-out on the renal pelvis. *F*, If more renal pelvis must be closed, the stitches are continued cephalad in a shoelace-type fashion. (*Modified from Eichel, L, Khonsari, S, Lee, DI et al: One-knot pyeloplasty. J Endourol 18:201, 2004.*)

Closure

Once the suturing of the anastomosis is complete, the traction suture is removed; depending on where it was placed, this will allow the perirenal fat to fall and subsequently cover the anastomosis or will release the upper pelvis. The pneumoperitoneum is dropped to a pressure of 5 mm Hg, and all dissected areas are inspected for signs of bleeding. A 5-mm round Jackson-Pratt (JP) is placed adjacent to the anastomosis and brought out through the lower, lateral 8-mm port. All trocars are removed under direct vision, and only the periumbilical 12-mm port site fascia is closed using a figure-of-eight absorbable braided suture. The skin of all port sites is closed using a subcuticular running 3-0 absorbable monofilament suture and a topical skin adhesive (Dermabond, Ethicon, Somerville, NJ).

If an external stent was placed at the outset of the procedure, then the patient is now turned supine and an indwelling 7-French stent is placed under fluoroscopic control.

RETROPERITONEAL APPROACH

In circumstances in which patients have had significant prior abdominal surgery or to minimize the time required to dissect the UPJ, the retroperitoneal approach may be used for UPJ repair. This approach is less popular because of the markedly diminished working space, such that some feel that the retroperitoneal approach is contraindicated for robotic pyeloplasty.[10] Despite these challenges, this approach has been described and in the largest series to date of five patients by Rubinstein et al.[19] This approach was deemed feasible. However, this represents just the earliest experience with this approach, and more time and further follow-up studies are needed; for the time being, the transperitoneal approach is recommended.

Technical Modifications and Variations

With the increasing popularity of the procedure and the availability of the da Vinci system, many variations of the procedure exist. Many perform the UPJ anastomosis using two running 4-0 absorbable braided (polyglactin-910 or polydioxanone) sutures closing an anterior and posterior suture line. Still others prefer to place an interrupted initial suture of 3-0 absorbable suture, followed by flanking running sutures of 4-0 absorbable suture either immediately or after placing two additional flanking interrupted sutures of 4-0.

There are also myriad port variations. Some prefer to place all three ports midline; however, this results in a middle, nonumbilical 12-mm port, which detracts from the cosmesis of the procedure. Another variation others use is the placement of a fourth standard subxiphoid or anterior axillary line assistant port.[15] The latter is difficult as the assistant is in competition with the robotic arms for access; however, it provides excellent entry for lateral retraction of the UPJ and for "following" a running suture. Others have moved to a standard three-port approach.[16]

POSTOPERATIVE CONSIDERATIONS

Postoperatively, pain control is achieved with intravenous Ketorolac and morphine sulfate for breakthrough pain during hospitalization. The Foley catheter is typically removed early on postoperative day 1, with subsequent JP drain removal if the outputs remain low. As a rule, we prefer to remove the Foley catheter only after the JP drainage has fallen to less than 50 mL for 8 hours; after Foley catheter removal, the JP drain is removed if the drainage continues at less than 50 mL for the next 8-hour period. If this is not the case, then the Foley catheter is replaced and the patient is discharged with both the Foley catheter and drain in place. The same regimen can be applied by the patient at home, with an office visit scheduled to remove the drain when the drainage has become scant.

Patients usually undergo ureteral stent removal 3 to 6 weeks after their procedure, followed by a nuclear renal scan within 1 to 2 weeks. Follow-up renal scans and analog pain scales are obtained at 1.5, 3, 6, and 12 months and then annually for the next 2 years.

RESULTS

Table 16A-1 lists all published reports of robotic-assisted laparoscopic pyeloplasty. The larger series note success rates between 89% and 100%, mean operative times from 124 to 300 minutes, and average hospital lengths of stay of 1 to 2 days. These results are comparable to those reported with conventional laparoscopic pyeloplasty.[3,4] In addition, reported complication rates of approximately 12%, including urinary tract infection, a urine leak, and gluteal compartment syndrome requiring fasciotomy, parallel those of the conventional laparoscopic experience.[3,17] However, it is important to note that among these series, only one has follow-up beyond 12 months, only five exceed 25 patients, and not one series exceeds 50 patients. As such, although preliminary results are as favorable as standard laparoscopy, longer follow-up is certainly needed to define the true value of this procedure in light of longer-term data on laparoscopic and open pyeloplasty.

CONCLUSIONS

Preliminary results in small series support the hypothesis that robotic-assisted pyeloplasty appears to provide equivalent results to standard laparoscopic and open approaches. We believe that the features of the robotic platform provide all but the most experienced laparoscopic surgeons with improved laparoscopic abilities that may prove invaluable for the dissemination of this less invasive technique to many of the urologists who are already skilled in open pyeloplasty.

REFERENCES

1. Schuessler WW, Grune MT, Tecuanhuey LV, et al: Laparoscopic dismembered pyeloplasty. J Urol 150:1795, 1993.
2. Kavoussi LR, Peters CA: Laparoscopic pyeloplasty. J Urol 150:1891, 1993.
3. Bauer JJ, Bishoff JT, Moore RG, et al: Laparoscopic versus open pyeloplasty: assessment of objective and subjective outcome. J Urol 162:692, 1999.
4. Jarrett TW, Chan DY, Charambura TC, et al: Laparoscopic pyeloplasty: the first 100 cases. J Urol 167:1253, 2002.
5. Sung GT, Gill IS: Robotic laparoscopic surgery: a comparison of the da Vinci and Zeus systems. Urology 58:893, 2001.
6. Graham RW, Graham, SD, Bokinsky GB, et al: Urological upper tract surgery with the da Vinci robotic system, pyeloplasty. J Urol 165(suppl):V74, 2001.
7. Guilloneau B, Cappele O, Vallancien G, et al: Robotic-assisted laparoscopic pyeloplasty. J Urol 165(suppl):V75, 2001.
8. Whitaker RH: Methods of assessing obstruction in dilated ureters. Br J Urol 45:15, 1973.
9. Gettman MT, Peschel R, Neururer R, et al: A comparison of laparoscopic pyeloplasty performed with the da Vinci robotic system versus standard laparoscopic techniques: initial clinical results. Eur Urol 42:453, 2002.
10. Gettman MT, Neururer R, Bartsch G, et al: Anderson-Hynes dismembered pyeloplasty performed using the da Vinci robotic system. Urology 60:509, 2002.
11. Peschel R, Neururer R, Bartsch G, et al: Robotic pyeloplasty: technique and results. Urol Clin North Am 31:737, 2004.
12. Hubert J: Robotic pyeloplasty. Curr Urol Rep 4:124, 2003.
13. Bentas W, Wolfram M, Brautigam R, et al: Da Vinci robot assisted Anderson-Hynes dismembered pyeloplasty: technique and 1 year follow-up. World J Urol 21:133, 2003.
14. Munver R, Del Pizzo JJ, Sosa RE, et al: Minimally invasive surgical management of ureteropelvic junction obstruction: laparoscopic and robot-assisted laparoscopic pyeloplasty. J Long Term Eff Med Implants 13:367, 2003.
15. Mendez-Torres F, Woods M, Thomas R: Technical modifications for robot-assisted laparoscopic pyeloplasty. J Endourol 19:393, 2005.
16. Siddiq FM, Leveillee RJ, Villicana P, et al: Computer-assisted laparoscopic pyeloplasty: University of Miami experience with the daVinci Surgical System. J Endourol 19:387, 2005.
17. Palese MA, Stifelman MD, Munver R, et al: Robot-assisted laparoscopic dismembered pyeloplasty: a combined experience. J Endourol 19:382, 2005.
18. Yohannes P, Burjonrappa SC: Rapid communication: laparoscopic Anderson-Hynes dismembered pyeloplasty using the da Vinci robot: technical considerations. J Endourol 17:79, 2003.
19. Rubinstein M, Moinzadeh A, Colombo J, et al: Robotic-assisted laparoscopic retroperitoneal pyeloplasty. J Urol 173 (suppl):V1150, 2005.
20. Patel V: Robotic-assisted laparoscopic dismembered pyeloplasty. Urology 66:45, 2005.
21. Luke PP, Girvan AR, Al Omar M, et al: Laparoscopic robotic pyeloplasty using the Zeus Telesurgical System. Can J Urol 11:2396, 2004.
22. Van Velthoven RF, Ahlering TE, Peltier A, et al: Technique for laparoscopic running urethrovesical anastomosis: the single knot method. Urology 61:699, 2003.
23. Eichel L, Khonsari S, Lee DI, et al: One-knot pyeloplasty. J Endourol 18:201, 2004.

CHAPTER 16B

Amy E. Krambeck • Matthew T. Gettman • Reinhard Peschel

Robotic Renal Surgery: Partial Nephrectomy and Nephropexy

INTRODUCTION

Robotic technology has been available in other surgical fields for many years, but it has only recently been introduced to urology. Current marketing of the robotic systems target urologist with minimal laparoscopic skills, claiming robotic technology makes laparoscopy available to all surgeons. However, the performance-enhancing features of telerobotics may also augment the performance of the most experienced laparoscopists. The six degrees of freedom at the distal end of the instruments, the three-dimensional stereoscopic vision, movement scale-down, and tremor filters can enhance any surgeon's skills. Robotic assistance has found a definite place in prostatectomy and pyeloplasty and is currently being applied to various other urologic procedures. This chapter discusses the application of telerobotics to laparoscopic partial nephrectomy and nephropexy, as well as potential benefits and downfalls based on our initial clinical experience.

ROBOTIC PARTIAL NEPHRECTOMY

Background

The treatment of renal masses has changed dramatically over the past two decades. The increased use of computed tomography (CT) and magnetic resonance imaging (MRI) has led to the incidental discovery of small renal masses amenable to partial nephrectomy. Nephron-sparing surgery is increasingly being performed in the presence of a normal contralateral kidney, with proven efficacy and long-term patient-related benefits.[1–3] Although laparoscopic nephrectomy has become widely accepted, the use of laparoscopic partial nephrectomy has been limited because of technical difficulty, mainly the ability to reliably provide effective hemostasis during the procedure. Current available hemostatic materials include argon beam coagulation, electrocautery, gelatin sponges, ultrasound dissection, radiofrequency ablation, and fibrin glue.[4–9] Laparoscopic techniques mimicking open partial nephrectomy provide more reliable hemostasis but require advanced laparoscopic skills in intracorporeal suturing to limit warm ischemia time. The introduction of robotics has been theorized to improve laparoscopic partial nephrectomy by allowing use of open partial nephrectomy hemostatic techniques with limited warm ischemia time through improving intracorporeal suturing.

Indication

We recommend the use of the robotic-assisted laparoscopic partial nephrectomy for predominantly exophytic renal lesions. Solitary, enhancing lesions or suspicious cystic renal lesions (Bosniak category III or IV) are acceptable candidates. These criteria are similar to those described for laparoscopic partial nephrectomy.[10] Endophytic or central renal lesions are not recommended for robotic-assisted laparoscopic partial nephrectomy because they prove difficult to dissect while preserving hilar structures. Patients with multiple prior abdominal surgeries should also be excluded because of possible bowel adhesions and distortion of anatomic landmarks. Approach to the renal mass should be based on its location. Anterior lesions can easily be approached through a transperitoneal approach, and posterior lesions can likewise be approached via a transperitoneal approach; however, direct access is also feasible robotically through a retroperitoneal approach. For surgeons new to robotic-assisted procedures, we recommend initially treating only anterolateral-based tumors and approaching these lesions in transperitoneal fashion. The transperitoneal approach provides more familiar anatomic landmarks and a larger working space. Both of these factors can provide technical advantages when performing robotic-assisted laparoscopic partial nephrectomy.

Preoperative Evaluation

A full history and physical is necessary, with specific focus on prior renal and abdominal surgeries. A history of prior abdominal surgery is not an absolute contraindication to laparoscopy and robotic-assisted surgery; however, access to the abdomen and performance of the planned procedure can be more challenging. All patients should be evaluated with a CT scan of the abdomen and pelvis. If there is question of tumor thrombus involvement of the renal vein, MRI should also be performed. Standard complete blood panel, serum electrolytes, chest x-ray films, liver function tests, and serum creatinine should also be performed. If there are questionable lung lesions on the chest x-ray film, a CT scan of the chest is needed to rule out pulmonary metastases.

Surgical Technique

The night before the procedure the patient should undergo a bowel-cleansing preparation. In the operating room after general anesthetic is administered, a Foley bladder catheter and nasogastric tube are placed. The robotic-assisted laparoscopic partial nephrectomy can be performed via a transperitoneal or retroperitoneal approach with or without an intra-arterial renal catheter for renal cooling. We describe both methods. If an intra-arterial renal catheter is to be used, it is placed prior to port placement by interventional radiology in the operating room. If a transperitoneal approach is to be used, the patient is placed in a 45-degree modified flank position. The ports are placed after pneumoperitoneum is established with a Veress needle. A 12-mm trocar is initially placed at the umbilicus to serve as the assistant port during the robotic procedure. Using the robotic endoscope through this initial port, the surgeon inspects the peritoneal cavity to determine the generalized location of the kidney and the renal lesion. An additional 12-mm trocar for the robotic endoscope is then placed at a midclavicular, infraumbilical position in line with the noted location of the renal tumor. Trocars for two additional robotic arms (8-mm ports, Intuitive Surgical, Sunnyvale, CA) are then placed medially and laterally such that the distance between the camera port and each working port is at least 7 cm. In addition, the robotic ports are ideally placed such that the angle created between the working ports and the camera port is obtuse (Figure 16B–1*A*). In more recent cases, we have modified our trocar placement with equivalent technical results. In the alternative trocar placement arrangement, the robotic endoscope is place at the umbilicus. Trocars for the two additional robotic arms (8-mm ports, Intuitive Surgical) are placed in the midline midway between the umbilicus and the xiphoid process and at an ipsilateral midclavicular position just below the level of the umbilicus. Using this trocar arrangement, the assistant port is placed in the midline approximately 5 to 7 cm below the umbilical port (Figure 16B–1*B*). For patients undergoing a retroperitoneal approach, a full flank position is used. After the working space is created, the camera port is placed below the tip of the 12th rib; the working ports are similarly placed such that the angle between the working ports and the camera is obtuse (Figure 16B–2).

The da Vinci–assisted laparoscopic partial nephrectomy follows the principles established for open partial nephrectomy and conventional laparoscopic partial nephrectomy.[10–14] The initial dissection is performed with a hook electrode on the lateral working robotic arm and a Prograsp or Cadiere forceps on the medial working robotic arm. The procedure can be performed entirely using the da Vinci robotic system. Alternatively, some surgeons have advocated performing the initial exposure of the renal lesion with standard laparoscopic techniques and then placing the robotic system to assist with the actual partial nephrectomy portion of the procedure. With a transperitoneal approach, the line

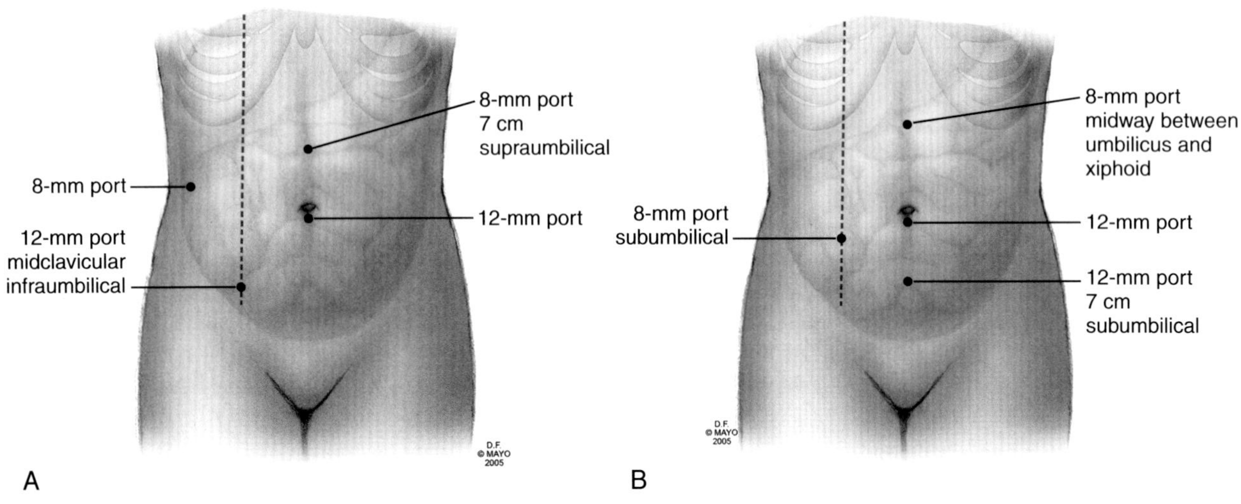

FIGURE 16B–1 Standard *(A)* and modified *(B)* port placement for transperitoneal da Vinci–assisted partial nephrectomy.

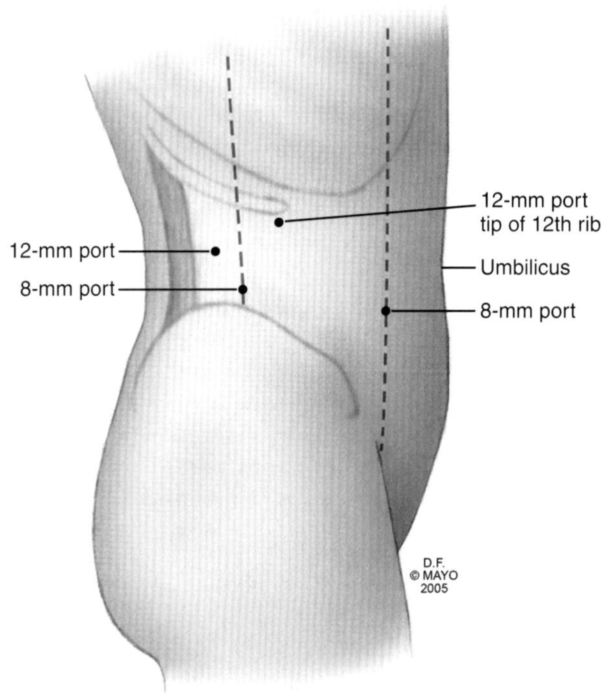

FIGURE 16B–2 Port placement for retroperitoneal da Vinci–assisted partial nephrectomy.

of Toldt is incised, the bowel is mobilized medially, and Gerota's fascia is incised. If a retroperitoneal approach is used, Gerota's fascia is identified and likewise incised. The surgical assistant facilitates dissection using conventional laparoscopic instruments to provide countertraction and suction. Initially the ureter and pedicle are identified and isolated. The kidney is completely mobilized within Gerota's fascia to identify the renal lesion and exclude additional lesions. Fat overlying the renal lesion is left in place and included as part of the pathologic specimen. The renal hilum is then dissected to allow occlusion during mass excision.

In preparation for the partial nephrectomy, the assistant introduces a 2-0 Vicryl suture (15–20 cm in length) through the 12-mm assistant port. A bolster composed of Gelfoam and Surgicel is also placed intra-abdominally in preparation for suturing after tumor excision. Mannitol 12.5 g is then administered intravenously. If no intra-arterial cooling catheter is to be used, the renal artery and vein are occluded using laparoscopic bulldog clamps. This requires that the surgeon at the console elevate the kidney and place the hilum on tension, while the assistant surgeon places the bulldog clamps laparoscopically. Alternatively, for patients undergoing intra-arterial catheter placement for delivery of iced saline, renal artery occlusion is achieved using the intra-arterial catheter balloon.[14,15] Cold ischemia is achieved by continuous infusion of iced saline, which also prevents venous backflow during resection. Using cold, round-tip scissors, the mass is then excised from the renal parenchyma. During tumor excision, the assistant uses a suction/irrigator or conventional laparoscopic graspers for countertraction and to optimize visualization of the surgical field. The excised mass is temporarily placed adjacent to the kidney, and the assistant places two large-needle drivers on the robotic arms. Damage to the collecting system and large bleeding vessels is controlled with 2-0 Vicryl sutures. Collecting system violations are identified by visual inspection of the renal defect after tumor excision. Suture closure of the renal defect is then performed using the Surgicel bolsters. After closure of the renal defect, the bulldog clamps are removed and the excised renal tumor is placed into a retrieval bag. If an intra-arterial cooling balloon is used, the balloon occluding the renal artery is released after suture closure of the renal defect. Frozen section evaluation is helpful in determining margin status at this point. Gerota's fascia is then reapproximated over the kidney with 2-0 Vicryl suture, and the bowel is brought back into anatomic position. A Jackson-Pratt drain is placed through the more lateral 8-mm trocar site, and the tumor is then retrieved intact. All ports are removed under direct vision, and trocar sites are closed in a standard fashion.

Postoperative Care

Standard serum chemistries as well as complete blood count are checked on postoperative day 1. Patients are encouraged to ambulate on this day, and diets are advanced as tolerated with the passage of flatus. The urinary catheter is removed when the patient is fully mobile. The drain is removed prior to discharge, pending no signs of active bleeding or urine leak.

Results

Two major series on robotic-assisted laparoscopic partial nephrectomy have been published to date. Our series from the Mayo Clinic, Rochester, and the University of Innsbruck, Austria, consisted of 13 patients and the series from Phillips et al.[16] from New York University consisted of 12 patients. Both techniques were similar; however, Phillips and colleagues did not use intra-arterial renal catheter for renal cooling.

In our series, eight patients underwent intra-arterial catheter renal cooling and the remaining five patients underwent standard renal hilar clamping. Mean operative time was 215 minutes (range, 130–262 minutes), which included time for installation/setup of the robot. Mean tumor diameter was 3.5 cm (range, 2.0–6.0 cm), and the mean estimated blood loss was 170 mL (range, 50–300 mL). Collecting system violations occurred in two cases and were closed at time of surgical procedure with no postoperative renal leaks noted.

For the five patients undergoing renal clamping, the overall mean warm ischemia time was 22 minutes (range, 15–29 minutes). For those with intra-arterial cooling catheter, the mean cold ischemia time was 33 minutes (range, 18–43 minutes). We had no difficulty with angiocatheter placement, and at no time during the procedure was it dislodged. Excellent hemostasis was obtained using this catheter device, and it did not appear to complicate excision of the renal mass.

We experienced no open conversions in our series and no intraoperative complications. One patient had a prolonged hospitalization of 7 days because of a postoperative ileus. However, overall mean hospital stay was 4.3 days (range, 2–7 days). A positive margin was noted in one case despite negative intraoperative frozen section analysis. Laparoscopic radical nephrectomy was subsequently performed in this patient and showed no evidence of residual tumor. Our follow-up is currently limited to 2 to 11 months, but no recurrences have been observed.[17]

Phillips and colleagues have experienced similar results. Their mean operative time was 265 minutes, which included robotic setup. Average tumor size was 1.8 cm. Mean estimated blood loss was 240 mL, with a mean decrease in hematocrit of 6.5%. Average warm ischemia time was 26 minutes, and cold ischemia was not used. Collecting-system repair was necessary in 25% of the patients in this series, and one patient did develop a urine leak requiring percutaneous drainage for 5 weeks.

Conversion to open technique was necessary in two patients in this series. In one case the robot malfunctioned; in the other, the vascular clamps dislodged during mass excision. A third patient required conversion to a hand-assisted laparoscopic technique because of bleeding after removal of the hilar clamps. Overall mean length of hospital stay for patients in this series was 2.7 days.[16]

Both series found robotic-assisted laparoscopic partial nephrectomy feasible, and suture closure of the renal defect was possible with the da Vinci. This approach demonstrates overall reliable hemostasis and operative times comparable to those for other laparoscopic partial nephrectomies. In our series we did find a retroperitoneal approach possible, but it required more frequent modifications of the robotic alignment by the assistant surgeon. For this reason we recommend a transperitoneal approach when possible, especially when first performing this technique. In addition, an emphasis on port placement should be made. For optimal function of the robot, the angle created between each working robotic port and the camera port should be obtuse and the trajectory to the renal tumor should bisect this angle. Endoscopic visualization of the surgical field at the beginning of the procedure prior to subsequent port placements is necessary to establish the appropriate trajectory; however, additional technical adjuncts or preoperative modeling based on cross-sectional imaging may optimize port placement in the future.

Both series recognized the importance of a team approach. Scrub assistants familiar with the robotic equipment and setup are essential for the procedure to run smoothly. In addition, an experienced surgical assistant or second surgeon is imperative. This individual is responsible for application of the pedicle clamps and introduction of suture and bolster material. It can be challenging for the scrubbed surgeon/assistant to provide optimal assistance with the ongoing movement of the robotic system. In the event of a rapid open conversion, the scrubbed surgeon/assistant will need to act quickly because he or she is the only person scrubbed and will need to initiate the conversion process.

If warm ischemia is to be used, tumor excision and repair should be less than 30 minutes to optimize renal function. The intra-arterial catheter with iced saline renal cooling can safely extend ischemia time beyond 30 minutes. We have started using the intra-arterial catheter in all recent cases. By removing the time constraint, a more relaxed, controlled working environment is maintained.

ROBOTIC NEPHROPEXY

Background

Nephropexy is the only available surgical procedure for the treatment of symptomatic nephroptosis. Nephroptosis is defined as downward renal descent of two vertebral bodies (or $\geq$5 cm) while standing in the upright position on intravenous pyelography (IVP) or nuclear medicine studies.[18] Ptotic kidneys occur in up to 20% of men and women at the time of routine IVP.[19,20] Only 10% to 20% of these cases are reported to be symptomatic, with women affected more frequently than men (5:1),[21] and slender women are more commonly affected because of minimal supportive perirenal fat.[22] Nephroptosis occurs more often on the right kidney (70%) than on the left (10%) and can be bilateral in 20% of the cases.[18–20] Although flank pain has been the hallmark symptom, other conditions such as recurrent urinary tract infection (UTI), hypertension, renal stone disease, renal ischemia or atrophy, hematuria, and proteinuria have also been attributed to this condition.[22,23] These symptoms are considered the result of altered renal perfusion, and it is known ptotic kidneys can demonstrate inaccurate split renal function on nuclear scans as well as obstruction.[24]

More than 170 different operative procedures for nephropexy have been described.[21,25,26] The Washington University group introduced laparoscopic transabdominal nephropexy in 1993 and reported early 1-year results of 100% resolution of symptoms.[27,28] This introduction of laparoscopy revived interest in nephropexy for the treatment of nephroptosis. The available treatment had become considerably less invasive, and more physicians were willing to attempt a repair to correct symptoms if morbidity could be limited. However, laparoscopic suturing can be challenging for even the most skilled laparoscopist. This led to the introduction of the robotic-assisted laparoscopic nephropexy. The da Vinci system greatly enhances intracorporeal suturing, which can decrease operative time and technical difficulty—a benefit for nephropexy.

Indications

Often the decision to treat these patients is made after all other etiologies for abdominal/flank pain are excluded. Boeminghaus[29] suggested a systematic categorization of these patients. He differentiated patients with nephroptosis into three groups: (1) ptosis without symptoms requiring no treatment, (2) patients with symptoms but no functional alterations, and (3) symptomatic patients with functional and sometimes morphologic alterations. Boeminghaus recommended treating only those patients in group 3. Rassweiler et al.[12] recommended surgical intervention only for those patients with renal descent of two or more vertebral bodies and the presence of two objective symptoms or one objective symptom and one subjective symptom. The majority of physicians who treat this condition are comfortable with performing the surgical procedure in symptomatic patients with demonstrable descent of the kidney after other etiologies have been ruled out.

Preoperative Evaluation

A complete history and physical examination focusing on prior abdominal surgeries should be performed. IVP in the supine and erect position demonstrating downward displacement of the kidney two or more vertebral lengths is necessary to make the diagnosis of nephroptosis. Dimercaptosuccinic acid (DMSA) renal scans have been suggested in the past but are unreliable in making the diagnosis of a ptotic kidney. Recent studies by Strohmeyer et al.[23] indicated color Doppler imaging measured resistive index (RI) to be a valuable tool in initial diagnosis. RI (peak systolic velocity − end diastolic velocity/peak systolic velocity) has been established as an excellent means to assess renal perfusion. This group found a reduction of RI of more than 0.10 in 88.5% of their patients with nephroptosis. Combining color Doppler ultrasound with IVP may be helpful in identifying which patient will be most benefited by surgical intervention.

Surgical Technique

The night before the procedure, the patient should undergo a bowel-cleansing preparation. In the operating room after general anesthetic is administered, a Foley bladder catheter and nasogastric tube are placed. For the transperitoneal approach, the patient is placed in the 45-degree modified lateral flank position. Using the Veress needle technique, the surgeon establishes a pneumoperitoneum and places a 12-mm trocar subumbilical. The robotic endoscope is introduced at this site. With an abdominal pressure of 12 mm Hg, three additional trocars are inserted: an 8-mm port at the level of the umbilicus in the midclavicular location, an 8-mm port subxiphoid, and an additional 5-mm port high midclavicular just inferior to the ribs. The angle between the working ports and the robotic camera port should be obtuse (Figure 16B–3). Alternatively, the trocar arrangement can be performed in similar fashion as that used for robotic-assisted laparoscopic partial nephrectomy (see Figure 16B–1). The retroperitoneum is opened along the line of Toldt, and the kidney is completely mobilized. The renal pelvis and ureter are exposed by opening the anterior Gerota's fascia and perirenal fat. A small area on the posterior, inferior surface of the kidney is fulgurated using cautery, as is a corresponding area on the quadratus lumborum or psoas muscle. Using 3-0 PDS suture, the surgeon fixes the fulgurated capsule of the kidney to the corresponding area on the muscle with several intracorporeal sutures. Care should be taken to ensure that only the renal capsule is incorporated into the suture, not large amounts of renal parenchyma. The bowel is reapproximated with 3-0 PDS, and a 5-mm drain is brought through one of the 8-mm ports. The rest of the ports are removed under direct vision and the incisions closed.

A retroperitoneal approach can alternatively be used. The patient is placed in a lateral decubitus position and the table flexed. A 15-mm skin incision is made in the midaxillary line at the level of the umbilicus. The retroperitoneal space is

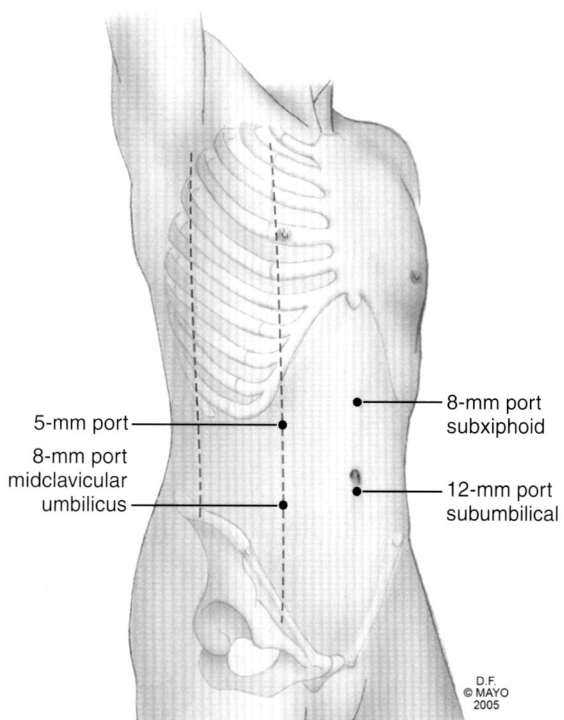

FIGURE 16B–3 Port placement for transperitoneal da Vinci–assisted nephropexy.

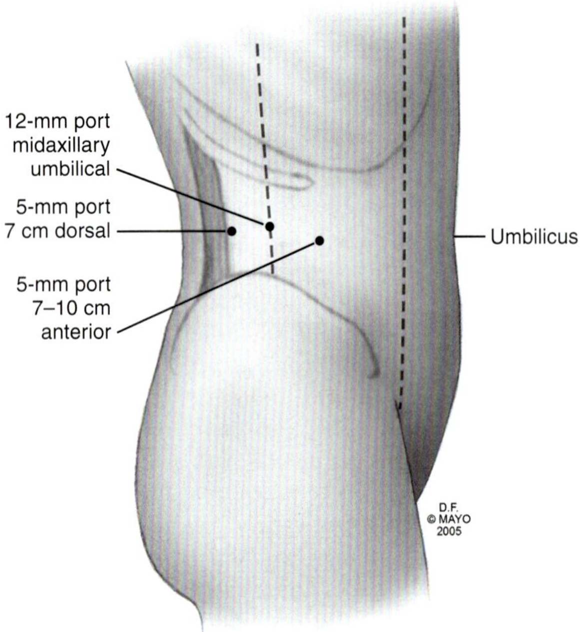

FIGURE 16B–4 Port placement for retroperitoneal da Vinci–assisted nephropexy.

entered and developed by blunt finger dissection. A balloon dissector is then introduced to develop a retroperitoneal working space. Next, a 12-mm port is introduced through the prior skin incision for the robotic endoscope. Pneumoretroperitoneum is maintained at a pressure of 8 mm Hg, and a 5 mm trocar is placed 7 to 10 cm dorsal to the first. The peritoneum is then dissected from the abdominal wall anteromedially. A third 10-mm trocar is placed 7 to 10 cm anterior to the first trocar. A fourth 5-mm trocar can be placed near the third trocar if necessary for retraction (Figure 16B–4). The rest of the procedure is as described for the transperitoneal approach.

Postoperative Care

Patients are allowed to ambulate on postoperative day 1, and pain medicine is administered accordingly. An IVP and ultrasound are performed during the hospitalization to rule out hydronephrosis and verify correct position of the kidney. The drain is removed before discharge home.

Results

Robotic-assisted laparoscopic nephropexy is currently performed at only a few institutions, and available outcome data are limited. An extensive series comparing laparoscopic nephropexy to robotic-assisted nephropexy has not been performed and is necessary before recommendations can be given as to the value of using the robotic system. Unlike robotic partial nephrectomy, nephropexy does not require a highly skilled assistant for vascular clamping. The core of the nephropexy procedure is suturing of the kidney to the psoas or quadratus lumborum muscle, which is aided by the robotic system. Therefore, robotics may prove successful for nephropexy, and there is potential for it to gain further acceptance.

CONCLUSION

Definitive roles of robotic-assisted laparoscopic partial nephrectomy and nephropexy in the general urologist's practice remain undefined. Robotic-assisted laparoscopic partial nephrectomy, although beneficial in that warm ischemia time is reduced by enhanced intracorporeal suturing, requires a skilled surgical assistant with a team approach. This may not be practical for most surgeons. Possibly, modifications in surgical technique will be necessary before robotic-assisted laparoscopic partial nephrectomy is feasible for general practice. On the other hand, robotic-assisted laparoscopic nephropexy is a new technique with limited data available. Further published series are necessary before this approach can be recommended over standard laparoscopic procedures. However, initial results are favorable, and it may find itself in the urologist's armamentarium next to robotic pyeloplasty.

REFERENCES

1. Lau W, Blute ML, Weaver AL, et al: Matched comparison of radical nephrectomy vs. nephron-sparing surgery in patients with unilateral renal cell carcinoma and a normal contralateral kidney. Mayo Clin Proc 75:1236–1242, 2000.
2. Herr HW: Partial nephrectomy for unilateral renal carcinoma and a normal contralateral kidney: 10-year followup. J Urol 161:33–34, 1999.
3. Fergany AF, Hafez KS, Novick AC: Long-term results of nephron sparing surgery for localized renal cell carcinoma: 10-year followup. J Urol 163:442–445, 2000.
4. Organ K, Cadeddu JA: Minimally invasive management of the small renal tumor: review of laparoscopic partial nephrectomy and ablative techniques. J Endourol 16:635–643, 2002.
5. Guillonneau B, Bermudez H, Gholami S, et al: Laparoscopic partial nephrectomy for renal tumor: single center experience comparing clamping and no clamping techniques of the renal vasculature. J Urol 169:483–486, 2003.
6. Simon SD, Ferrigni RG, Novicki DE, et al: Mayo Clinic Scottsdale experience with laparoscopic nephron sparing surgery for renal tumors. J Urol 169:2059–2062, 2003.

7. Janetschek G, Daffner P, Peschel R, et al: Laparoscopic nephron sparing surgery for small renal cell carcinoma. J Urol 159:1152–1155, 1998.
8. Harmon WJ, Kavoussi LR, Bishoff JT: Laparoscopic nephron-sparing surgery for solid renal masses. Urology 56:754–759, 2000.
9. Richter F, Schnorr D, Deger S, et al: Improvement of hemostasis in open and laparoscopically performed partial nephrectomy using a gelatin matrix-thrombin tissue sealant (FloSeal). Urology 61:73–77, 2003.
10. Gill IS, Desai MM, Kaouk JH, et al: Laparoscopic partial nephrectomy for renal tumor: duplicating open surgical techniques. J Urol 167:469–476, 2002.
11. Desai MM, Gill IS, Kaoul JH, et al: Laparoscopic partial nephrectomy with suture repair of the pelvicaliceal system. Urology 61:99–104, 2003.
12. Rassweiler JJ, Frede T, Recker F, et al: Retroperitoneal laparoscopic nephropexy. Urol Clin North Am 28:137–144, 2001.
13. Bermudez H, Guillonneau B, Gupta R, et al: Initial experience in laparoscopic partial nephrectomy for renal tumor with clamping of renal vessels. J Endourol 17:373–378, 2003.
14. Janetschek G, Abdelmaksoud A, Bagheri F, et al: Laparoscopic partial nephrectomy in cold ischemia: renal artery perfusion. J Urol 171:68–71, 2004.
15. Marberger M, Georgi M, Guenther R, et al: Simultaneous balloon occlusion of the renal artery and hypothermic perfusion in in situ surgery of the kidney. J Urol 119:463–467, 1978.
16. Phillips CK, Taneja SS, Stifelman MD: Robot-assisted laparoscopic partial nephrectomy: the NYU technique. J Endourol 19:441–445, 2005.
17. Gettman MT, Blute ML, Chow GK, et al: Robotic-assisted laparoscopic partial nephrectomy: technique and initial clinical experience with daVinci robotic system. Urology 64:914–918, 2004.
18. Young HH, Davis DM: Malformation and abnormalities of the urogenital tract. In: Young's Practice of Urology, Vol. 2. Philadelphia, WB Saunders, 1926, pp 1–36.
19. Kelly HA: Moveable kidney and neurasthenia. Trans Am Surg Assoc 28:513, 1910.
20. Hoenig DM, Hemal AK, Shaihav AL, et al: Nephroptosis; a disparaged condition revisited. Urology 54:590–596, 1999.
21. Hubner WA, Schlarp O, Riedl C, et al: Laparoscopic nephropexy using tension-free vaginal tape for symptomatic nephroptosis. Urology 64:372–374, 2004.
22. Barber NJ, Thompson PM: Nephroptosis and nephropexy—hung up on the past? Eur Urol 46:428–433, 2004.
23. Strohmeyer DM, Peschel R, Effert P, et al: Changes of renal blood flow in nephroptosis: assessment by color Doppler imaging, isotope renography and correlation with clinical outcome after laparoscopic nephropexy. Eur Urol 45:790–793, 2004.
24. O-Reilly PH, Pollard AJ: Nephroptosis: a cause of renal pain and a potential cause of inaccurate split renal function determination. Br J Urol 61:284–288, 1998.
25. Mayor G, Bandhauer K, Zingg EJ: Urologic Surgery: Diagnosis, Techniques, and Postoperative Treatment. New York, John Wiley & Sons, 1976, p 32.
26. Wandshneider G, Haas P, Leb G, et al: Establishment of need for and evaluation of results of nephropexy with the aid of the combined-isotope study of the kidneys. Urologe A 5:161–169, 1972.
27. Urban DA, Clayman RV, Kerbl K, et al: Laparoscopic nephropexy for symptomatic nephroptosis: initial case report. J Endourol 7:27–30, 1993.
28. Elashry OM, Nakada SY, McDougall EM, et al: Laparoscopic nephropexy: Washington University experience. J Urol 154:165–169, 1995.
29. Boeminghas H: Nephropexie. In Banascheski WG (ed): Urologie-Operative Therapie, Klinik-Indikation. Munick, Banaschewski, 1960, vol 1, pp 46–52

CHAPTER 17

J. Del Pizzo

Miscellaneous Adult Robotic Surgery

INTRODUCTION

The past decade has witnessed tremendous growth and evolution in the field of robotic urology. With continued technologic advancement and surgeon familiarity with robotic systems, the urologic applications of robotic surgery will surely continue to expand. In this chapter we discuss several of the more recent urologic applications of robotic surgery, including adrenalectomy, vasovasostomy, and urinary diversion.

ADRENALECTOMY

Background

Adrenalectomy is indicated for incidentally detected adrenal lesions meeting size criteria, hyperfunctioning adrenal tumors, select cases of bilateral adrenal hyperplasia, adrenocortical carcinoma, and additional miscellaneous lesions. The open approach to adrenal surgery has long been the standard of care; however, minimally invasive approaches have rapidly become the preferred approach since laparoscopic adrenalectomy was first reported in 1992 by Gagner et al.[1] Minimally invasive techniques avoid the need for a large morbid incision for the removal of a comparably small organ, improving aesthetic results. Retrospective comparisons have demonstrated reduced postoperative pain, disability, length of hospital stay, faster recovery, and lower rate of complications compared with open adrenalectomy.[1,2]

More recently, robotic adrenalectomy has been demonstrated to be a feasible minimally invasive approach. Robotic adrenalectomy was first reported in an animal model by Gill et al.[3] and in humans shortly thereafter.[4] Subsequently, several other groups have demonstrated robotic adrenalectomy to be a safe and effective approach.[5–7] Robotic adrenalectomy offers reduced morbidity and disfigurement to the patient while allowing conventionally trained urologic surgeons to perform this minimally invasive operation successfully.[7] The six degrees of freedom in movement, fine scaling, and superb three-dimensional optics offered by the da Vinci system are of benefit during the meticulous dissection around the great vessels and viscera that is required during adrenalectomy.

Technique—Left-Sided Adrenalectomy

For left-sided robotic adrenalectomy, the patient is placed in the right lateral decubitus position with a 45-degree tilt and slight Trendelenburg, similar to standard flank positioning for open retroperitoneal surgery. The kidney rest may be used. A transperitoneal approach is preferred. After access is gained via a Veress needle or with the open Hasson technique, pneumoperitoneum is established. For left-sided adrenalectomy, three ports for the robotic arms (two robotic working ports and one camera port) are used. One additional port is used for the bedside assistant. Specifically, a 12-mm port is placed in the paramedian position, approximately halfway between the costal margin and umbilicus for the 30-degree robotic laparoscope. Two 8-mm robotic instrument ports are placed: 2 cm inferior to the costal margin at the midaxillary line, and approximately 2 cm cephalad to the anterior superior iliac spine in the iliac fossa. A 10-mm port, positioned superolateral to the umbilicus, is placed for the use of retractors, suction, and clip-applying devices by the bedside assistant (Figure 17–1). The robot is then brought into the operative field and positioned on the patient's left at a 45-degree angle to the long axis of the operating table. The robotic laparoscope and instruments are engaged.

After the peritoneal cavity is inspected and any necessary lysis of adhesions is performed, the white line of Toldt is incised from the level of the iliac vessels to above the spleen. The lienocolic, splenorenal, and splenophrenic attachments are incised using electrocautery hook or scissors to completely mobilize the spleen medially. The tail of the pancreas is carefully dissected off Gerota's fascia to enable the pancreas to fall medially with the spleen. This provides excellent exposure of the adrenal and upper pole of the left kidney. The adrenal is then dissected circumferentially beginning with the upper border; branches from

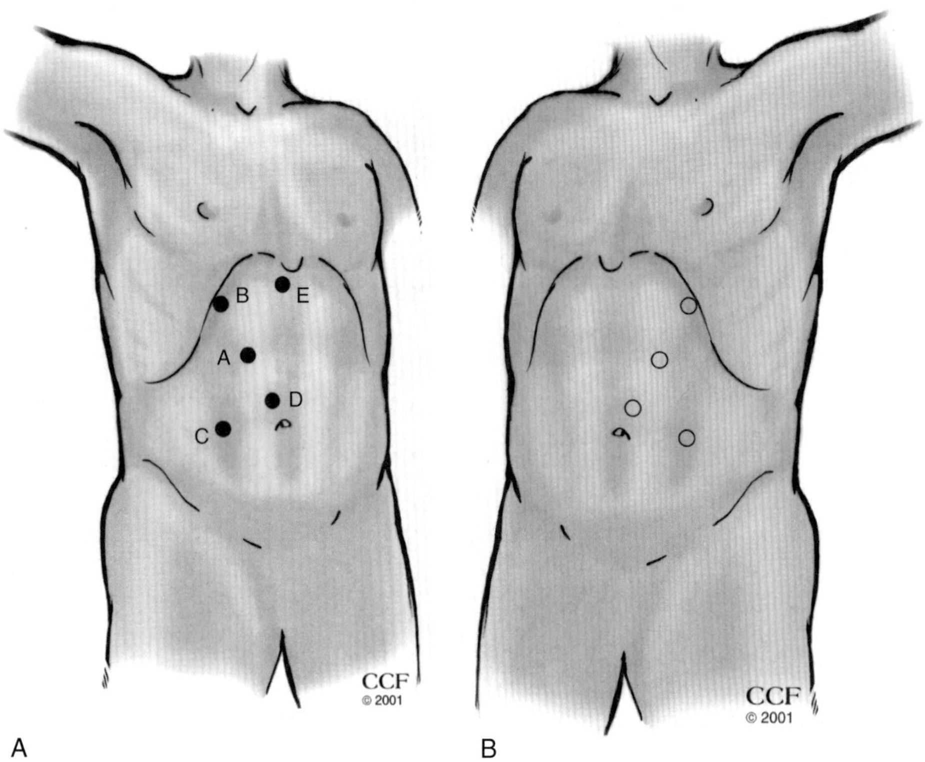

FIGURE 17–1 *A*, Port placement for the robotic-assisted laparoscopic right adrenalectomy. The right-sided procedure was performed with five ports. Primary (12-mm) camera port *(A)*; right (8-mm) *(B)* and left (8-mm) *(C)* robotic working ports; assistant (12-mm) port *(D)*; liver retraction (5-mm) port *(E)*. *B*, Port placement for robotic-assisted left adrenalectomy. The left-sided procedure was performed through four ports, which was similar to the right-sided port placement, minus the 5-mm liver retraction port. *(From Desai MM, Gill IS, Kaouk JH, et al: Robotic-assisted laparoscopic adrenalectomy. Urology 60:1104–1107, 2002.)*

the inferior phrenic vessels are controlled with cautery or clips. Next, the medial aspect of the gland is approached, taking care to control small vessels emanating from the aorta. At this point, the adrenal vein is identified and divided between clips. Gerota's fascia is incised at the junction of the upper pole of the kidney and the adrenal vein to complete the inferior dissection; care should be taken to identify additional venous/arterial branches arising from the renal vein and/or artery. Last, the remaining lateral attachments of the adrenal are released, freeing the specimen completely. A laparoscopic retrieval sac is used to extract the specimen in its entirety. The field is irrigated and inspected with reduced insufflation pressures, hemostasis ensured, and port sites closed as appropriate.

Technique—Right-Sided Adrenalectomy

Right-sided robotic adrenalectomy is typically performed via five ports; an additional 5-mm port for the bedside assistant is used for liver retraction (see Figure 17–1). Exposure of the right adrenalis dependent on adequate hepatic mobilization; complete mobilization of the ascending colon and hepatic flexure is unnecessary. The liver is mobilized by incising the posterior peritoneum along the undersurface of the liver and the triangular ligament laterally. The liver is retracted with a self-retaining retractor or with the assistance of bedside assistant. The inferior vena cava is identified, which may require Kocherization of the second portion of the duodenum. Careful dissection along the lateral wall of the vena cava will allow for the identification of the right adrenal vein, which is divided between clips. As described for left adrenalectomy, dissection proceeds circumferentially, clipping and/or cauterizing the stellate arterial supply. The relatively avascular lateral attachments are the last to be divided, allowing for removal of the specimen via a retrieval bag.

Summary

Robotic adrenalectomy has been demonstrated to be feasible, safe, and effective. Multiple reports document acceptable operative times and low estimated blood loss and rates of complications.[5–9] The multiple attributes of the da Vinci system, including superb optics, tremor reduction, and six degrees of freedom afforded by EndoWrist technology, aid in the delicate dissection required during adrenalectomy. With the further integration of robotics into everyday urologic practice, the robotic approach will have an expanding role in the future.

VASOVASOSTOMY AND VASOEPIDIDYMOSTOMY

Background

The number of vasectomies performed each year in the United States is approximately 500,000, and it is estimated that between 2% and 6% of these men will ultimately seek reversal.[10] Although the success rate of microsurgical vasectomy reversal has been reported to be high, with patency rates of up to 99.5% for vasovasostomy[11] and 84% for vasoepididymostomy,[12] these procedures have widely been considered among the most technically challenging in urology, with long learning curves.

Robotic technology, specifically use of the da Vinci surgical robotic system, offers several advantages that may be particularly suited for performing vasectomy reversal. Specifically, the robot provides motion reduction and improved stability during suturing by eliminating the surgeon's normal physiologic tremor.[13] Moreover, the robot possesses scale setting, with an ultrafine 5:1 reduction gear that reduces the surgeon's movements at the console at the ends of the robot arms.[13] In addition, the six degrees of freedom in movement offered by the da Vinci system facilitates suture placement and knot tying with both the dominant and nondominant hands. Together, these features may increase the precision of an anastomosis, such as during vasectomy reversal.

Technique

Robotic-assisted vasovasostomy begins according to steps previously described for the microsurgical multilayer microdot method.[10] Briefly, a high vertical scrotal incision is performed approximately 1 cm lateral to the base of the penis, and the testis is delivered into the incision with the tunica vaginalis left intact. The vas deferens is identified above and below the site of obstruction and mobilized to allow a tension-free anastomosis. Patency of the testicular and abdominal ends of the vas is then confirmed as the ends are cut, dilated, and stabilized with a Microspike approximating clamp. A microtip marking pen is used on both the testicular and abdominal ends of the vas to map out the six needle exit points for the mucosal sutures, halfway between the mucosal ring and the outer edge of the muscle layer.

At this point, the robot is brought into the operating field on the left side of the patient, while the first assistant remains on the patient's right side. The arms of the robot are positioned at an approximately 10-degree angle in relation to each other and to the patient's abdominal surface (Figure 17–2). Microforceps are loaded into each arm of the robot, and the 0-degree lens is used in the camera. Motion scaling is set to the maximum 5:1 downscaling ratio.

Both one-layer[14] and two-layer[15,16] robotic-assisted anastomotic techniques have been described, and the order of suture placement and knot tying depends on the surgeon. We perform a two-layer anastomosis with the first layer consisting of six equally spaced mucosal sutures, using 10-0 nylon, double-armed with 70-μm diameter taper-point needles bent into a fishhook configuration (available from Sharpoint and Ethicon). The double-armed configuration allows all sutures to be placed in an inside-out fashion, with the needle exiting through the center of each dot. We prefer to place all three posterior sutures, tie, then place the three anterior sutures and tie these. Next, the outer muscularis layer is brought together to support the anastomosis with six 9-0 nylon sutures placed between the mucosal sutures. We then approximate the vasal sheath with six interrupted 7-0 PDS sutures to cover the anastomosis and relieve tension. All sutures are cut by the assistant, who is wearing surgical loupes.

After the anastomosis is completed, the robot is removed from the operating table. The dartos layer is approximated with interrupted 4-0 absorbable sutures, and the skin is closed with subcuticular sutures of 5-0 Monocryl. An identical procedure is performed on the contralateral side. At the conclusion of the procedure, fluff gauze dressings are placed over the scrotum and a scrotal supporter is applied. Patients are discharged home on the day of surgery, and no intercourse or ejaculation is allowed for 4 weeks. Semen analyses are obtained at 1, 3, and 6 months postoperatively.

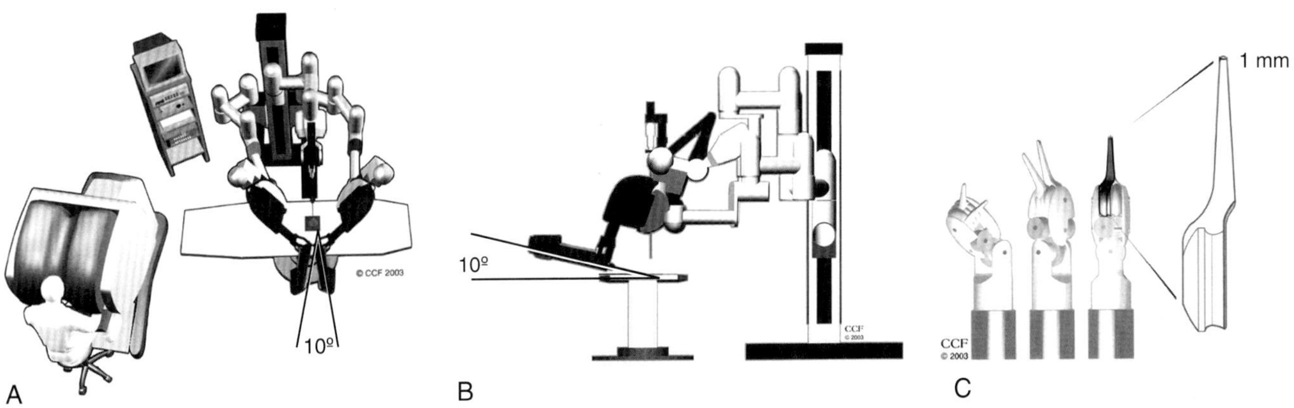

FIGURE 17–2 *A*, Top view. *B*, Lateral view *C*, Microforceps used for robotic vasovasostomy.

Vasoepididymostomy represents the most technically challenging procedure in microsurgery. We perform robotic-assisted vasoepididymostomy using a longitudinal intussusception pull-through technique.[10] First, the epididymis is examined under the Zeiss operating microscope (Carl Zeiss, Oberkochen, Germany) to select a dilated epididymal tubule. The vasal end is then secured to the epididymal tunic with a single 9-0 nylon suture. The microscope is removed, the robot brought to the operating table, and the longitudinal intussusception pull-through vasoepididymostomy performed with two 10-0 double-armed nylon sutures placed parallel and longitudinal into the epididymal tubule and inside-out into the vasal end (Figure 17–3). Eight to ten interrupted 10-0 nylon sutures are then used to approximate the epididymal tunic to the vasal muscle, thereby reinforcing the anastomosis. The robot is then removed, and wound closure performed as described for vasovasostomy earlier.

Summary

The feasibility of robotic vasectomy reversal has been well demonstrated with in vitro and animal studies.[14–16] Investigators have found no difference in patency rates or complications for robotic vasovasostomy compared with microscope-assisted reconstruction,[15,16] and they have reported a decrease in sperm granuloma formation after robotic vasovasostomy, which may be attributed to improved precision of the anastamosis.[15] Operative times have been variably reported as longer[14,16] and shorter[15] using the robot compared with the conventional microscopic approach. Studies comparing outcomes from traditional microsurgical and robotic-assisted vasovasostomy in humans are pending. Currently, robotic-assisted vasoepididymostomy has been described in a single animal study,[15] in which operative time, sperm granuloma rate, and patency rate were not significantly different from the conventional microsurgical technique.

One limitation of robotic surgery that has been cited is a lack of tactile feedback. In vasectomy reversal, this may be particularly relevant for determining the tension necessary to pull up on the anastomotic stitches without breaking the suture. Therefore, visual cues such as the curling of the suture must be used in robotics to help guide the amount of tension to apply.[13] Moreover, the usual magnification of the microscope is 16× to 25×, whereas the da Vinci robot system has a 10× lens. Magnification of up to 30× is possible with the robot by moving the camera lens to 1 cm from the operative field[14]; however, improvements in the system may allow the working distance to be increased, thereby creating more space for instrument movements and minimizing any thermal effects on the vas.[14]

Overall, use of the robot may result in improved precision of suturing for vasovasostomy and vasoepididymostomy, resulting in more watertight anastomoses and improved outcomes. Elimination of the physiologic tremor

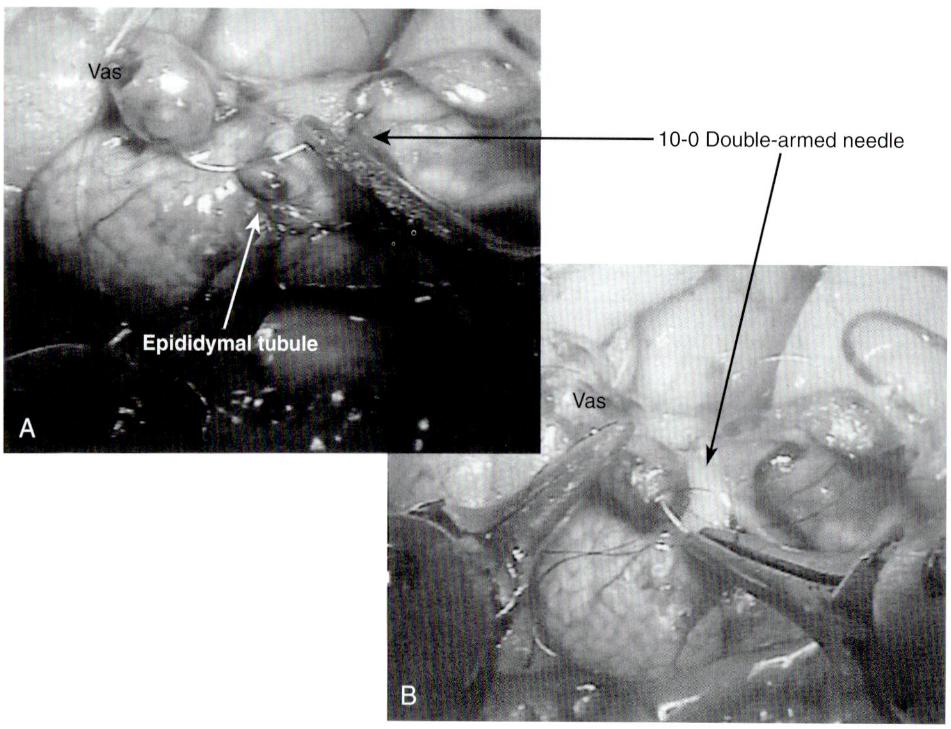

FIGURE 17–3 Robotic microsurgical longitudinal intussusception vasoepididymostomy. Pull-through vasoepididymostomy was done with two 10-0 nylon double-armed sutures placed parallel and longitudinal into epididymal tubule *(A)*, and then placed inside out into vaval end using robot *(B)*. *(From Schiff J, Li PS, Goldstein M: Robotic microsurgical vasovasostomy and vasoepididymostomy: a prospective randomized study in a rat model. J Urol 171:1720–1725, 2004.)*

may in fact make the procedures less challenging and thereby shorten the learning curve. Continued advancements in robotic technology, including improved magnification and the development of finer instruments, will further facilitate the use of robotics in vasectomy reversal.

URINARY DIVERSION

Background

Urinary diversion may be indicated either for benign or malignant disease and may take the form of an orthotopic neobladder, continent catheterizable pouch, or conduit. The application of minimally invasive techniques for urinary diversion has been undertaken with the goals of decreasing morbidity and improving cosmesis, while maintaining functionally equivalent outcomes to open surgery. However, these procedures involve the creation of multiple anastomoses and are therefore among the most difficult of laparoscopic cases, as intracorporeal suturing is technically challenging. Robotic technology, with three-dimensional stereoscopic visualization and fine control of surgical instruments with six degrees of freedom, facilitates dissection, suturing, and knot tying, and thus may be applied to urinary diversion to facilitate a minimally invasive approach.

Technique

Several techniques have been described for using the robot in urinary diversion. The most widely used approach to date has been for patients with bladder cancer who undergo robotic radical cystectomy with extracorporeal diversion performed through the incision made for extraction of the specimen.[17–20] Using this approach, either an ileal conduit or orthotopic neobladder may be created. The technique of robotic radical cystectomy is described elsewhere in the text. After the specimen is placed in an EndoCatch bag, a 5- to 6-cm incision is made midway between the umbilicus and pubic symphysis, through which a segment of ileum may be isolated. For an ileal conduit, the ureterointestinal anastomoses are performed in an open fashion and the ileum is brought to the right lower quadrant for creation of a stoma. The midline incision is then closed.

For an orthotopic neobladder, the ileum is extracted, detubularized, and reconfigured extracorporeally according to the surgeon's preference. The neobladder neck is created, and the ureterointestinal anastomoses are performed. At this point, the pouch is returned to the pelvis, a catheter is then passed through the urethra and into the pouch, the balloon of the catheter is inflated, and the pouch is pulled down to the urethral stump. The abdominal incision is then closed, and the robot is redocked for anastomosis of the neobladder to the urethra. The anastomosis is completed with a continuous running double-armed 3-0 polydioxane suture, which is prepared by tying together the ends of two 5-inch sutures of 3-0 polydioxane, one dyed and one undyed.[17–20]

An alternative approach to urinary diversion has been to perform the mobilization and dissection laparoscopically and then to use the robot for suturing.[21,22] For example, the robot may be used to construct the ureterointestinal anastomoses during laparoscopic ileal conduit diversion.[21] For this procedure, five 12-mm ports are positioned (Figure 17–4).

The left colon is first dissected laparoscopically with a harmonic scalpel by incising the line of Toldt, exposing the left ureter at the level of the iliac bifurcation. The ureter is mobilized proximally and distally to the ureterovesical junction, where it is divided and then brought under the sigmoid mesentery. The right ureter is then identified, mobilized, and divided after reflecting the right colon. An approximately 15-cm segment of ileum is isolated for the conduit 15 cm proximal to the ileocecal valve and is divided using the Endo-GIA 60-3.5 stapler (U.S. Surgical, Norwalk, CT). A side-to-side ileoileal anastomosis is completed using the Endo-GIA stapler.

At this point, the robot is docked, a needle driver is placed in each of the robot arms, and the mesenteric window is closed using interrupted 3-0 silk sutures. Scissors and Debakey forceps are then placed into the robot arms, and the ureters are spatulated for several centimeters. Needle drivers are again placed into the robot arms, and the ureters are reimplanted into the ileal loop according to

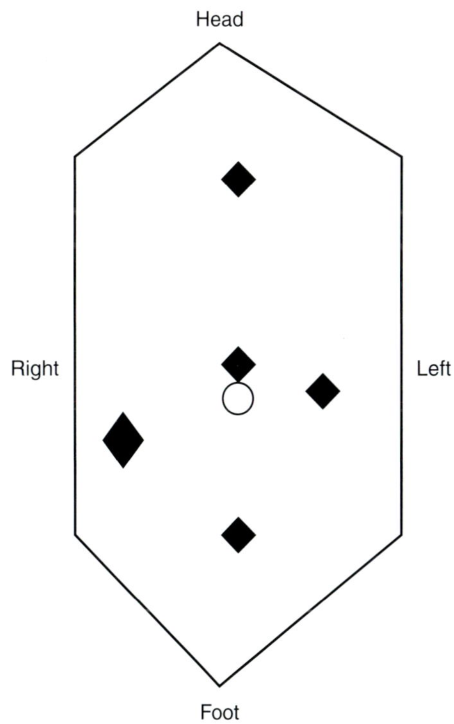

FIGURE 17–4 Diamond-shaped abdominal five-port placement. Circle indicates umbilicus; small dark diamonds indicate port sites; and large dark diamond, port and ileal conduit stoma site. *(From Balaji KC, Yohannes P, McBride CL, et al: Feasibility of robot-assisted totally intracorporeal laparoscopic ileal conduit urinary diversion: initial results of a single institutional pilot study. Urology 63:51–55, 2004.)*

the surgeon's technique of choice. We favor a Bricker-type anastomosis, with interrupted 4-0 Vicryl sutures, completed over a stent that is brought out to the skin within the conduit. After the ureteroileal anastomoses are completed, the proximal end of the conduit is tacked to the parietal peritoneum using two to three silk sutures, and the distal end is brought out through the anterior abdominal wall at the site of the right lower quadrant port and matured using interrupted 2-0 Vicryl sutures. At the conclusion of the procedure, a suction drain may be left through the left periumbilical port.

The technique of using the robot for suturing during an otherwise laparoscopic diversion has also been used for appendicovesicostomy, using a 12-mm laparoscopic camera port through the umbilicus and two 10-mm robotic laparoscopic ports, one in the left lower quadrant and one in the right midaxillary line at the level of the umbilicus, as well as a fourth port in the left midaxillary line.[22] After the appendix and right colon are mobilized laparoscopically, an Endo-GIA stapler is used to divide the appendix at its base. A vertical cystotomy is then made in the posterior wall of the bladder, and the robot is brought in to anastomose the appendix to the bladder using interrupted 4-0 Vicryl sutures.[22] The appendix is then brought up to the umbilicus, and a stoma is created.

A third approach to robotic-assisted urinary diversion is to perform the entire procedure, including mobilization, dissection, and anastomoses, using the da Vinci robot. This technique has been described both for ileal conduit diversion[23] and for orthotopic neobladder.[24] To construct an ileal conduit, three robotic ports are placed in a horizontal line just above the umbilicus (a 12-mm port for the laparoscope and two 10-mm instrument ports), and three additional ports are inserted to pass laparoscopic instruments (a 12-mm left subcostal trocar, a 12-mm right lower quadrant trocar, and a 5-mm suprapubic port). The ureters are first identified, dissected free, and divided, with the left ureter passed under the base of the sigmoid mesentery into the right lower quadrant. An ileal segment approximately 15 cm in length is isolated 15 cm proximal to the ileocecal valve and divided using the Endo-GIA stapler, using a 70-degree cystoscope inserted through the suprapubic port to identify mesenteric vessels. The mesenteric window is closed using 3-0 silk sutures. The ureters are then spatulated for several centimeters on the anterior aspect of the distal ureter and reimplanted into the ileal loop according to the surgeon's technique of choice. We favor a Bricker-type anastomosis, with interrupted 4-0 Vicryl sutures, completed over a stent that is brought out to the skin within the stoma of the conduit. The proximal end of the conduit is then tacked to the parietal peritoneum using two to three silk sutures, and the distal end is brought out through the anterior abdominal wall at the site of the 12-mm right lower quadrant port. A rosebud stoma is secured to the skin using interrupted 2-0 Vicryl sutures. A suction drain may be left through the left subcostal port.

A W-shaped ileal neobladder may similarly be constructed completely robotically, using the ports shown in Figure 17–5. After radical cystectomy and pelvic lymph node dissection, the specimens are placed into a large organ bag and stored in the abdominal cavity. A 60-cm segment of terminal ileum is then isolated starting approximately 15 cm proximal to the ileocecal valve and divided using an Endo-GIA stapler. The position of the neobladder neck is defined in the aboral dependent limb of the W, and an incision is made over the antimesenteric portion of this segment. A catheter is inserted through the urethra and guided into the newly created neobladder neck, and the anastomosis is completed with a continuous running double-armed 3-0 polydioxane suture, prepared as described previously. The remainder of the bowel segment is then incised along the antimesenteric portion, leaving the oral end tubularized as a chimney for the ureteral anastomoses. The neobladder is then aligned in a W configuration, and the posterior wall of the neobladder is

A
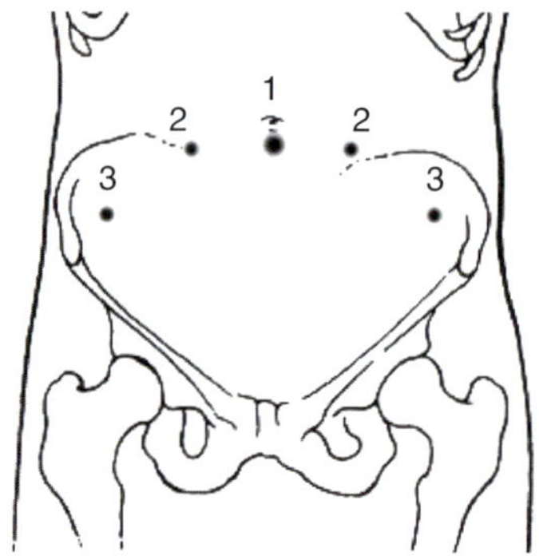

B
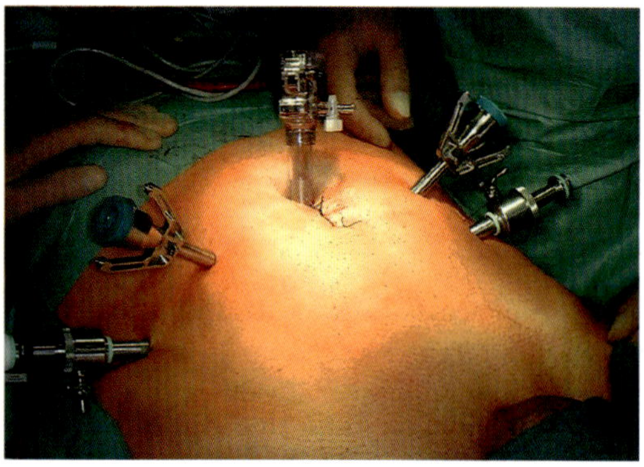

FIGURE 17–5 A, Cartoon of trocar positions. B, Photo of typical trocar positions. Initially, a standard 12-mm trocar is inserted paraumbilically for access of three-dimensional (3D) laparoscope *(1)*; two special 8-mm trocars are placed pararectally for the access of the endowristed laparoscopic tools *(2)*. During the procedure, two additional 10-mm trocars *(3)* were inserted bilaterally into the lower abdomen to allow access of standard laparoscopic tools as bipolar graspers, suction/irrigation device, clip applier, and bowel stapler. *(From Beecken WD, Wolfram M, Engl T, et al: Robotic-assisted laparoscopic radical cystectomy and intra-abdominal formation of an orthotopic ileal neobladder. Eur Urol 44:337–339, 2003; Urology 63:51–55, 2004.)*

constructed by suturing the detubularized segments together with two layers of 2-0 Vicryl, the first a running layer and the second interrupted. Next, the ureters are spatulated and reimplanted into the tubularized chimney as for an ileal conduit, described previously. Single-J stents inserted into the ureters are brought out through the lateral wall of the neobladder and through the skin of the right lower quadrant. The anterior wall of the neobladder is then closed in two layers. Last, the specimen is extracted through by extending the midline incision, and the ileal ends are brought through the extraction incision to perform a side-to-side bowel anastomosis.

SUMMARY

The application of minimally invasive techniques in urology continues to expand to the most complex of procedures, including urinary diversion. The improved visualization, increased degree of movement, and elimination of physiologic tremors afforded by the robot allow the surgeon to achieve equivalent functional outcomes to open surgery while minimizing morbidity and improving cosmesis. The role for robotics in urinary diversion continues to evolve with increased experience with robotic surgery and improvements in robotic technology and instrumentation.

REFERENCES

1. Gagner M, Lacroix A, Bolte E: Laparoscopic adrenalectomy in Cushing's syndrome and pheochromocytoma. N Engl J Med 327:1033, 1992.
2. Brunaud L, Bresler L, Zarnegar R, et al: Does robotic adrenalectomy improve patient quality of life when compared to laparoscopic adrenalectomy? World J Surg 28:1180–1185, 2004.
3. Gill IS, Sung GT, Hsu TH, Meraney AM: Robotic remote laparoscopic nephrectomy and adrenalectomy: the initial experience. J Urol 164:2082–2085, 2000.
4. Horgan S, Vanuno D: Robots in laparoscopic surgery. J Laparoendosc Adv Surg Tech A 11:415–419, 2001.
5. Young JA, Chapman WH 3rd, Kim VB, et al: Robotic-assisted adrenalectomy for adrenal incidentaloma: case and review of the technique. Surg Laparosc Endosc Percutan Tech 12:126–130, 2002.
6. Desai MM, Gill IS, Kaouk JH, et al: Robotic-assisted laparoscopic adrenalectomy. Urology 60:1104–1107, 2002.
7. Bentas W, Wolfram M, Brautigam R, et al: Laparoscopic transperitoneal adrenalectomy using a remote-controlled robotic surgical system. J Endourol 16:373–376, 2002.
8. Undre S, Munz Y, Moorthy K, et al: Robot-assisted laparoscopic adrenalectomy: preliminary UK results. BJU Int 93:357–359, 2004.
9. D'Annibale A, Fiscon V, Trevisan P, et al: The da Vinci robot in right adrenalectomy: considerations on technique. Surg Laparosc Endosc Percutan Tech 14:38–41, 2004.
10. Goldstein M: Surgical management of male infertility and other scrotal disorders. In Walsh PC, Retik AB, Wein AJ, et al (eds): Campbell's Urology, 8 edition. Philadelphia, WB Saunders, 2002, pp 1532–1587.
11. Goldstein M, Li PS, Matthews GJ: Microsurgical vasovasostomy: the microdot technique of precision suture placement. J Urol 159:188–190, 1998.
12. Chan PT, Brandell RA, Goldstein M: Prospective analysis of outcomes after microsurgical intussusception vasoepididymostomy. BJU Int 96:598–601, 2005.
13. Fleming C: Robotic-assisted vasovasostomy. Urol Clin North Am 31:769–772, 2004.
14. Kuang W, Shin PR, Matin S, et al: Initial evaluation of robotic technology for microsurgical vasovasostomy. J Urol 171:300–303, 2004.
15. Schiff J, Li PS, Goldstein M: Robotic microsurgical vasovasostomy and vasoepididymostomy: a prospective randomized study in a rat model. J Urol 171:1720–1725, 2004.
16. Kuang W, Shin PR, Oder M, et al: Robotic-assisted vasovasostomy: a two-layer technique in an animal model. Urology 65:811–814, 2005.
17. Hemal AK, Abol-Enein H, Tewari A, et al: Robotic radical cystectomy and urinary diversion in the management of bladder cancer. Urol Clin North Am 31:719–729, 2004.
18. Menon M, Hemal AK, Tewari A, et al: Nerve-sparing robot-assisted radical cystoprostatectomy and urinary diversion. BJU Int 92:232–236, 2003.
19. Menon M, Hemal AK, Tewari A, et al: Robot-assisted radical cystectomy and urinary diversion in female patients: technique with preservation of the uterus and vagina. J Am Coll Surg 198:386–393, 2004.
20. Shah NL, Hemal AK, Menon M: Robot-assisted radical cystectomy and urinary diversion. Curr Urol Rep 6:122–125, 2005.
21. Balaji KC, Yohannes P, McBride CL, et al: Feasibility of robot-assisted totally intracorporeal laparoscopic ileal conduit urinary diversion: initial results of a single institutional pilot study. Urology 63:51–55, 2004.
22. Pedraza R, Weiser A, Franco I: Laparoscopic appendicovesicostomy (Mitrofanoff procedure) in a child using the Da Vinci robotic system. J Urol 171:1652–1653, 2004.
23. Hubert J, Feuillu B, Beis JM, et al: Laparoscopic robotic-assisted ileal conduit urinary diversion in a quadriplegic woman. Urology 62:1121, 2003.
24. Beecken WD, Wolfram M, Engl T, et al: Robotic-assisted laparoscopic radical cystectomy and intra-abdominal formation of an orthotopic ileal neobladder. Eur Urol 44:337–339, 2003.

CHAPTER 18

Glen W. Barrisford • Craig A. Peters

Robotically Assisted Techniques in Pediatric Urology

INTRODUCTION

Minimally invasive surgical techniques have evolved over the past several decades in an effort to reduce surgical morbidity associated with incisional size, length of stay, and recovery. The emergence of new technology has allowed for the development of innovative instrumentation and new surgical approaches. As surgical optics improve and as instruments contract in size while expanding in capability, surgeons are better equipped to develop novel surgical strategies.

As a result of information widely available on the Internet and in the media, an increasingly knowledgeable patient population has become more resistant to surgical procedures that require large incisions and extended recovery periods. Given patient preference and commercial pressures, minimally invasive surgery has found an expanding niche despite incompletely defined benefits. As technology evolves and as laparoscopic experience improves, the merits of minimally invasive surgery will likely become more clearly defined. Despite the availability of specialty training programs, minimally invasive surgery is generally recognized as a tool that serves as an adjunct to patient care across many surgical disciplines.[1]

Initially, laparoscopy was performed for diagnostic purposes. Among pediatric urologists, orchidopexy was performed following laparoscopic localization of the maldescended testis. Subsequent development of operative laparoscopy occurred when competency and equipment improved, as well as the breakdown of attitudinal barriers. Once laparoscopy was demonstrated as a safe and effective alternative, its application became more widespread. Despite the range of presumptive advantages associated with the use of laparoscopy, its major limitations have been those associated with reduced dexterity/precision, difficult intracorporal suturing, and a steep learning curve. In an effort to overcome some of these restrictions, novel devices were developed.

The boundaries of minimally invasive surgery were greatly expanded with the development of robotic surgical systems. Robotic surgical technology was initially developed by military research teams in an effort to expedite medical care for battlefield soldiers. The original concept was envisioned as a self-contained mobile robotic surgical suite. This unit was to be staffed by trained medics and operated remotely by a surgeon. This system was focused on providing rapid operative care while protecting a limited number of experienced surgeons. Although this technology has to date not been widely used, it has given rise to several derivative applications. Perhaps the most significant advances made through robotic surgical technology have been the addition of high-resolution three-dimensional vision, dexterous wristlike movement capabilities, and tremor filtration with geometric scaling of movements. In addition, the development of more advanced computer and robotic technology has given rise to a concept referred to as "telecollaboration."

At a workshop designed to evaluate the future of surgical technology and its application in the operating suite, a group of physicians, "OR2020," defined several terms associated with telecollaboration[2]:

- *Tele-evaluation:* The appraisal, typically including some type of physical examination, of a patient distant from the health care professional. The most common media type used for this process is audio-video teleconferencing.
- *Telementoring / teleproctoring:* The teaching and supervision of a less experienced surgeon by a remotely located expert surgeon. Telementoring includes giving real-time advice about the various mechanical steps of a particular operation. Audio-video teleconferencing is fundamental to this activity. Often, telementoring is enhanced with the use of telestration devices.
- *Telemonitoring:* The observation of another surgeon's or surgeon-in-training's performance during a surgical procedure. This practice can be thought of as "telegrading" that is typically done in real time but can be accomplished via store-and-forward technology. Telemonitoring usually includes some assessment of the operating surgeon by the expert, but without the real-time expression of that assessment.

- *Telemanipulation:* The remote operation of a device (e.g., camera, needle, instrument) for a specific purpose (e.g., visualization, biopsy). This activity necessitates that control signals be sent across telecommunications lines to move the device. Telemanipulation is a limited subset of telesurgery (defined next).
- *Telesurgery / telepresence surgery:* The performance of surgery (including all tasks typically assigned to a surgeon) at a distance using remote control of surgical robots over telecommunications networks. Telesurgery is bimanual remote manipulation of the tissue being operated on with complete real-time visual access to the operative field. When using telesurgery to operate in conjunction with a local surgeon, telesurgery allows the remotely located expert or consultant surgeon to "take over" as necessary to demonstrate the "next move" or to actually perform the surgery."

With the use of real-time video, audio, and data streaming, the U.S. Navy demonstrated the application of telementoring in a series of five laparoscopic inguinal hernia repairs aboard the aircraft carrier USS *Abraham Lincoln.*[3] Similarly, a less experienced laparoscopic surgeon in Singapore was telementored by a more experienced surgeon from the United States during a radical nephrectomy and a bilateral varicocelectomy.[4] In an example of telemanipulation, surgeons demonstrated feasibility in animal experiments by remotely manipulating an endoscope during urologic surgical procedures in a porcine model.[5]

Although several aspects of robotic surgery have been successfully demonstrated, several limiting factors have been identified that have prevented the more widespread application of telesurgery. The OR2020 group defined four major limitations of remote robotic surgery: control latency, visual discrepancy, round trip delay, and jitter.[2] *Control latency* refers to the time delay that occurs between initiation of movement and the response. *Visual discrepancy* indicates the delay that occurs between the movement of an object in the operative field and the appreciation of the visual image by the remote surgeon. *Round trip delay* is the sum of the control latency and visual discrepancy. It represents the time that it takes for a remote surgeon to initiate movement of an instrument and for the visual appreciation to occur. Finally, *jitter* refers to variable delays that occur as a result of fluctuations in traffic along telecommunications networks. It is expected that as telecommunications networks and robotic equipment improve, many of the difficulties associated with latency and bandwidth of data will improve substantially. Until then, proximately located surgeons will be able to use the improved vision and manipulative aspects associated with robotic surgery without having to face the challenges associated with a remote location.

Pediatric urologists represent a relatively small group of highly specialized surgeons who are generally located in large urban centers. For pediatric urologists not in practices with high-laparoscopic volumes, the development of operative proficiency remains challenging. In addition to the visual and manipulative improvements associated with robotic technology, the advantage of a foreshortened learning curve and the potential for telecollaboration with remotely located experts makes pediatric urology an ideal specialty for the continued development and use of robotic technology.

ROBOTIC EQUIPMENT

Among the multiple robotic surgical systems that are currently commercially available, the most widely used is the da Vinci (Intuitive Surgical, Sunnyvale, CA). It was the first robotic surgical system to receive U.S. Food and Drug Administration approval (July 11, 2000), offering it a clear marketplace advantage. To date, more than 320 systems have been sold worldwide. The approximate purchase price is $1.4 million, with an annual maintenance cost of approximately $35,000. This system is composed of three main components: robot, surgeon's console, and instrument tower. The robot is composed of a large pedestal, two (or three) manipulative arms, and a three-dimensional endoscopic camera. This robot is draped in a sterile fashion and placed at the patient's bedside. The surgeon's console is a large unit with manipulative hand controls, foot pedals, and a view port with a three-dimensional display. This is generally located in the same operating room (OR) but is placed away from the patient's bedside. The instrument tower provides a monitor for the patient side surgeon, a light source for the camera, and appropriate space and connections for video recording equipment.

OPERATING ROOM AND SURGICAL TEAM

When using new equipment and technology, patient safety remains the utmost priority. It is important to properly train and coordinate the surgical team. Nowhere is this more critical than when working with pediatric patients. Team coordination is essential for the safe performance of robotic procedures. All members of the team have participated in dry laboratory training to understand the movements of the system, the mode of action, and the methods involved in instrument changes. The team is composed of the operating surgeon, patient side surgeon, scrub nurse, circulating nurse, and anesthesia team. The operating surgeon remains nonsterile and sits at the surgeon's console. The patient side surgeon wears sterile surgical attire and is located at the patient's bedside. This surgeon generally changes instruments and makes adjustments to the robotic arms. In our institution, this role is generally filled by a urologic resident who is interested in participating. The scrub nurse assists the patient side surgeon with instrument changes. A dedicated nursing team is essential and should be provided.

The robotic equipment is set up while the patient is anesthetized and while cystoscopy is performed as the procedure may require. In addition to the required robotic equipment, a few basic reusable conventional laparoscopic instruments are available in the room. In addition, a surgical tray is set up in the room in the event of the need for conversion to open surgery. As with laparoscopy, the conversion of a robotic to an open surgical procedure is a decision that is made to maximize patient safety. Most robotic procedures that are converted are performed under nonemergent controlled circumstances. However, in an extremely rare number of cases, large vessel injury during trocar placement can be an emergent reason to open. Although this is very uncommon, an appropriate contingency plan should be in place.

Before the initiation of the procedure, the robotic system is "powered up" and checked. When performed in an efficient manner, this process takes approximately 20 minutes and is concurrent with anesthetic induction and cystoscopy when necessary. A rectal catheter is placed to decompress the bowel, and a bladder catheter is used to fill or empty the bladder depending on the procedure. Appropriate coordination with the anesthesia team provides awareness of patient and equipment positioning. Impaired communication can result in a loss of situational awareness and patient injuries.

PATIENT POSITIONING AND ACCESS

With any surgical procedure, patient positioning can greatly influence the progress and level of difficulty of the case. The patient should be appropriately positioned, cushioned at all pressure points, and secured to the operating table. Prior to draping the patient, we verify patient immobility by cycling the operating table with a large degree of tilt in each direction (Figure 18–1). When performing renal procedures, the kidney can be exposed transmesenterically or by reflecting the colon. When reflecting the colon, the patient should be tilted approximately 60 degrees. However, transmesenteric access requires only 30 degrees of tilt. For deep pelvic and bladder procedures, the robot is placed at the foot of the bed and the patient is placed in the Trendelenburg position for improved exposure. With open and standard laparoscopy, patient position can be adjusted throughout the procedure. However, once the robot is engaged, the patient is not able to be moved without disengaging the robot. Attention to the details of positioning will maximize efficiency, exposure, and patient safety.

Once the patient is appropriately positioned, placement of surgical cannulae can begin. Proper port location is of paramount importance in pediatric patients given the limited working space. In adult patients, a distance of four fingerbreadths is generally placed between ports. This is not practical in a child whose abdomen cannot accommodate this. Consequently, symmetry rather than spacing is crucial. The camera is placed along the central axis, and the instrument ports are located laterally in uniform positions. When the ports are not placed evenly, the instrument movement may be limited or the instruments may entangle with the camera. The safe placement of ports cannot be overemphasized because vascular injury at this time represents one of the few catastrophic complications that can occur.[6]

Port placement can be performed using the open Hasson technique[7] or with a Veress needle.[8] Although the Hassan technique allows direct visualization, ports can be safely placed using the Veress needle. The saline drop test can be

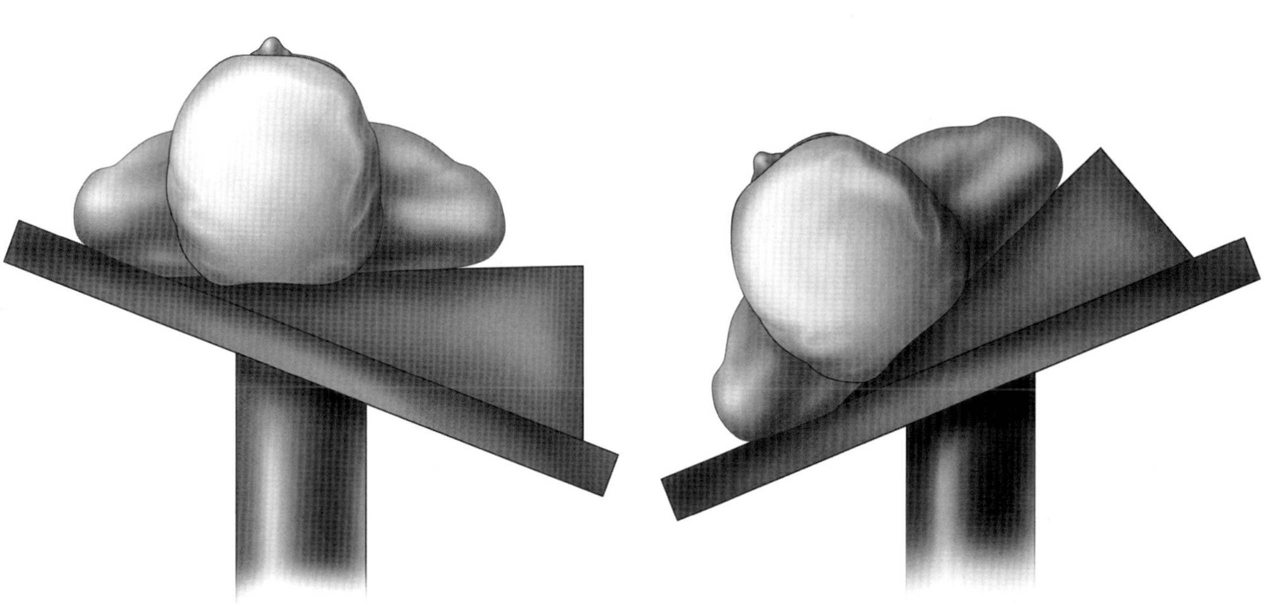

Position for access | Position for procedure

FIGURE 18–1 Positioning for robotic renal surgery.

performed when using the Veress needle. In the event that the Veress needle has been inadvertently inserted into a vessel, insufflation can result in a carbon dioxide embolus. This can be avoided if one initially aspirates through the Veress needle and then uses the saline drop test. Working ports are placed under direct vision with preplaced fascial sutures in a box-stitch fashion to permit rapid closure at the end of the procedure.

When the cannulae have been placed, the robotic arms are positioned and the instruments inserted (Figure 18–2). When appropriate position is established, instrument changes are performed quickly and safely. If properly replaced, the newly inserted instrument will not travel past the location of the original instrument. Surgical instruments are available in 5- or 8-mm sizes, with a 12-mm three-dimensional endoscopic camera. Although the 5-mm instruments are smaller and more delicate, the tip is longer and they require a larger operative field to manipulate the instrument into a right-angled position. This often limits movement of 5-mm instruments when in confined spaces. The most commonly used instruments for urologic procedures include DeBakey forceps, Maryland dissectors, hook electrocautery, scissors, and large and fine-tip needle drivers. It is important to anticipate and minimize instrument changes because they tend to disrupt the continuity of the procedure.

The development of multifunctional instruments would greatly enhance the procedural flow. Perhaps the most notable deficiency is the inability to place suture in an interrupted fashion without the repetitive exchange of needle driver for scissors. The development of a needle driver capable of cutting suture would improve this deficiency. However, in procedures with four or five cannulae, an assistant can use a handheld laparoscopic scissor to cut suture for the operating surgeon. In general, we limit the number of ports because of space constraints and to limit morbidity. Another inadequacy is the absence of cutting current on the hook electrocautery. At this time, only coagulating current is available. When attempting to divide tissue, the process is slow, with a great deal of tissue damage. In an effort to rectify this problem, the newly available electrified 8-mm scissors have been developed.

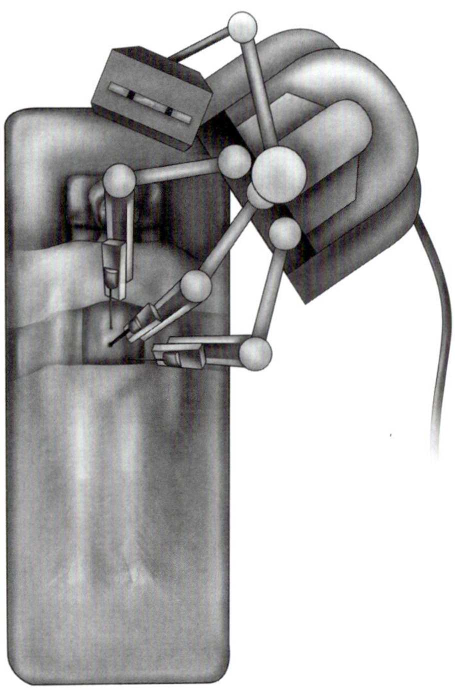

FIGURE 18–2 Robotic positioning for renal surgery.

RENAL SURGERY

Nephrectomy

Nephrectomy is a procedure that can be performed proficiently with standard laparoscopic equipment securing hilar vessels with surgical clips. However, the enhanced vision and improved dexterity associated with robotic systems offer a greater advantage to the surgeon. We favor a three-port technique, with improved hilar exposure via the use of ureteral traction. A fourth port is occasionally required for adequate exposure. It is our preference to obtain vascular control prior to the complete mobilization of the kidney. Once the kidney has been mobilized, it can often impair hilar exposure and increase the level of procedural difficulty. In adult patients, hand-assisted techniques are often preferred given the tactile feedback and hand dissection available to the surgeon.[9,10] In the pediatric population, hand ports would often be larger than the requisite open surgical incision. Thus, robotic-assisted techniques may offer an advantage to purely laparoscopic nephrectomy.

Partial Nephrectomy

Robotic-assisted partial nephrectomy has been reported in adult patients.[11,12] Gettman and colleagues[11] successfully performed both transperitoneal and retroperitoneal techniques. In the pediatric literature the only reports of partial nephrectomy have been made by Peters[13] and by Pedraza et al.[14] Pedraza et al. reported the performance of a bilateral hemi-nephroureterectomy in a 4-year-old girl. The control provided by the robot facilitated the delicate dissection of the polar vessel without excess traction on the remaining vessels. The enhanced visualization is an advantage when separating the two poles. Our experience has been with a nonarticulating harmonic scalpel that has been adapted for the robot. An articulating version would be advantageous. In the absence of this device, monopolar electrocautery can be used. Hemostasis and suturing of the cut surface in the residual pole should be adequate to prevent the formation of hematoma or urinoma. Occurrences of these complications have been reported in the literature following partial nephrectomies with standard laparoscopic techniques.[15] Adequate repair of the defect, as in open surgery, is easily performed with the robot. Consequently, reports of this complication are infrequent.

Pyeloplasty

Robotic-assisted pyeloplasty was first reported in adult patients in 1995 using the Aesop (Computer Motion, Goleta, CA) scope-holder system.[16] Subsequent to initial reports, several studies appeared in the literature.[17–23] To date, the pediatric literature exhibits few reports of robotic-assisted techniques.[13,17,18,24–30] However, several accounts of laparoscopic pyeloplasty appear, reflecting widespread interest in a minimally invasive approach.[31–35] This procedure can be performed in a transperitoneal or retroperitoneal fashion. It requires suturing with great precision and control, which has been technically challenging with traditional laparoscopic equipment. Use of the robotic precision and enhanced vision combined with a hitch stitch as described by Tan[36] provides optimal exposure of the renal pelvis and anastomotic site. The hitch stitch is secured to the abdominal wall before the ureteropelvic junction (UPJ) is dismembered. This stabilizes the tissues and keeps the visual field free from blood. Alternatively, the hitch stitch can be delivered through the abdominal wall and can be used to provide external tension.

The anastomosis is performed with monofilament and can be placed in a running or interrupted fashion (Figure 18–3). The posterior aspect of the anastomosis is completed first. The repair can be stented or a separate drain may be placed.[13] As we have previously noted, interrupted sutures can be time consuming and slow procedural flow. Intentional tearing of the suture with the robotic arms is not recommended because this may damage the anastomosis. Suture length should range from 12 to 16 cm. Working with a longer piece of suture in an effort to be efficient can often make suturing awkward and inefficient. When the knots are tied, the free end should be kept short to make more ergonomic movements. Careful tension should be applied to the suture when securing knots because the resistance the surgeon senses does not reflect the true tension applied to the suture. Overly aggressive movements can tear delicate suture. Drainage is achieved with either retrograde or antegrade double-J ureteral stent placement. Retrograde stent placement allows use of a withdrawal string to avoid the need for cystoscopic removal of a stent (Figure 18–4). Our results with pyeloplasty have been good, with significant reduction in postoperative analgesic requirements and shorter hospital stays compared with an age-matched open pyeloplasty control group. Operative times are longer on average, but the most recent cases have equaled the total OR time as age-matched open cases.[30]

Pyelolithotomy

Laparoscopic pyelolithotomy has been described in pediatric patients.[37,38] However, robotic-assisted techniques have not been reported. When urinary calculi are of a size and composition that is not suitable for ureteroscopic or shock wave treatment, percutaneous treatment becomes the therapy of choice. However, the establishment of percutaneous access in a nondilated renal pelvis can be a difficult procedure. Laparoscopic treatment has been described as an alternative in patients with failed access.[39] In addition, laparoscopic pyeloplasty with concomitant pyelolithotomy has been described.[40] We have noted the advantage of robotic assistance for the repair of an obstructed UPJ. Most approaches to laparoscopic

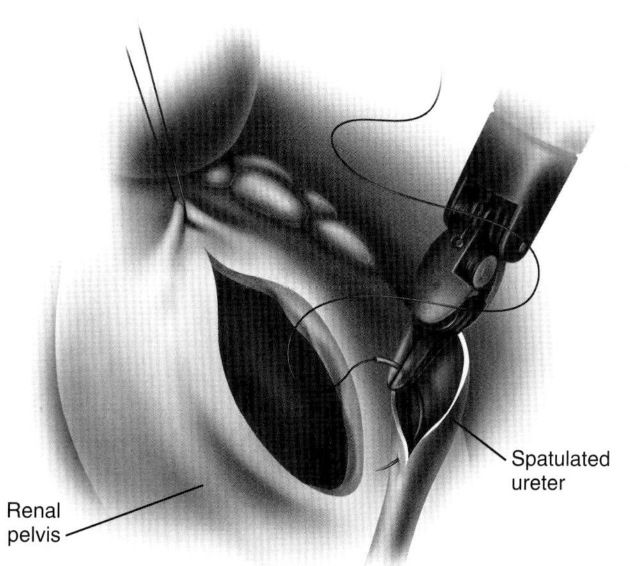

FIGURE 18–3 Initial anastomotic suture placement in robotic pyeloplasty.

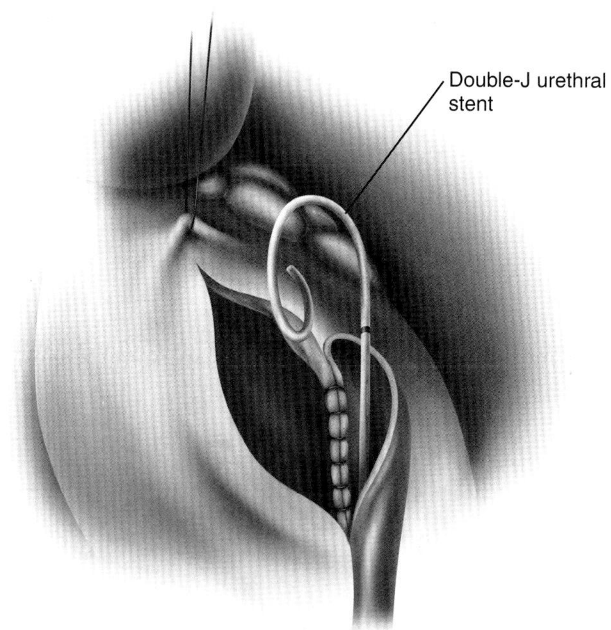

FIGURE 18–4 Double-J ureteral stent has been placed across anastomosis after completion of the back wall closure and prior to the anterior closure.

pyelolithotomy have been described using flexible endoscopic equipment,[41] and these have been adapted to the robotic system by passing a 15-French flexible cystoscope through the working cannula to remove calyceal stones under both robotic and endoscopic guidance. Robotic-assisted suturing provided for efficient closure of the renal pelvis. We have used this approach in patients with a large stone burden, particularly with harder cystine stones for which the therapeutic efficacy of alternative modalities are limited. In patients requiring combined procedures (pyelolithotomy/pyeloplasty), robotic assistance appears to offer advantages.

PELVIC SURGERY

Although we have demonstrated that robotic surgery offers many clear assets to renal surgery, robotic surgery is particularly advantageous for procedures deep within the pelvis. Pelvic surgery is typically known for poor visualization with awkward approaches during retrovesical procedures. The vision and working space is greatly enhanced with robotic assistance. Access to the seminal vesicles, Müllerian remnants, and bladder neck is excellent when approached with a 30-degree upwardly directed camera. Laparoscopic approaches to Müllerian remnants have been described,[42,43] but to date, there are no published accounts of robotic techniques. Our experience has been encouraging, and the exceptional vision and the ability to perform delicate manipulations behind the bladder have provided remarkable results (Figure 18–5).

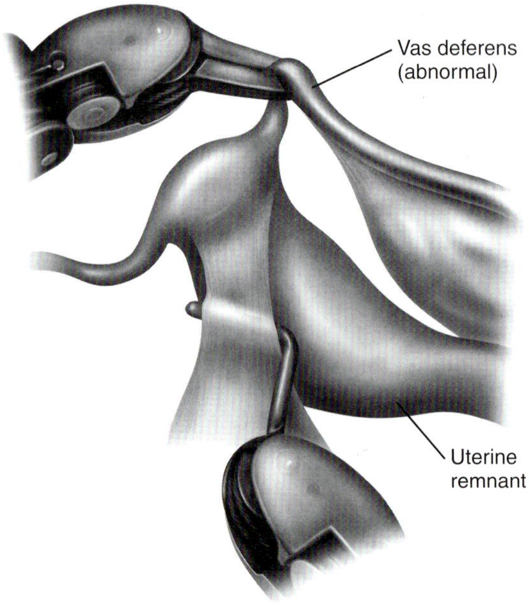

FIGURE 18–5 Robotic excision of a Müllerian remnant in a boy with a ring-Y chromosomal anomaly, dysgenetic right gonad, and recurrent epididymitis of the left testis. The vas deferens entered into the Müllerian structure that resembled a uterus and vagina.

BLADDER SURGERY

Minimally invasive bladder surgery was initially described over a decade ago. However, the difficult dissection and suturing served as a barrier to more widespread application. It was reintroduced in the new millennium but remained a technologic challenge.[44] Initial laparoscopic antireflux procedures were performed in an extravesical fashion using the Lich-Gregoir technique. Unfortunately, bilateral extravesical reimplantation had been associated with an increased risk of transient urinary retention.[45] The laparoscopic approach was thought to reduce this risk,[44] although this issue has not yet been decisively resolved. It is likely that some risk exists when using laparoscopic techniques. Given the potential for transient urinary retention, a laparoscopic transvesical approach was demonstrated in three patients.[46] More recently, a robotic approach was demonstrated in a porcine model.[47] Both approaches used Cohen cross-trigonal techniques. Our institutional experience has been with extravesical and transvesical.[48]

When performing unilateral repairs, an extravesical three-port approach is used. The robotic pedestal is positioned at the foot of the bed with the arms facing toward the feet. A pneumoperitoneum is established (12 mm Hg), and the three-dimensional endoscopic camera (30-degree angle downward) is placed at the umbilicus through a 12-mm port using the Hassan technique.[7] The working ports (5 or 8 mm) are placed just inferior to and equidistant from the camera port along the midinguinal line. In females, the ureter is identified cephalad to the uterus and its orientation can be determined. The ureter is exposed by incising the peritoneum anterior to the uterus and sweeping the uterine ligament and pedicle posteriorly. The ureter is seen outside the bladder, mobilized, and cleared for approximately 4 or 5 cm. Care is taken to avoid too extensive a degree of mobilization. The posterior bladder wall is then cleared, and the bladder is partially filled. A hitch stitch can be used to move the bladder upward to aid in exposure, and the camera is switched to the 30-degree upward orientation. A detrusor incision is made and taken to the level of the mucosa for approximately 2.5 to 3 cm (Figure 18–6). It is best to peel the detrusor off the mucosa laterally to facilitate wrapping of the ureter. A Y-shaped mobilization around the hiatus of the ureter is executed but not completed circumferentially. The detrusor is then sutured over the ureter using 3-0 or 4-0 Polydiozanone or Vicryl suture. The muscle can be brought around the ureter and closed in either direction (Figure 18–7). Working in a distal to proximal fashion permits clear visualization of all structures but requires passing the needle under the ureter during closure. Postoperative care includes bladder catheterization for 1 to 2 days. However, recent cases have been performed

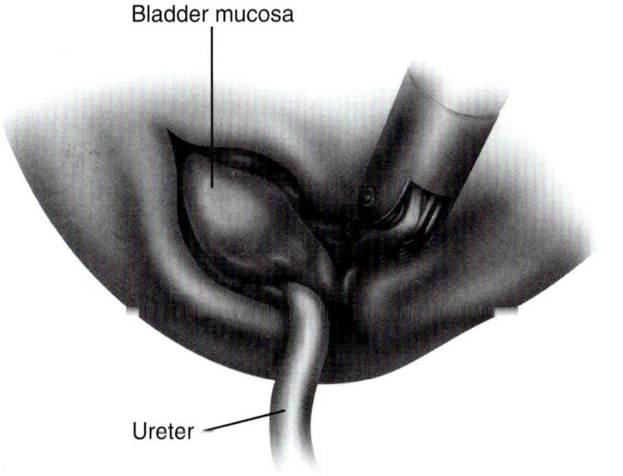

FIGURE 18–6 Extravesical ureteral reimplant for reflux showing exposure of the bladder mucosa in the creation of the detrusor trough.

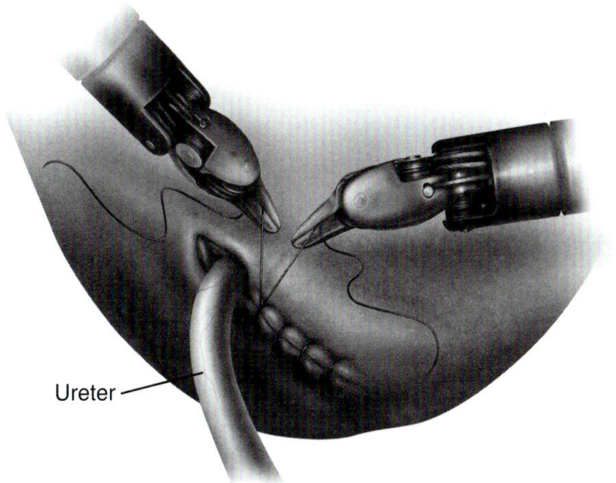

FIGURE 18–7 Completion of the ureteral reimplant with the ureter now passing through the detrusor tunnel.

without catheterization and with discharge in the evening or the following morning.

The transvesical approach is performed in a fashion similar to the open Cohen cross-trigonal approach as described by Yeung et al.[49] When access to the bladder is obtained, the puncture sites must be sealed. Once access is established, the bladder is filled with carbon dioxide. In the event of a port site leak, the gas will fill the retroperitoneum. Under these circumstances, the operative field will be reduced. If this occurs, the leaks must be sealed and the extraperitoneal gas is vented with a needle or plastic catheter. Our approach has included placing ports just above the level of a Pfannenstiel incision and to begin with a bladder filled with saline. Blunt dissection through the umbilical port site is used to free the bladder dome. Sutures are placed to lift and secure the bladder. These sutures will be used to close the bladder at the completion of the procedure. The camera is then placed into the bladder and used to insert the working ports under vision. After all three ports are placed and the bladder is sealed, the saline is drained and the bladder is filled with carbon dioxide. At this point, the procedure continues similarly to an open reimplantation. Five-centimeter segments of feeding tubes are inserted into the ureters and sutured in place to provide traction. A feeding tube is placed in the urethra to suction blood and urine. Dissection and development of tunnels can be performed more proficiently than the open approach, given the dexterity of the instruments. The ureters are brought through the tunnels and secured using 4-0 or 5-0 Monocryl or chromic suture. The path of the ureter is checked with a feeding tube to demonstrate patency. The bladder is closed with the previously placed sutures, and fascia and skin are closed at the port sites. A bladder catheter is left in place for 1 to 2 days, and the patients discharged when voiding. Our initial results have not been as positive as those reported by Yeung et al.,[49] with some residual reflux. The robotic system offers excellent dexterity and control, but the challenge of gaining and maintaining access in the bladder remains to be fully met.

RECONSTRUCTIVE SURGERY

The performance of complicated reconstructive procedures using laparoscopic techniques represents a major challenge to pediatric urologists. The requirement of precise efficient suturing has served as an obstacle, even for the most experienced laparoscopic surgeons. Robotic technology has provided an alternative for this technical challenge.

Continent Diversion and Enterocystoplasty

The ability to create a continent catheterizable stoma using laparoscopic techniques was demonstrated in a case report by Jordan and Winslow[50] (Mitrofanoff procedure) and in a porcine model by Siqueria et al.[51] (Monti procedure). Despite the limited number of reports that followed Jordan, the demonstration of feasibility encouraged Docimo and colleagues to develop techniques that integrated laparoscopic mobilization with extended port site incisions. These incisions were used to construct the augmented bladder and reanastomose the bowel externally.[52–54] These techniques have served as a bridge to develop the skills required to perform these complicated reconstructions in a minimally invasive fashion. The addition of endoscopic stapling and suturing devices has decreased procedural difficulty and operative time, but these complicated reconstructions remain technically challenging. Pedraza et al.[55] performed a robotic appendicovesicostomy (Mitrofanoff procedure) in a 7-year-old boy using the da Vinci system. The report described a four-port transperitoneal technique, free from intraoperative and postoperative complications that required 6 hours of operative time. This group noted a great advantage when creating the appendicovesical anastomosis. Using this technique, we adapted this procedure for the da Vinci robotic system and have performed two de novo and one revision appendicovesicostomy with excellent results. In addition, Elliot and colleagues[56] described a complete laparoscopic ileal cystoplasty. At present, we are currently evaluating technical aspects in a porcine model. Although we are at the initial stages in our evaluation, our progress thus far is promising. Surgeons in our group with limited laparoscopic/robotic experience have successfully performed this challenging reconstruction.

CONCLUSIONS

Robotically assisted laparoscopic surgery continues to gain favor within pediatric urology. The assets associated with improved vision, dexterous instrumentation, a foreshortened learning curve (as compared with traditional laparoscopy), and the potential for various methods of telecollaboration offer many advantages to the pediatric urologist. Despite the many advantages of robotic technology, the main disadvantage remains the poor tactile sensation when handling tissue or suture. As haptic technology improves, this will become less of a disadvantage in newer generations of robotic surgical systems.

At this time, it is unclear if minimally invasive techniques have more to offer than open or traditional laparoscopic techniques in pediatric patients. Given the economic pressures imposed on health care systems worldwide, robotically assisted surgery may appear to be an extravagant expense for procedures that are well tolerated by traditional open approaches. However, as robotic technology becomes more widely available, economies of scale and technologic development will reduce costs. If prudent application of this novel technology can demonstrate a clinical and economic advantage, then robotic surgery may become the gold standard rather than a forgotten technologic whim.

REFERENCES

1. Peters CA: Laparoscopic and robotic approach to genitourinary anomalies in children. Urol Clin North Am 31:595–605, xi, 2004.
2. Cleary K, Mun SK, Kinsella A: OR2020: The operating room of the future. Turf Valley Conference Center; Ellicot, MD, 2004.
3. Cubano M, Poulose BK, Talamini MA, et al: Long distance telementoring. A novel tool for laparoscopy aboard the USS Abraham Lincoln. Surg Endosc 13:673–678, 1999.
4. Lee BR, Png DJ, Liew L, et al: Laparoscopic telesurgery between the United States and Singapore. Ann Acad Med Singapore 29:665–668, 2000.
5. Bowersox JC, Cornum RL: Remote operative urology using a surgical telemanipulator system: preliminary observations. Urology 52:17–22, 1998.
6. Peters C: Complications of retroperitoneal laparoscopy in pediatric urology: prevention, recognition, and management. In Caione P, Kavoussi LR, Micalli F (eds): Retroperitoneoscopy and Extraperitoneal Laparoscopy in Pediatric and Adult Urology. Milano, Springer, 2003, pp 203–210.
7. Hasson HM: A modified instrument and method for laparoscopy. Am J Obstet Gynecol 110:886–887, 1971.
8. Veress J: [A needle for the safe use of pneumoperitoneum]. Gastroenterologia 96:150–152, 1961.
9. Wolf JS Jr, Moon TD, Nakada SY: Hand-assisted laparoscopic nephrectomy: technical considerations. Tech Urol 3(3):123–128, 1997.
10. Nakada SY: Hand-assisted laparoscopic nephrectomy. J Endourol 13:9–14, 1999; discussion 14–15.
11. Gettman MT, Blute ML, Chow GK, et al: Robotic-assisted laparoscopic partial nephrectomy: technique and initial clinical experience with DaVinci robotic system. Urology 64:914–918, 2004.
12. Phillips CK, Taneja SS, Stifelman MD: Robot-assisted laparoscopic partial nephrectomy: the NYU technique. J Endourol 19:441–445, 2005.
13. Peters CA: Robotically assisted surgery in pediatric urology. Urol Clin North Am 31:743–752, 2004.
14. Pedraza R, Palmer L, Moss V, et al: Bilateral robotic assisted laparoscopic heminephroureterectomy. J Urol 171(6 pt 1):2394–2395, 2004.
15. Valla JS, Breaud J, Carfagna L, et al: Treatment of ureterocele on duplex ureter: upper pole nephrectomy by retroperitoneoscopy in children based on a series of 24 cases. Eur Urol 43:426–429, 2003.
16. Partin AW, Adams JB, Moore RG, et al: Complete robot-assisted laparoscopic urologic surgery: a preliminary report. J Am Coll Surg 181:552–557, 1995.
17. Mendez-Torres F, Woods M, Thomas R: Technical modifications for robot-assisted laparoscopic pyeloplasty. J Endourol 19:393–396, 2005.
18. Palese MA, Stifelman MD, Munver R, et al: Robot-assisted laparoscopic dismembered pyeloplasty: a combined experience. J Endourol 19:382–386, 2005.
19. Peschel R, Neururer R, Bartsch G, et al: Robotic pyeloplasty: technique and results. Urol Clin North Am 31:737–741, 2004.
20. Clayman RV: Anderson-Hynes dismembered pyeloplasty performed using the da Vinci robotic system. J Urol 170(2 pt 1):691–692, 2003.
21. Hubert J: Robotic pyeloplasty. Curr Urol Rep 4:124–129, 2003.
22. Gettman MT, Neururer R, Bartsch G, et al: Anderson-Hynes dismembered pyeloplasty performed using the da Vinci robotic system. Urology 60: 509–513, 2002.
23. Sung GT, Gill IS: Robotic laparoscopic surgery: a comparison of the DA Vinci and Zeus systems. Urology 58:893–898, 2001.
24. Atug F, Woods M, Burgess SV, et al: Robotic assisted laparoscopic pyeloplasty in children. J Urol 174(4 pt 1):1440–1442, 2005.
25. Bernie JE, Venkatesh R, Brown J, et al: Comparison of laparoscopic pyeloplasty with and without robotic assistance. JSLS 9:258–261, 2005.
26. Palese MA, Munver R, Phillips CK, et al: Robot-assisted laparoscopic dismembered pyeloplasty. JSLS 9:252–257, 2005.
27. Patel V: Robotic-assisted laparoscopic dismembered pyeloplasty. Urology 66:45–49, 2005.
28. Razdan S, Bagley DH, McGinnis DE: Minimizing minimally invasive surgery: the 5-mm trocar laparoscopic pyeloplasty. J Endourol 19:533–536, 2005.
29. Lorincz A, Knight CG, Kant AJ, et al: Totally minimally invasive robot-assisted unstented pyeloplasty using the Zeus Microwrist Surgical System: an animal study. J Pediatr Surg 40:418–422, 2005.
30. Lee R, Retik AB, Borer JG, et al: Pediatric robotic assisted laparoscopic dismembered pyeloplasty: comparison with a cohort of open surgery. J Urol 175:683–687, 2006.
31. Bonnard A, Fouquet V, Carricaburu E, et al: Retroperitoneal laparoscopic versus open pyeloplasty in children. J Urol 173:1710–1713, 2005. discussion 1713.

32. Peters CA: Laparoscopy in pediatric urology. Curr Opin Urol 14:67–73, 2004.
33. Valla JS, Al-Mohaidaly M, Tursini S, et al: Use of laparoscopy techniques in pediatric urology. Saudi Med J 24(5 suppl):S30, 2003.
34. Schier F: Laparoscopic Anderson-Hynes pyeloplasty in children. Pediatr Surg Int 13:497–500, 1998.
35. Peters CA, Schlussel RN, Retik AB: Pediatric laparoscopic dismembered pyeloplasty. J Urol 153:1962–1965, 1995.
36. Tan HL: Laparoscopic Anderson-Hynes dismembered pyeloplasty in children. J Urol 162(3 pt 2):1045–1047; discussion 1048, 1999.
37. Micali S, Caione P, Virgili G, et al: Retroperitoneal laparoscopic access in children using a direct vision technique. J Urol 165:1229–1232, 2001.
38. El-Ghoneimi A, Valla JS, Steyaert H, et al: Laparoscopic renal surgery via a retroperitoneal approach in children. J Urol 160(3 pt 2):1138–1141, 1998.
39. Casale P, Grady RW, Joyner BD, et al: Transperitoneal laparoscopic pyelolithotomy after failed percutaneous access in the pediatric patient. J Urol 172:680–683, 2004. discussion 683.
40. Ramakumar S, Lancini V, Chan DY, et al: Laparoscopic pyeloplasty with concomitant pyelolithotomy. J Urol 167:1378–1380, 2002.
41. Whelan JP, Wiesenthal JD: Laparoscopic pyeloplasty with simultaneous pyelolithotomy using a flexible ureteroscope. Can J Urol 11:2207–2209, 2004.
42. McDougall EM, Clayman RV, Bowles WT: Laparoscopic excision of mullerian duct remnant. J Urol 152(2 pt 1):482–484, 1994.
43. Willetts IE, Roberts JP, MacKinnon AE: Laparoscopic excision of a prostatic utricle in a child. Pediatr Surg Int 19:557–558, 2003.
44. Lakshmanan Y, Fung LC: Laparoscopic extravesicular ureteral reimplantation for vesicoureteral reflux: recent technical advances. J Endourol 14:589–593, 2000. discussion 593–594.
45. Lipski BA, Mitchell ME, Burns MW: Voiding dysfunction after bilateral extravesical ureteral reimplantation. J Urol 159:1019–1021, 1998.
46. Gill IS, Ponsky LE, Desai M, et al: Laparoscopic cross-trigonal Cohen ureteroneocystostomy: novel technique. J Urol 166:1811–1814, 2001.
47. Olsen LH, Deding D, Yeung CK, et al: Computer assisted laparoscopic pneumovesical ureter reimplantation a.m. Cohen: initial experience in a pig model. APMIS Suppl (109):23–25, 2003.
48. Peters CA, Woo R: Intravesical robotically assisted bilateral ureteral reimplantation. J Endourol 19:618–621, 2005. discussion 621–622.
49. Yeung CK, Sihoe JD, Borzi PA: Endoscopic cross-trigonal ureteral reimplantation under carbon dioxide bladder insufflation: a novel technique. J Endourol 19:295–299, 2005.
50. Jordan GH, Winslow BH: Laparoscopically assisted continent catheterizable cutaneous appendicovesicostomy. J Endourol 7:517–520, 1993.
51. Siqueria TM Jr, Paterson RF, Kuo RL, et al: Laparoscopic ileocytoplasty and continent ileovesicostomy in a porcine model. J Endourol 17:301–305, 2003.
52. Hedican SP, Schulam PG, Docimo SG: Laparoscopic assisted reconstructive surgery. J Urol 161:267–270, 1999.
53. Cadeddu JA, Docimo SG: Laparoscopic-assisted continent stoma procedures: our new standard. Urology 54:909–912, 1999.
54. Docimo SG, Moore RG, Adams J, et al: Laparoscopic bladder augmentation using stomach. Urology 46:565–569, 1995.
55. Pedraza R, Weiser A, Franco I: Laparoscopic appendicovesicostomy (Mitrofanoff procedure) in a child using the da Vinci robotic system. J Urol 171:1652–1653, 2004.
56. Elliott SP, Meng MV, Anwar HP, et al: Complete laparoscopic ileal cystoplasty. Urology 59:939–943, 2002.

CHAPTER 19

Simon C. Moten • Alan P. Kypson • W. Randolph Chitwood, Jr.

Use of Robotics in Other Surgical Specialties

INTRODUCTION

Recently, there has been an explosion in the use of robotics in multiple surgical specialties. After a realization of the persistent limitations of laparoscopic surgery combined with the real advantages of robotic surgery, being spectacular high-definition vision with depth perception, intuitive instrument motion with handlike degrees of freedom of movement, and ergonomic posturing for the surgeon, there has been a frenetic interest in and adoption of robotic techniques in surgery. Today the da Vinci surgical system (Intuitive Surgical, Sunnyvale, CA) remains the sole telemanipulative (robotic) system on the market. Its initial application focused on cardiac surgery; however, subsequently, it has made progressive strides into other specialties. Its application to urologic surgery is well documented. In this chapter we review its application to cardiac, general, and gynecologic surgery.

Currently, telemanipulation systems are beginning to revolutionize the way surgery is performed by overcoming limitations inherent in current endoscopic procedures. This has enabled surgeons to perform operations through even smaller incisions. More important, it has retained manual dexterity by translating fine hand motions through computer-controlled instrument arms placed inside the patient. Complex reconstructive surgery necessitating extensive suturing and intricate anastomoses, particularly when performed in a relatively limited space, have to date shown the greatest benefit with robotic surgery. Already this exciting technology has affected the way many surgical procedures are being performed. Although currently expensive, robotic telemanipulation of tissues and organs is necessary to pave the way for future technologic breakthroughs. Both robotics and adjunctive technology will be required for the evolution of minimally invasive surgery from extirpative and ablative procedures to full tissue reconstructions and accurate anastomoses. Advanced surgical robotic systems offer the promise of a unique combination of advantages over open and conventional laparoscopic approaches, including precise intricate instrument articulation, magnified three-dimensional (3D) visualization, camera stabilization and direct control, tremor filtration, motion scaling, and improved ergonomics. Despite widespread surgeon and patient enthusiasm for these procedures, we need to critically evaluate their impact, effectiveness, and clinical and economic benefit.

ROBOTIC TECHNOLOGY

Computer-assisted or robotic surgery has been developed to facilitate surgeon hand motions in limited operating spaces. These devices offer advantages such as improved access, magnified vision, and stabilized instrument implementation. Standard endoscopic instruments, with only four degrees of freedom, reduce operative dexterity significantly. When working through a fixed-entry trocar, fulcrum-dependent motion ensues, requiring the operator to reverse hand motions. At the same time, instrument shaft shear in the trocar, or resistive drag, induces higher forces needed to manipulate the operating tips leading to hand muscle fatigue. Also, human motor skills deteriorate with visual-motor incompatibility associated with most endoscopic surgery.

Computer-enhanced instrumentation systems can overcome these and other limitations. The surgeon operates from a console (Figure 19–1*A*), immersed in a 3D operative field. Through a computer interface, his or her motions are reproduced in scaled proportion through "microwrist" instruments that are mounted on robotic arms inserted through the body wall (Figure 19–1*B*). These instruments (Figure 19–2) emulate human X-Y-Z axis wrist activity throughout a full seven degrees of ergonomic freedom. Tremor filtering and motion scaling are translated into enhanced dexterity in confined operating spaces.

Initially, there were two competing robotic systems, Zeus (Computer Motion, Goleta, CA) and da Vinci. These devices differed from each other considerably. The advantages of the da Vinci system include integrated 3D visualization and a robotic wrist. The Zeus system lacks a fully articulated wrist, and the visualization system is two-dimensional; however, it was used in combination with 3D visualization

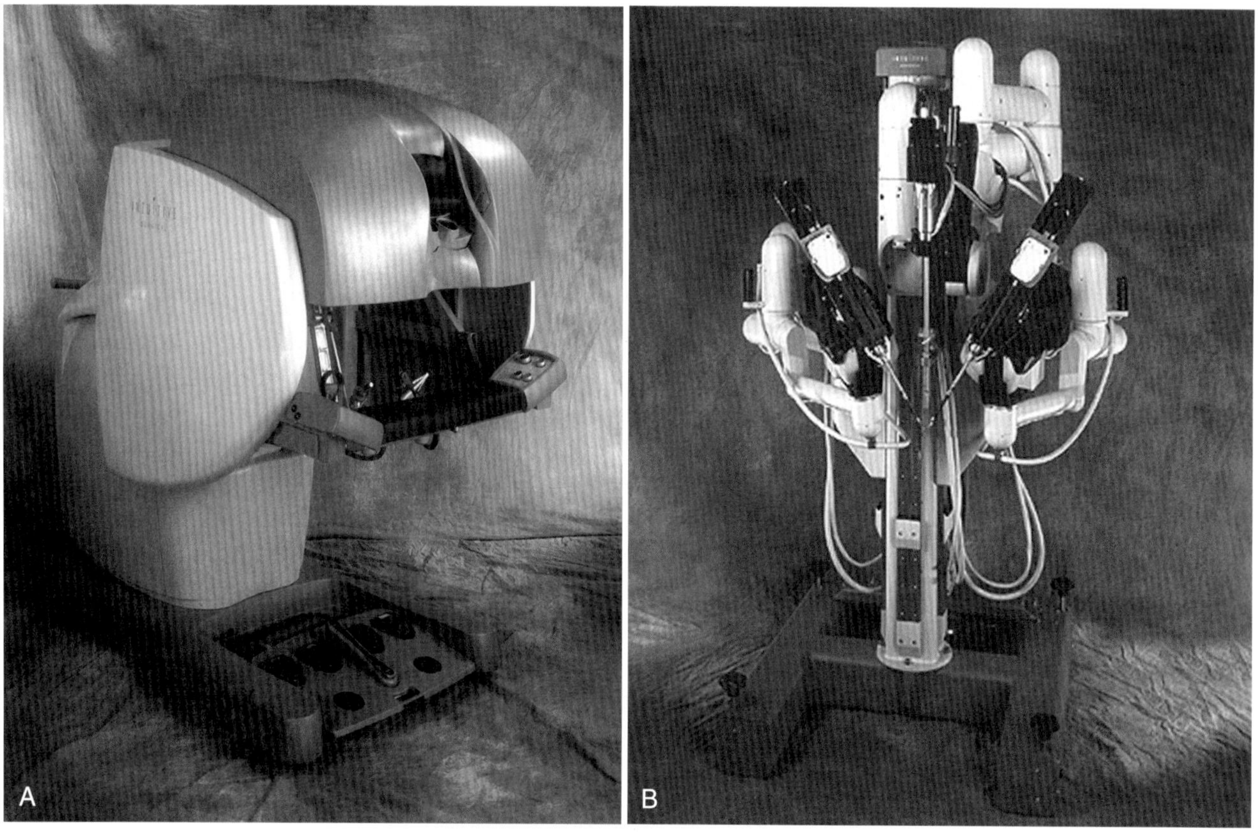

FIGURE 19–1 *A,* da Vinci Robotic Tele-manipulation System: the operative console where the surgeon is seated. *B,* da Vinci Robotic Tele-manipulation System: the instrument cart with two instrument arms and a camera arm that stands next to the operating room table.

systems developed independently. Interestingly, in 2003, Intuitive Surgical, Inc., acquired Zeus technology, leaving one robotic platform approved by the U.S. Food and Drug Administration (FDA) for clinical use. The FDA approved da Vinci for use in abdominal operations in 2000 and more recently for cardiac procedures.

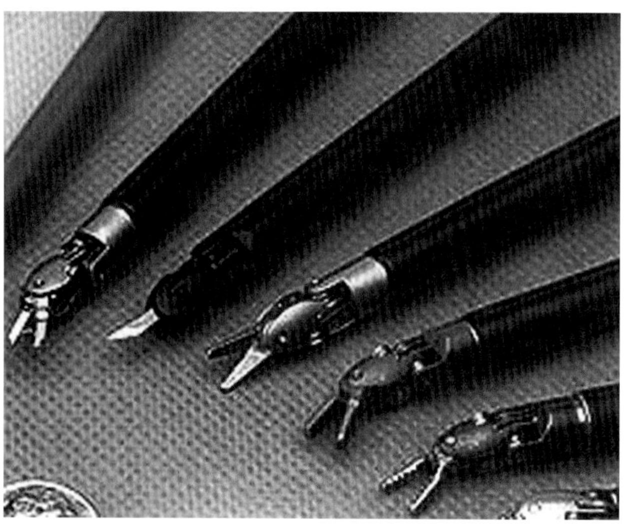

FIGURE 19–2 Various instrument arms that can be used in the da Vinci robotic system. Note the dime in the lower left-hand corner for scale.

ROBOTICS IN GENERAL SURGERY

As a whole, abdominal surgeons possess excellent videoendoscopic surgical skills. However, the limitations of laparoscopy, such as reduced range of motion, loss of instrument dexterity, and a two-dimensional view of the operative field, have inspired even the most accomplished laparoscopists to investigate the potential of surgical robotics to broaden their application of the minimally invasive surgery paradigm.

Compared with conventional endoscopy, a magnified 3D operative field with associated intuitively controlled articulating instruments should enhance surgeon precision and dexterity, presumably leading to better outcomes. Compared with cardiac surgery, where no real laparoscopic equivalent has existed, general surgeons have been less compelled to embrace robotics because of efficient conventional laparoscopic skills with the current level of technology and experience. Robotic telemanipulative systems have evolved to overcome some of the difficulties associated with handling long laparoscopic instruments, being limited instrument tip dexterity, less flexible tissue handling, reduced depth perception, and poor ergonomics and surgeon discomfort. Nevertheless, experience with robotics in abdominal surgery remains limited, and current approaches and setup are not standardized, reflecting the evolving nature of this field. Instrumentation for robotic abdominal surgery does not currently match the complement of laparoscopic instruments available. This affects operative times and further limits its wider application. Despite this, various units have demonstrated early success with robotic general surgery as detailed in the following.

Antireflux Surgery

Laparoscopic Nissen fundoplication has become increasingly popular since its introduction in the early 1990s, and by the time robotics were introduced into laparoscopic surgery in the late 1990s, laparoscopic fundoplication for gastroesophageal reflux had already proved effective. Because of these successes and decreased costs with laparoscopic technology, robotic applications for reflux surgery still remain limited. Because laparoscopic fundoplication does not require fine movement within a confined space to perform extensive suturing and/or knot tying, robotic-assisted fundoplication has, to date, provided few clinical advantages. Robotic operative times are longer, with little difference in outcomes from laparoscopic techniques. Typical port placement and setup for robotic Nissen fundoplication is shown in Figure 19–3. Despite this slow adoption, antireflux operations remain the only robotic application in general surgery that has randomized controlled clinical trial data.

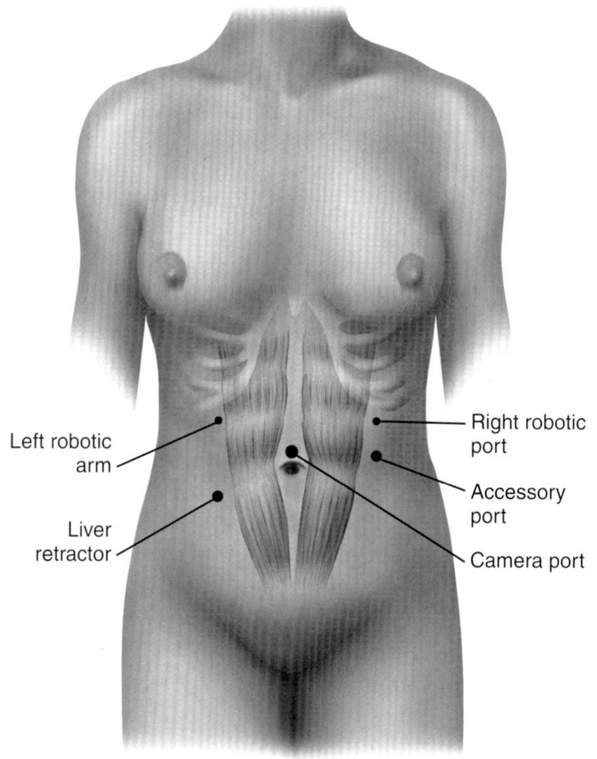

FIGURE 19–3 Schematic representation of port placement for robotic Nissen fundoplication. The camera port is placed approximately 2 cm above the umbilicus in the midline. Four additional ports are then placed under direct vision. A fan retractor is placed through a right-sided port. Ultrasonic dissectors and additional graspers can be placed through the accessory port.

In 2000, Chapman et al.[1] reported the first robotic Nissen fundoplication in a 56-year-old woman. Subsequently, Melvin et al.[2] compared 20 consecutive robotic Nissen fundoplications to 20 performed laparoscopically. The operative times in the robotic cohort averaged 45 minutes longer and had similar clinical outcomes. Cadiere et al.[3] prospectively randomized 21 patients undergoing Nissen fundoplication into laparoscopic ($n = 11$) and robotic operations ($n = 10$). Operative times were 52 minutes (range, 45–62 minutes) in the laparoscopic group and 76 minutes (range, 59–130 minutes) in the robotic group ($P < .01$). The mean time for hiatal dissection was 9 minutes (range, 5–14) in the laparoscopic group and 15 minutes (range, 8–27 minutes) in the robotic group ($P < .05$). Similarly, the mean suturing time for the fundal wrap was 6.5 minutes (range, 4–12 minutes) in the laparoscopic group and 8 minutes (range, 6–13 minutes) in the robotic group ($P = .151$). There were no conversions to an open operation, and a trocar stomach perforation was the single-study (robotic) complication. There was no difference in hospital length of stay. Each group experienced similar blood loss and perioperative morbidity. Recently, Hanly and Talamini[4] reported 57 robotic fundoplications with similar results. These studies demonstrated feasibility and safety with robotic fundoplications, and the general consensus among most groups has been that the da Vinci robotic system enables surgeons to perform advanced laparoscopic procedures with ease, safety, and precision, whereas comparisons with conventional laparoscopic techniques have shown longer operative times and increased cost with the same clinical benefit.[5,6] Despite these early successes, the reports of robotic fundoplication procedures remain limited to small series and isolated cases. To date, there is no clear clinical benefit from robotic fundoplication procedures compared with conventional laparoscopic procedures that have established excellent results.

Bariatric Surgery

Although great strides have been made in laparoscopic bariatric surgery, these operations still can be quite challenging. Because of the difficulty of insufflation and passage of instruments through the abdominal wall, a number of groups have explored the potential role of robotics.[7–9] The gastrojejunal anastomosis is a technically challenging step in laparoscopic gastric bypass. Different techniques have been described, including a circular-stapled, a linear-stapled, and a hand-sewn anastomosis in laparoscopic surgery. The da Vinci system, with its multiarticulated instruments, may help make a sewn gastrojejunostomy more plausible for surgeons. The system may be used for Roux-en-Y gastric bypass, for laparoscopic adjustable gastric banding, or for biliary pancreatic diversion. The da Vinci system offers a superior mechanical advantage over traditional laparoscopic instruments, particularly in extremely obese patients with body mass index greater than 60 kg/m^2. The depth of the abdominal wall creates increased torque on straight laparoscopic instruments, thereby making precise movements difficult, but this is overcome by the power of the robotic system.

In September 1998, Cadiere et al.[7] performed the first robotic-assisted gastric band procedure. They reported 10 robotic-assisted gastroplasties done for morbid obesity. The mean operative time was 60 minutes, with no complications. The main benefit was to improve ergonomics to improve surgeon dexterity during tissue manipulation. No differences were found in outcomes when compared with conventional laparoscopic gastric banding.

Horgan and Vanuno[8] performed the first robotic-assisted gastric bypass in September 2000. Thereafter, they reported seven successful robotic gastric bypass operations as well as two other gastrojejunostomies, proving evidence for feasibility in bariatric procedures.[8] The authors surmised that the microprecision articulating instruments and 3D view facilitated the hand-sewn (robotic-sewn) anastomosis significantly. Furthermore, the robotic system minimized surgeon fatigue by decreasing instrument radial torque at the trocar, which often causes a conflict to maintain instrument position. Recently, Jacobsen and colleagues[9] published a multicenter series of 107 robotically assisted gastric bypass operations. Outcomes were excellent, and there were no postoperative gastric leaks or mortality. There were four complications: two improper port placements, one imaging system malfunction, and one robotic arm movement difficulty.

Totally robotic laparoscopic Roux-en-Y gastric bypass procedure using the da Vinci surgical system has been safely performed in 10 patients.[10] This report is rare in that it documented reduced surgical time with use of the robotic surgical procedure versus conventional laparoscopic Roux-en-Y gastric bypass surgery (169 versus 208 minutes). Additional prospective, randomized studies are needed to assess the advantages of robotically assisted bariatric surgery.

Biliary Surgery

Multiple series have been published establishing the feasibility of the robotic cholecystectomy. These reports show that the method is learned readily and results are at least equivalent to the laparoscopic cholecystectomy. The first robotic-assisted cholecystectomy was performed by Himpens in 1997.[11] Later studies[12–16] reported similar successes despite longer operative times. Nevertheless, clinical outcomes were no different from conventional endoscopic operations. Of the total 127 robotic-assisted cases reported in the literature, there were only 3 complications and no mortality.

Preoperative setup of the robot requires additional time. Typical robot positioning and port placement is shown in Figure 19–4. Robotic cholecystectomy operative technique is similar to that for laparoscopic techniques (Figure 19–5). In reported series, setup times averaged an additional 14 minutes. Ballantyne and colleagues[14] have reported on 25 da Vinci operations. The total operative times were increased initially but decreased with experience. The robotic mean operative time was 110 ± 33 minutes compared with 99 ± 28 in an endoscopic control group ($P < .05$). There were no open conversions, and clinical outcomes were similar to those for the control group. The hospital length of stay was similar between groups (1.2 ± 0.6 versus 1.6 ± 1.6; P = NS). Kim et al.[12] reported 10 patients who underwent robotic cholecystectomy with an operative time of 60 ± 25 minutes. Ruurda and colleagues[13] reported 35 cases with a median 82-minute surgical time. Length of stay was similar in all of these studies, and there was no operative mortality. In all

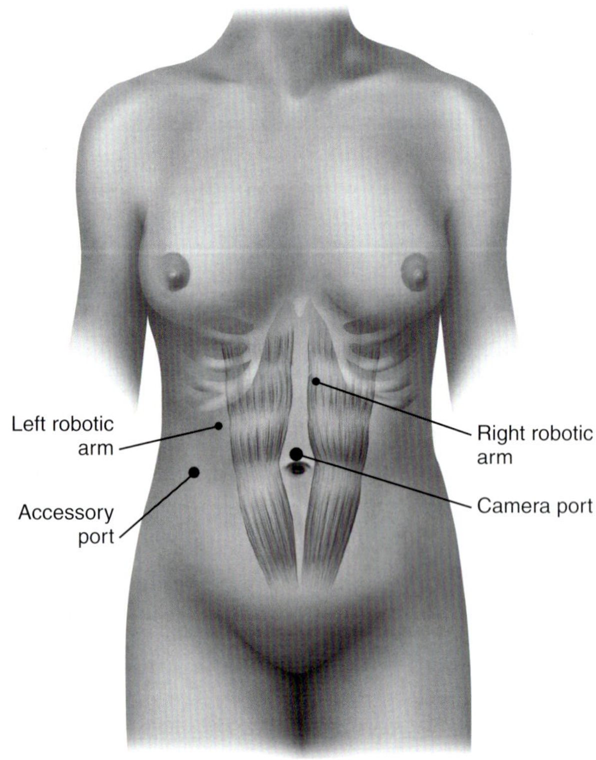

FIGURE 19–4 Diagram of port placement for robotic cholecystectomy. The camera port is placed cephalad to the umbilicus. Under direct vision, the robotic arm ports are placed in the right upper quadrant (midclavicular line) and just to the left of midline in the epigastric region. An accessory port is used as necessary.

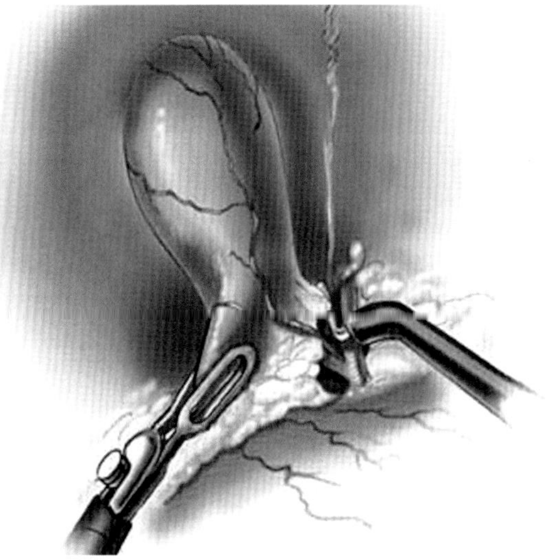

FIGURE 19–5 Robotic cholecystectomy performed with da Vinci. Dissection of the gallbladder is performed in similar fashion to laparoscopic surgery.

of these series, the ductal anatomy was seen much better because of the magnified 3D image. Furthermore, all authors agreed that robotic assistance facilitated dissection. Whether using robotic systems with improved dexterity and better anatomic visualization will translate into a reduction in bile duct injuries will not be known until large, multicenter trials are conducted.

Splenic Surgery

Robotically assisted splenectomies have been performed more frequently than other general surgical procedures; however, only a few published series exist.[17,18] The high-definition, magnified 3D view associated with da Vinci improves the ability to identify vessel architecture and topographic relationships to the pancreas. Robotic instruments allow precise manipulation of the fragile splenic hilum and exposure of the vessels. Chapman et al.[18] described the first robotically assisted splenectomy for idiopathic thrombocytopenic purpura. Complete dissection of the spleen took 31 minutes. The total operating time was 90 minutes, and the robot setup time was only 9 minutes. The patient was discharged less than 24 hours after admission. Hanly and Talamini.[4] reported 16 cases with operative times ranging from 90 to 240 minutes, with no complications.

In a recent critical assessment of minimally invasive splenectomies, Bodner et al.[19] reported that using either conventional laparoscopic techniques or the da Vinci robotic system are feasible; however, the robotic system resulted in prolonged overall operative time and significantly higher procedural costs. No relevant benefit could be attributed to the robotic system for laparoscopic splenectomy, thereby making its use unjustifiable at present.

Pancreatic Surgery

Just as with computer-assisted splenic operations, there are few reports that detail robotic pancreatic resections.[4,20–22] Melvin et al.[20] reported the first robotic resection of a pancreatic lesion (neuroendocrine tumor in the tail of the pancreas). Subsequently, he described five patients (one developed a pancreatic fistula that healed without further treatment) who underwent robotic sutured pancreaticojejunostomy after an open pancreaticoduodenectomy. Melvin[21] concluded that precise tissue manipulation and 3D imaging may allow a better surgical approach to a complex task such as reconstruction of the pancreatic duct as compared with open or laparoscopic-assisted surgery. Furthermore, Giulianotti et al.[22] have performed three full robotic pancreatoduodenectomies and eight full robotic left pancreatectomies. One death occurred in this small series. Results, thus far, have been encouraging. However, concern over robotic resection of pancreatic head tumors has been raised[4] because of the lack of haptic feedback inherent in today's robotic systems.

Adrenal Glands

In most centers, open adrenalectomies have been supplanted by laparoscopic methods. Reports describing robotically assisted adrenalectomies exist,[23–25] but no clinical trials have been performed comparing robotic adrenalectomy with either an open or a laparoscopic adrenalectomy. In 1999, Piazza et al.[26] first published a robotic-assisted adrenalectomy that took 3 hours and had no complications. Since then, Hanly and Talamini[4] have performed 30 robotic adrenalectomies for adrenal masses ($n = 18$), pheochromocytomas ($n = 9$), and aldosteronomas ($n = 3$) without an open conversion. Robotic visualization and instrumentation greatly facilitate identification of the small adrenal vessels and the posterior and lateral dissection of the adrenal gland. The wristlike movements of the instrument's tip facilitate detachment of surrounding organs from the gland and vessel isolation, while the 3D vision facilitates dissection of the veins from the vena cava. Young et al.[25] found that the ability to control the camera from the console and zoom in on pertinent structures enabled a very precise dissection. They concluded that the robotic dissection was more accurate than a standard laparoscopic dissection.

Colorectal Surgery

The first two robotically assisted colectomies were performed in 2001.[27] Since then, groups have published studies comparing laparoscopic to robotically assisted colon surgery. Delaney et al.[28] compared patients undergoing right hemicolectomies, sigmoid colectomies, and proctopexy to matched laparoscopic controls. Although the robotic system facilitated the performance of intricate colonic mobilization and accurate vascular ligation, only operative time and cost differed significantly between the groups (robotic: >1 hour and $350 more per case). Operative times increased from a median time of 108 minutes for standard laparoscopic colorectal surgery to 165 minutes for robotic-assisted laparoscopic surgeries. Munz et al.[29] compared robotic nonresectional proctopexies with historical laparoscopic controls. Robotic repairs had no perioperative morbidity, recurrent prolapse, or constipation. Comparatively, 19% of control patients had one of these complications. In contrast, D'Annibale et al.[30] compared retrospectively 53 patients operated using traditional laparoscopic techniques to an equal cohort done robotically. His group found no significant differences in operative times, specimen length, number of lymph nodes retrieved, bowel function recovery, or length of hospital stay (Table 19–1). The only significant difference seen was longer times to prepare the operating room for robotic surgery. Other groups have limited their robotic applications to patients with benign disease, such as recurrent diverticular disease and laparoscopically unresectable polyps.[4]

The da Vinci system was initially designed for use in cardiac surgery. The requirements of abdominal surgery were not initially contemplated in the original design. As such, the range of instrumentation for abdominal surgery is limited. The large bulky robot arms are not attached to the operating table and must therefore be removed during maneuvers to reposition the patient, thereby delaying complex abdominal procedures. The large excursions of the arms on the exterior often lead to collisions and restricted internal motion.

ROBOTICS IN THORACIC SURGERY

There are relatively few reports describing noncardiac robotic thoracic surgery. The number of operations performed at any one institution has often been insufficient to achieve adequate experience. Transthoracic robotic surgery requires different planning than other robotic procedures because of the rigidity of the chest wall and potential external conflict with surrounding structures, in particular the patient's shoulder. Preoperative chest computed tomography is integral to the successful placement of trocars, which require careful positioning to optimally use the rotational degrees of freedom inherent in da Vinci.

Robotic technology can be used to perform advanced intrathoracic maneuvers thoracoscopically. The da Vinci robot allows precise dissection in remote and difficult-to-reach areas, making the rigid anatomy of the chest an ideal condition for robotic surgery. A major limitation for robotic thoracic surgery remains the lack of more appropriate instruments.

Heller Cardiomyotomy

Laparoscopic Heller myotomy is the treatment of choice for achalasia. Recent data suggest that computer-enhanced robotic techniques provide an advantage over standard laparoscopy for the operative treatment of achalasia.[31] Robotic Heller cardiomyotomies have been described by several groups who demonstrated excellent outcomes with minimal to no complications[32–34] (Table 19–2). The superior imaging qualities provide excellent visualization of esophageal muscle fibers, facilitating differentiation from the submucosal plane. This seems helpful in avoiding mucosal perforations. Also, the articulated instrument tips may facilitate myotomy extension and reduce cautery tip injury of the mucosa.

In a large series of 104 patients by Melvin et al.[31] who underwent robotic Heller myotomy with partial fundoplication, there were no esophageal perforations, only eight minor complications, and one conversion to open procedure. Thus, the application of computer-enhanced operative techniques appears to provide superior outcomes in selected esophageal procedures; however, avoidance of mucosal perforation has not been shown in all series but can be managed successfully robotically.[33] In addition, other potential benefits of robotic Heller myotomy may be the avoidance of the need for an antireflux procedure because of the minimal lateral and posterior dissection with the use of wristed instruments.[33]

Table 19–1 Surgical Parameters

	VLS (Mean ± SD)	ROB (Mean ± SD)	*P* Value
da Vinci system and patient setup time	18 ± 7	24 ± 12	0.002
Operating time (min)	222 ± 77	240 ± 61	NS
Specimen length (cm)	29 ± 11	27 ± 13	NS
No. of lymph nodes	16 ± 9	17 ± 10	NS
Intraoperative blood loss (ml)	37 ± 102	21 ± 80	NS

NS, not significant; ROB, robotic group; SD, standard deviation; VLS, conventional laparoscopic group.

Modified from D'Annibale A, Morpurgo E, Fiscon V, et al: Robotic and laparoscopic surgery for treatment of colorectal diseases. Dis Colon Rectum 47:2162, 2004.

Table 19–2 Initial Experience in Foregut Procedures

	Nissen	Heller	Toupet	Diagnostic Laparoscopy	Distal Pancreatectomy	Esophagectomy	Pyloroplasty
Number	20	9	2	1	1	1	1
Average patient age (yr)	44	49	50.5	64	44	53	56
Average robot use time (min)	84	84	125	16	185	108	42
Average total operating time (min)	140	139	174	190	275	462	128
Average length of hospital stay (days)	1.4	1	1	7	4	12	3

Modified from Melvin WS, Needleman BJ, Krause KR, et al: Computer-enhanced robotic telesurgery: initial experience in foregut surgery. Surg Endosc 16:1790, 2002.

Esophageal Resection

Dissection of the intrathoracic esophagus and adjacent lymph nodes is feasible using a robotic-assisted thoracoscopic approach. Resections of both malignant and benign tumors are feasible. In 2004, Elli and colleagues[35] reported two patients with esophageal leiomyomas who underwent right-sided robotic extirpation with operative times of 2 hours. Tumor removal was performed without mucosal perforation.

An entirely robotic esophagectomy was reported by Melvin et al.[32] Surgeons robotically completed both the thoracic esophageal dissection with gastric mobilization and then performed the esophagogastrostomy using a modified Ivor-Lewis technique. The procedure took 7.5 hours, and the patient was discharged 12 days later without any complications.[32] Operative times continue to improve, and Bodner et al.[36] reported their series of six patients with esophageal tumors. Median overall operating time was 173 minutes in the four oncologic cases and 121 minutes in the two benign cases. No intraoperative complications were encountered. Nevertheless, robotic-assisted esophageal resections are still prone to complications associated with laparoscopic and open approaches, such as operative mortality, anastomotic leaks, chylous leaks, and vocal cord paralysis[37]; however, direct comparison in a randomized trial has not been performed.

Robotic transhiatal resections have also been described.[38,39] In nine patients, the mean operative time was 312 minutes (range, 245–360 minutes). The estimated blood loss was less than 60 mL per procedure, and the intensive care unit stay was between 1 and 5 days.[39] No operative deaths occurred, and the average length of hospital stay was 8 days. Other more recent series substantiate these outcomes as well.[40]

Thymectomy

The first robotic thymectomy was performed in January of 2001 by Yoshino et al.[41] Using a combined robotic and mediastinotomy approach, a 2.5-cm thymoma was resected in a little more than 2 hours. Patients with myasthenia gravis also have had excellent results with this approach.[40,41] In a series of 21 myasthenic patients, 40% were discharged on the same day of surgery, with an additional 40% discharged within 24 hours.[40] No postoperative cases of myasthenic crisis have been described, and this may relate to the reduced surgery-induced acute phase response. Savitt and coworkers[42] reported their series of 18 robotic-assisted resections of anterior mediastinal masses, which included 14 patients who underwent successful robotic-assisted thymectomy. No conversions, intraoperative complications, or deaths occurred. The mean operative time was 96 minutes (range, 62–132 minutes), with a mean robotic time of 48 minutes (range, 22–76 minutes) and a median hospital stay of 2 days.

Pulmonary Lobectomies

In 2001, initial reports of robotic pulmonary lobectomies emerged.[43,44] Operative times approached 6 hours in some early cases. The largest series of robotic lobectomies described 19 patients.[45] All had peripheral, small (<3 cm) tumors. Operative time ranged from 2.5 to 5.9 hours (median, 3.5 hours), and the hospital length of stay was 2 to 8 days (median, 4 days). Further details of robotic pulmonary resections are limited to case reports.[46,47] Currently, a major limitation of robotic surgery in this field is the lack of appropriate instruments, such as bronchial and vascular staplers. To date, there have been no reports of robotic segmentectomy, metastasectomy, tracheal, or bronchial procedures.

Resection of Mediastinal Masses

Several case reports of mediastinal mass resection exist, including posterior mediastinal masses[41,47,48] and other benign mediastinal masses.[46] Advantages over thorascopic or open procedures are not assessable at this time because of the limited numbers.

ROBOTICS IN CARDIAC SURGERY

Coronary Artery Bypass Grafting

Endoscopic coronary artery bypass surgery is limited to only a few centers, and the results are highly controlled. Coronary surgery depends on multiple, complex steps culminating in the creation of a vascular anastomosis. As such, most clinical series introduced robotically assisted coronary surgery in a step-by-step fashion. Initial experience was therefore limited to endoscopic left internal mammary artery (LIMA) harvesting (Figure 19–6), followed by a robotically assisted anastomosis through a median sternotomy, and finally a totally endoscopic procedure performed on an arrested heart followed by a beating heart operation.

In May 1998, Mohr et al.[50] and Falk et al.[50] harvested a LITA with da Vinci and performed the first clinical coronary anastomosis through a small left anterior thoracotomy incision. Carpentier's group in Broussais[51] described the first two totally endoscopic coronary operations in June 1998. The Leipzig group attempted a total closed chest approached for LIMA to left anterior descending artery (LAD) grafting of the arrested heart in 27 patients and was successful in 22.[52]

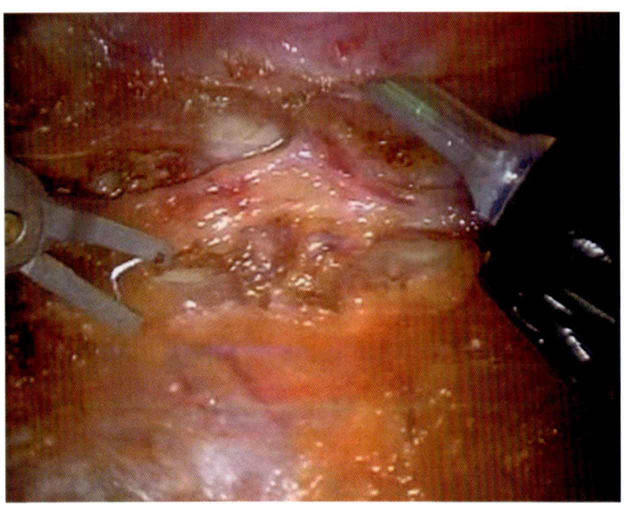

FIGURE 19–6 Left internal thoracic artery harvest using the da Vinci system. Robotic clip applicator shown in the left arm and electrocautery in the right arm. Harvesting techniques are similar to traditional methods.

Internal mammary artery harvesting can be performed in the range of 25 to 40 minutes for both the LIMA and the right internal mammary artery (IMA) following an initial learning curve. Harvesting of the pedicled or skeletonized IMA[53,54] is possible for both left and right mammary arteries, from a unilateral port placement, using the da Vinci system. Coronary anastomoses can then be performed, incorporating cardiac stabilizers, through a small lateral thoracotomy, without cardiopulmonary bypass.[49] Srivastava et al.[55] have published results from their first 200 cases using a similar approach, with good early results. Planned complete revascularization was achieved in all patients, with an average of 2.9 ± 1.1 grafts per patient. Conversion to cardiopulmonary bypass was required in two patients (1%). At East Carolina University, we have used this approach to robotic coronary surgery in conjunction with robotic mitral valve procedures.[56]

Furthermore, surgeons in Europe improved the initial da Vinci coronary method and were eventually able to complete bilateral IMA grafts off-pump to the anterior descending and right coronary arteries while working from one side of the chest.[57,58] Total endoscopic coronary artery bypass (TECAB) is now feasible and safe. Nevertheless, with current technology, these operations are usually performed on single-vessel (LAD) disease with either an arrested heart using the port access system or a beating heart using a specially designed endoscopic stabilizer.[59] Clinical trials are currently underway in Europe and North America.

The largest published series of TECAB comes from Wimmer-Greinnecker's group in Frankfurt, which includes 45 patients who underwent TECAB on an arrested heart.[60] Most of these (82%) were single-vessel bypass (either LIMA-LAD or right IMA to the right coronary artery). The first 22 patients had angiograms prior to discharge, revealing a 100% patency rate. Mean operative time for single-vessel TECAB was 4.2 ± 0.9 hours and 6.3 ± 1.0 hours for double-vessel bypass procedures (Table 19–3). Average cross-clamp time for single bypass was 61 ± 16 minutes and 99 ± 55 minutes for double bypass. The initial conversion rate of 22% decreased to 5% in the last 20 patients, reflecting an obvious learning curve.

Kappert and coworkers[61] described TECAB in 37 patients, of which 29 were performed on a beating heart. Double-vessel bypass using bilateral mammary arteries was performed in 29 of these, with the remainder receiving a LIMA to LAD. As experience was gained, the duration of surgery decreased noticeably from 280 ± 80.2 minutes to 186 ± 58.6 minutes. An average of 30 ± 6.5 minutes for robotically performed anastomosis versus 12 ± 3 minutes

Table 19–3 Intraoperative Data of Totally Endoscopic Coronary Procedures

Patient Groups	Operating Time (hr)	Port Placement (min)	IMA Takedown (min)	Anastomosis (min)	CPB Time (min)	Cross-Clamp Time (min)
Single vessel (*n* = 37) (LIMA-LAD, RIMA-RCA)	4.2 ± 0.9	15.4 ± 5.7	65 ± 21	18.4 ± 3.8	136 ± 32	61 ± 16
Double vessel (*n* = 8) (LIMA-DB-LAD, BIMA)	6.3 ± 1.0	18.4 ± 4.9	118 ± 12.3	21.1 ± 6.3	197 ± 63	90 ± 55

Values are mean ± SD. BIMA, bilateral internal mammary artery; CPB, cardiac bypass; DB, diagonal branch artery; IMA, internal mammary artery; LAD, left anterior descending coronary artery; LIMA, left internal mammary artery; RCA, right coronary artery; RIMA, right internal mammary artery. Modified from Dogan S, Aybek T, Andreßen E, et al: Totally endoscopic coronary artery bypass grafting on cardiopulmonary bypass with robotically enhanced telemanipulation: report of forty-five cases. J Thorac Cardiovasc Surg 123:1125–1131, 2002.

for directly hand-sewn anastomoses was observed. Currently, the midterm follow-up angiography is being performed to assess graft patency.

Mitral Valve Surgery

In May 1998, Carpentier et al.[62] performed the first mitral valve repair using da Vinci. In May 2000, under an FDA safety and efficacy trial, our group performed the first complete robotic mitral valve repair in North America.[63] Using the articulated wrist instruments, a trapezoidal resection of a large P_2 was performed with the defect closed using multiple interrupted sutures, followed by implantation of an annuloplasty band. In the early series of 20 patients, quadrangular leaflet resections, leaflet sliding plasties, chord transfers, polytetrafluoroethylene chord replacements, reduction annuloplasties, and annuloplasty band insertions were successfully performed (Figures 19–7 and 19–8). The mean total arrest time was 150 minutes, with 52 minutes used for leaflet repairs. Of the total arrest time, a mean of 42 minutes was needed to place an average of 7.5 annuloplasty band sutures. Total operating room times averaged 4.8 hours. There were no device-related complications and only one complication—a reexploration for bleeding from an atrial pacing wire. The average postoperative stay was 4 days (range, 3–7 days). At 3-month follow-up, echocardiography revealed nothing more than trace mitral regurgitation. All patients returned to normal activity by 1 month after surgery.[64]

We have published our results for the first 38 mitral repairs with the da Vinci system.[65] Patients were divided into two cohorts of 19 patients (early experience and late experience) for data analysis and comparison. Total robotic times represent the exact time of robot deployment after valve exposure up until the end of the annuloplasty band placement.

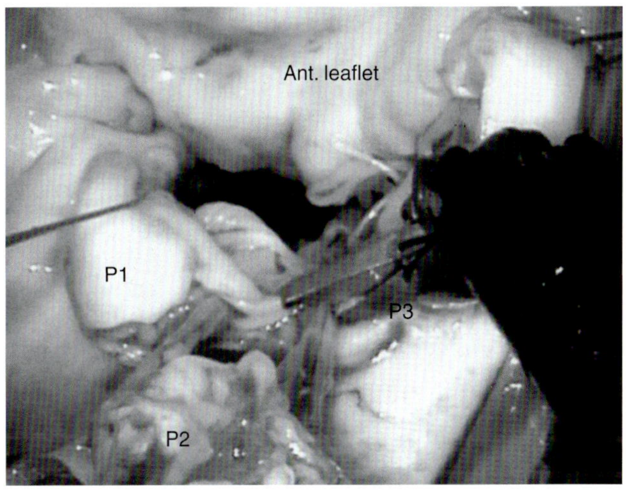

FIGURE 19–7 da Vinci mitral valve repair: The P_2 segment of the posterior leaflet is being resected by robotic microscissors. The annulus is reduced and both P_1 and P_3 approximated.

This time decreased significantly from 1.9 ± 0.1 hours in the first group to 1.5 ± 0.1 hours in the second group (P = .002). Concurrently, leaflet repair time decreased significantly, from 1.0 ± 0.1 hour in the first group to 0.6 ± 0.1 hour in the second group (P = .004). Total operating time decreased significantly from 5.1 ± 0.1 hours to 4.4 ± 0.1 hours in the second group. Furthermore, both cross-clamp and bypass times decreased significantly with experience. Similar time trends were reported in a later publication that reviewed subsequent da Vinci patient data.[66] The only time that did not change between the two groups was the annuloplasty band placement time, related to suture knot tying times. For the entire group of 38 patients, the mean length of stay was 3.8 days, with no difference between the two groups. For all patients in the study, 84% demonstrated a reduction of three or more grades in mitral regurgitation at follow-up. There were no

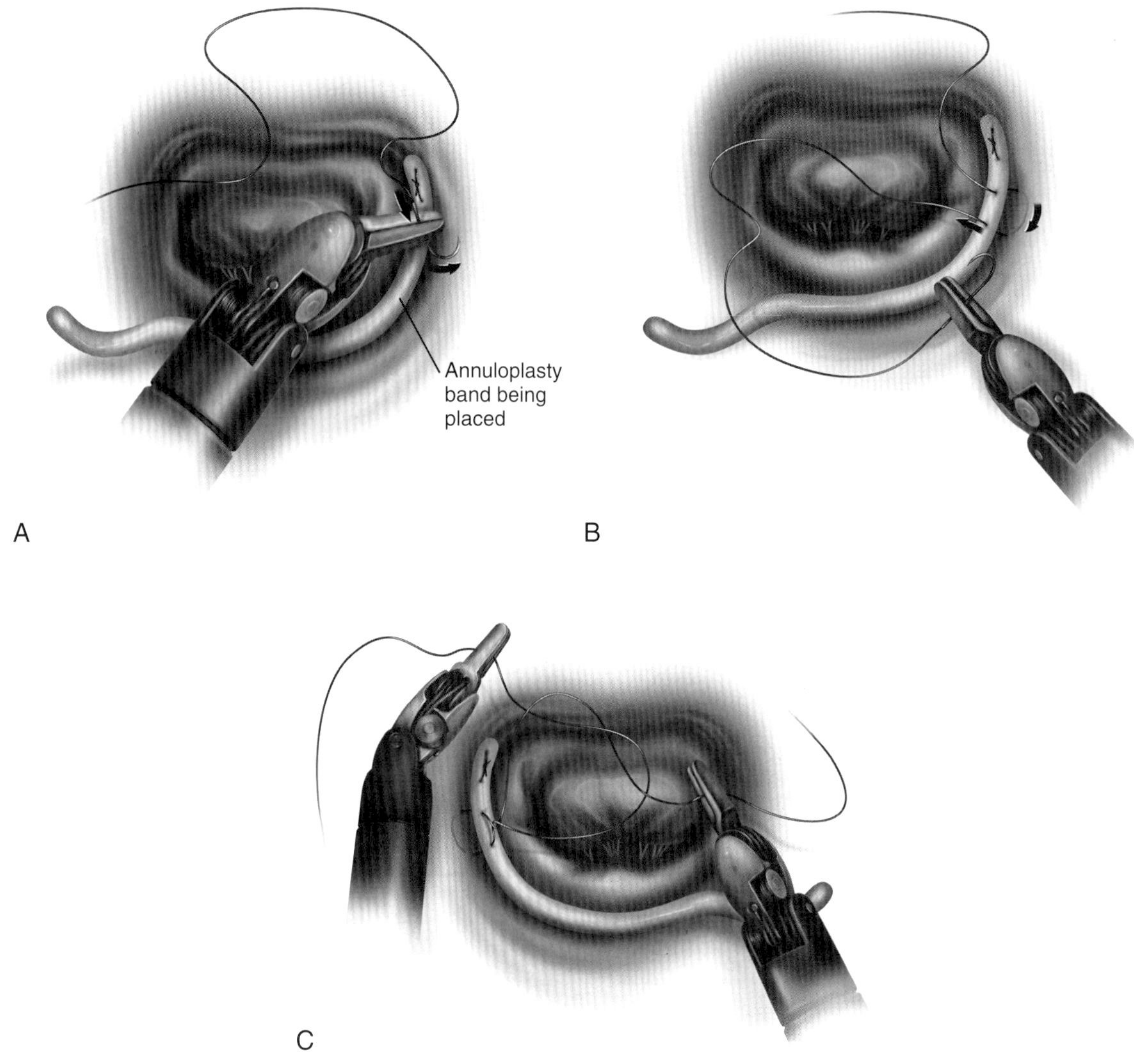

FIGURE 19–8 Robotic suture placement for a mitral band annuloplasty. Ten-centimeter 2-0 Ti-Cron sutures are placed and tied serially. Using a robotic needle holder, this single arm suture is placed first through the band *(A)* and then through the annulus *(B)*, and back through the band. Six knots generally will secure the band tightly with the proper amount of annular compression *(C)*.

device-related complications or operative deaths. One of the valves was replaced at 19 days because of hemolysis secondary to a leak directed against a prosthetic chord.

In addition to our own experience, results from a prospective multicenter phase II FDA trial have been published.[67] In this trial involving 10 institutions, da Vinci was used to perform mitral valve repairs in 112 patients. Valve repairs included quadrangular resections, sliding-plasties, edge-to-edge approximations, and both chordal transfers and replacements. Leaflet repair times averaged 36.7 ± 0.2 minutes with annuloplasty times of 39.6 ± 0.1 minutes. Total robot, aortic cross-clamp, and cardiopulmonary bypass times were 77.9 ± 0.3 minutes, 2.1 ± 0.1 hours, and 2.8 ± 0.1 hours, respectively. At 1-month follow-up, transthoracic echocardiography revealed nine patients (8.0%) had grade 2 or higher mitral regurgitation and six (5.4%) of these had reoperations (five replacements, one repair). There were no deaths, strokes, or device-related complications. This study demonstrated that multiple surgical teams could perform robotic mitral valve surgery safely early in the development of this technique.

To date, we have performed more than 240 robotic mitral valve repairs with the da Vinci system. One operative death occurred as a result of a protamine reaction, and two late deaths occurred more than 60 days after surgery. We have had no device-related injuries or alterations in the operative approach. Four patients required late reoperations secondary to hemolysis or an increasing leak. Operative times have progressively fallen, and new technology, such as the nitinol clips, has been a major factor in streamlining these operations. Moreover, we now are able to focus on more complex operations in patients with bileaflet prolapse, in which multiple chordal transfers and leaflet tailoring are mandatory.

The anchoring of annuloplasty bands with interrupted mattress sutures was initially a long part of the total repair time.[65] With the introduction of nitinol U-clips (Medtronic, Minneapolis MN) for annuloplasty band insertion, this time has been reduced significantly.[68,69] At East Carolina University, we have recently introduced use of a fourth robotic arm that is used to control a new left atrial retractor. Improved and simpler exposure, that is adjustable, has further led to ease of robotic valve repair.

Minimally invasive mitral valve repair can be performed with similar operative times compared with standard techniques using a median sternotomy.[70] Current experience demonstrates that robotically assisted mitral valve repair can also be performed safely and with satisfactory early results.[71] Early extubation and early hospital discharge, within 24 hours of surgery, are possible. Our group has demonstrated fewer pulmonary complications and reoperations for bleeding.[65,72] Reduced surgical trauma, decreased pain, fewer complications, improved cosmesis, shorter length of stay, and earlier return to a normal daily activity for the patient has been consistently reported with robotic and minimally invasive mitral procedures.[72] Patient satisfaction with minimally invasive mitral valve repair is also improved through better cosmetic results.[73]

Left Ventricular Lead Placement

Cardiac resynchronization therapy via left ventricular (LV) and right ventricular (RV) pacing is an effective therapy for heart failure.[74–76] Current percutaneous LV lead placement techniques, via the coronary sinus, are associated with a 10% to 15% failure rate.[76,77] Lead dislodgement contributes to an additional 5% to 10% late failure rate of LV lead capture.[78] Furthermore, procedure time for implantation often remains prolonged. Appropriate LV site stimulation also remains critical for complete LV resynchronization. Epicardial left ventricular pacing leads for cardiac resynchronization therapy can be accurately and expeditiously attached on a beating heart using the da Vinci robot system.[79,80]

Congenital Heart Disease

Totally endoscopic closed chest atrial septal defect (ASD) repair, including sinus venosus defects, is readily achievable with an almost identical approach to mitral valve repair.[81,82] Robotic-assisted closure enables direct suture closure under direct vision, using standard repair techniques, while providing an alternative for patients desiring a minimally invasive ASD repair who may not be eligible for or reluctant to consider catheter-based interventions (which remain investigational in the United States). ASD repair or closure of patent foramen ovale can be performed endoscopically, using three-port incisions and a small working incision. Pericardiotomy, bicaval occlusion, right atriotomy, atrial septopexy (direct suture or patch closure), and atrial closure can be performed with the da Vinci system. Early series have reported favorable results with median cross-clamp times of 32 minutes and CPB times of 122 minutes.[83] Robotic ASD closure gained FDA approval in 2003.

GYNECOLOGY

The first gynecologic procedure performed with a robot was a tubal anastomosis. This was performed in 1998 with the Zeus robot.[84] With the development of current robotic technology, other robotic gynecologic procedures have been performed. As this technology develops, the applications for its use in gynecology and gynecologic oncology will increase.

Hysterectomy

The use of a computer-enhanced surgical robot for performing hysterectomy in humans was first reported in 2002 by Diaz-Arrastia and colleagues.[85] In this series, 11 patients underwent laparoscopic hysterectomy and bilateral salpingo-oophorectomy using a surgical robot. Operative time ranged from 4.5 to 10 hours. Subsequent reports of laparoscopic hysterectomies with da Vinci have shown similar operative results to those of standard laparoscopic hysterectomy.[86] In this series of 10 patients, lysis of adhesions, suturing, and knot tying were enhanced with the robotic system, prompting the authors to conclude that the robotic hysterectomy offered unique advantages over existing standard laparoscopic techniques.

Robotic-assisted hysterectomy has also been shown to provide a tool to overcome the surgical limitations seen with conventional laparoscopy in difficult cases in which variations in anatomy may limit laparoscopic techniques, such as pelvic adhesive disease with a scarred or obliterated anterior cul de sac.[87]

Complex Procedures

Further experience with robotic systems has allowed more complex procedures to be performed. Melamud et al.[88] reported the first case of robotic-assisted laparoscopic repair of a vesicovaginal fistula. Total operative time was 280 minutes, which included placement of ureteral catheters and repositioning. The fistula was repaired using robot-assisted laparoscopic techniques without complications, and the patient was discharged on the second postoperative day. Reports such as this suggested that robotic systems could successfully gain wider acceptance over more technically difficult laparoscopic procedures.

The use and benefit of robotic-assisted laparoscopic sacrocolpopexy in the treatment of posthysterectomy vaginal vault prolapse has also been reported, with facilitation of precise intracorporeal suture placement so that the procedure could be done in a fashion similar to that of the open method. Robotic-assisted laparoscopic sacrocolpopexy may therefore provide the same long-term durability of open sacrocolpopexy with the benefit of a minimally invasive approach.[89]

Tubal Anastomosis

Laparoscopic microsurgical tubal anastomosis may be performed with or without robotic assistance. In a comparison of the two techniques, operative times were 2 hours longer with robotic assistance, using the Zeus robotic system, and there was increased estimated blood loss. No benefit in patient recovery was shown with the robotic approach. Therefore, although robotic assistance is feasible, no appreciable improvement in patient recovery or clinical outcomes has been shown as compared with laparoscopic anastomosis.[90]

LIMITATIONS AND FUTURE DIRECTIONS

The early clinical experience with computer-enhanced telemanipulation systems has defined many limitations despite rapid procedural success. In the past, most surgeons believed that operations could not be done without optimal tactility or force feedback. When deformational or material characteristics are translated through long instruments and especially robotic arms, this response is either muted or absent. The level of fidelity required for an effective haptic response is an area of active research. This is especially true as it pertains to quantitative feedback needed to interface the visual input to the "touch" of the system. Specialized software has been developed to simulate the impact of pushing, pulling, and cutting the skin and underlying tissue. This software analyzes contact forces in soft tissues surrounding the wound and translates these characteristics into the graded user tactility.[91] This technology should enhance abilities to perform realistic operations more precisely. For example, Sutherland is developing haptic robotic technology that can distinguish brain tumors from surrounding normal neural tissue. He is planning to combine this with intraoperative magnetic resonance imaging (MRI) modeling during neurosurgical procedures.[92]

The way in which surgeons will visualize the operative field is changing as well. Future imaging modalities will include 3D reconstruction and modeling using composite images from computed tomography (CT), MRI, and/or ultrasound. Image-guided surgical technology may provide real-time data acquisition of pathologic tissue and structural characteristics. This alone may help surgeons guide optimal delivery of percutaneous therapy. Research being conducted in France and Germany is focusing on simulating and planning robotic procedures. From biplanar angiography, Falk and Coste-Maniere have created dynamic models of coronary anatomy and superimposed them on reconstituted magnetic resonance and CT images of the heart. This virtual model is designed to analyze and plan optimal topographic port site placement to optimize instrument arm convergence at the operative plane.[93] For robotic surgery, this adjunctive technology should provide ideal ergonomic dexterity at the operative plane.[94,95] Similar systems have already been introduced in craniomaxillofacial and orthopedic surgery.[96] The challenges are greater for moving targets such as off-pump coronary surgery.

Ultimately, all of these advances will enable "virtual reality" to be an integral part of the operating room and in the training of surgeons. Future surgeons will practice techniques through virtual reality eyewear or holographic monitors and feel the tension of moving through human tissue as they manipulate surgical tools in lifelike situations. These systems already are proving to be of an educational benefit.[97] Recently, it has been shown that the use of virtual reality surgical stimulation significantly improves operating room performance of residents during a laparoscopic cholecystectomy.[98] It is conceivable that future systems may allow surgeons to enter all preoperative imaging data on a patient, perform the operation first on a virtual simulator, and then reconstruct it digitally in a volumetric grid. This digital operative onlay grid could be transferred to a robotic telemanipulation system to facilitate flawless performance of the operation. This would not be "automatic surgery"; simply the surgeon would have experienced and corrected all ergonomic conflicts, avoided vital structures, and mapped out the best operative plan prospectively.

CONCLUSIONS

Critical appraisal of surgical techniques and outcomes has advanced our knowledge of robotic surgery dramatically. In its current state, the robotic platform is well suited to complex procedures with limited access and those requiring delicate precise dissection or suturing; however, this must be critically compared with well-established traditional and more recent laparoscopic operations that enjoy long-term success. Our current techniques and experience in laparoscopic surgery are well advanced. Despite more than 5 years of experience with the robotic system, there are no concrete outcome data to justify the cost of these systems. Surgeon and patient testimonials are encouraging but lack rigorous testing. Consequently, although robotic-assisted surgery is technically feasible in a wide variety of cases, there is often little evidence in a variety of fields to suggest it is beneficial or justifiable in a number of these, when compared with laparoscopic techniques. Most reports of robotic surgery are limited to small series from dedicated units with a special interest in the field. Large, randomized, multicenter trials are lacking. We must temper our enthusiasm for new techniques with a conscious respect for what is desirable for the patient and acceptable from an economic view. At the same time, we must maintain an inquisitive and adaptive approach to this expanding field. Advances in robotic surgery are being made slowly but in a progressive manner. Often it is the adoption by surgeons that slows any progress. However, of those reluctant, most have concerns that an adequate operation cannot be done without the benefits of human tactility, free range of motion, and visualization—rightly so, as they want the best for their patient. Nevertheless, advancements in technology are beginning to get us closer to a better operation using robotics. Well-constructed randomized trials by surgeons experienced in conventional and robotic techniques are needed to provide answers on the reasonable use of robotic surgery.

This new science is a trek and not a destination. Fueling this drive is the challenge and desire to reclaim conventional surgical capability in a minimally invasive intervention. Ongoing technologic advances in robotic technology, computing power, and optic re-creation continue to stimulate our imagination and desire for comprehensive surgery with minimal morbidity and superior results, thereby extending its application and reach for the greater population. In this era of outcomes-based medicine, surgical scientists must continue to evaluate robotics and all new technology critically. Despite enthusiasm, caution cannot be overemphasized. Surgeons must proceed carefully because indices of operative safety, speed of recovery, level of discomfort, procedural cost, and long-term operative quality remain poorly defined. Traditional operations still enjoy long-term success with ever-decreasing morbidity and mortality and remain our measure for comparison. However, robotic-assisted surgery has developed to become a safe and successful modality that surely will be modified with technologic advances in all surgical disciplines.

REFERENCES

1. Chapman WH, Young JA, Albrecht RJ, et al: Robotic Nissen fundoplication: alternative surgical technique for the treatment of gastroesophageal reflux disease. J Laparoendosc Adv Surg Tech A 1:27, 2001.
2. Melvin WS, Needleman BJ, Krause KR, et al: Computer-enhanced vs. standard laparoscopic antireflux surgery. J Gastrointest Surg 6:11, 2002.
3. Cadiere GB, Himpens J, Bruyns J, et al: Evaluation of telesurgical (robotic) Nissen fundoplication. Surg Endosc 15:918, 2001.
4. Hanly EJ, Talamini MA: Robotic abdominal surgery. Am J Surg 188:19S, 2004.
5. Ayav A, Bresler L, Brunaud L, et al: Early results of one-year robotic surgery using the Da Vinci system to perform advanced laparoscopic procedures. J Gastrointest Surg 8:720–726, 2004.
6. Stefanidis D, Korndorffer JR, Scott DJ: Robotic laparoscopic fundoplication. Curr Treat Options Gastroenterol 8:71–83, 2005.
7. Cadiere GB, Himpens J, Vertruyen M, et al: The world's first obesity surgery performed by a surgeon at a distance. Obes Surg 9:206, 1999.
8. Horgan S, Vanuno D: Robots in laparoscopic surgery. J Laparoendosc Adv Surg Tech A 11:415, 2001.
9. Jacobsen G, Berger R, Horgan S: The role of robotic surgery in morbid obesity. J Laparoendosc Adv Surg Tech A 13:279, 2003.
10. Mohr CJ, Nadzam GS, Curet MJ: Totally robotic Roux-en-Y gastric bypass. Arch Surg 140:779–786, 2005.
11. Himpens J, Leman G, Cadiere GB: Telesurgical laparoscopic cholecystectomy [letter to the editor]. Surg Endosc 12:1091, 1998.
12. Kim VB, Chapman WH, Albrecht RJ, et al: Early experience with telemanipulative robot-assisted laparoscopic cholecystectomy using da Vinci. Surg Laparosc Endosc Percut Tech 12:33, 2002.
13. Ruurda J, Broeders I, Simmermacher R, et al: An evaluation of 35 robot-assisted laparoscopic cholecystectomies. Surg Laparosc Endosc Percutan Tech 12:41, 2002.
14. Hourmont K, Chung W, Pereira S, et al: Robotic versus telerobotic laparoscopic cholecystectomy: duration of surgery and outcomes. Surg Clin North Am 83:1445, 2003.
15. Marescaux J, Smith MK, Folscher D, et al: Telerobotic laparoscopic cholecystectomy: initial clinical experience with 25 patients. Ann Surg 234:1, 2001.
16. Smith M, Rubino F, Leroy J, et al: Robot-assisted biliary surgery. Osp Ital Chir 7:397, 2001.
17. Hashizume M, Shimada M, Tomikawa M, et al: Early experiences of endoscopic procedures in general surgery assisted by a computer-enhanced surgical system. Surg Endosc 16:1187, 2002.
18. Chapman WH, Albrecht RJ, Kim VB, et al: Computer-assisted laparoscopic splenectomy with the da Vinci surgical robot. J Laparoendosc Adv Surg Tech A 12:155, 2002.
19. Bodner J, Kafka-Ritsch R, Lucciarini P, et al: A critical comparison of robotic versus conventional laparoscopic splenectomies. World J Surg 29:982–1085, 2005. discussion 985–986.
20. Melvin WS, Needleman BJ, Krause KR, et al: Robotic resection of pancreatic neuroendocrine tumor. J Laparoendosc Adv Surg Tech A 13:33, 2003.
21. Melvin WS: Minimally invasive pancreatic surgery. Am J Surg 186:274, 2003.
22. Giulianotti PC, Coratti A, Angelini M, et al: Robotics in general surgery: personal experience in a large community hospital. Arch Surg 138:777, 2003.
23. Desai MM, Gill IS, Kaouk JH, et al: Robotic-assisted laparoscopic adrenalectomy. Urology 60:1104, 2002.
24. Bentas W, Wolfram M, Brautigam R, et al: Laparoscopic transperitoneal adrenalectomy using a remote-controlled robotic surgical system. J Endourol 16:373, 2002.
25. Young JA, Chapman WH, Kim VB, et al: Robotic-assisted adrenalectomy for adrenal incidentaloma: case and review of the technique. Surg Laparosc Endosc Percutan Tech 12:126, 2002.
26. Piazza L, Caragliano P, Scardilli M, et al: Laparoscopic robot-assisted right adrenalectomy and left ovariectomy (case reports). Chir Ital 51:465, 1999.
27. Weber PA, Merola S, Wasielewski A, et al: Telerobotic-assisted laparoscopic right and sigmoid colectomies for benign disease. Dis Colon Rectum 45:1689, 2002.
28. Delaney CP, Lynch AC, Senagore AJ, et al: Comparison of robotically performed and traditional laparoscopic colorectal surgery. Dis Colon Rectum 46:1633, 2003.
29. Munz Y, Moorthy K, Kudchadkar R, et al: Robotic assisted rectopexy. Am J Surg 187:88, 2004.

30. D'Annibale A, Morpurgo E, Fiscon V, et al: Robotic and laparoscopic surgery for treatment of colorectal diseases. Dis Colon Rectum 47:2162, 2004.
31. Melvin WS, Dundon JM, Talamini M, et al: Computer-enhanced robotic telesurgery minimizes esophageal perforation during Heller myotomy. Surgery 138:553–558, 2005. discussion 558–559.
32. Melvin WS, Needleman BJ, Krause KR, et al: Computer-enhanced robotic telesurgery: initial experience in foregut surgery. Surg Endosc 16:1790, 2002.
33. Undre S, Moorthy K, Munz Y, et al: Robot-assisted laparoscopic Heller cardiomyotomy: preliminary UK results. Dig Surg 21:396-400, 2004.
34. Talamini MA, Chapman S, Horgan S, et al: A prospective analysis of 211 robotic-assisted surgical procedures. Surg Endosc 17:1521, 2003.
35. Elli E, Espat NJ, Berger R, et al: Robotic-assisted thoracoscopic resection of esophageal leiomyoma. Surg Endosc 18:713, 2004.
36. Bodner JC, Zitt M, Ott H, et al: Robotic-assisted thoracoscopic surgery (RATS) for benign and malignant esophageal tumors. Ann Thorac Surg 80:1202–1206, 2005.
37. Ruurda JP, Draaisma WA, van Hillegersberg R, et al: Robot-assisted endoscopic surgery: a four-year single-center experience. Dig Surg 22:313–320, 2005.
38. Horgan S, Berger RA, Elli EF, et al: Robotic-assisted minimally invasive transhiatal esophagectomy. Am Surg 69:624, 2003.
39. Jacobsen G, Espat NJ, Berger R, et al: A single institution experience with robotically assisted transhiatal total esophagectomy [abstract]. SAGES 2004 Scientific and Postgraduate Courses March 31–April 3, 2004. Denver, CO.
40. Kernstine KH: Robotics in thoracic surgery. Am J Surg 188:89S, 2004.
41. Yoshino I, Hashizume M, Shimada M, et al: Thoracoscopic thymomectomy with the da Vinci computer-enhanced surgical system. J Thorac Cardiovasc Surg 122:783, 2001.
42. Savitt MA, Gao G, Furnary AP, et al: Application of robotic-assisted techniques to the surgical evaluation and treatment of the anterior mediastinum. Ann Thorac Surg 79:450–455, 2005. discussion 455.
43. Menconi G, Melfi FM, Angeletti CA: Robotic technology in thoracoscopic surgery. Osp Ital Chir 7:413, 2001.
44. Melfi FM, Menconi GF, Mariani AM, et al: Early experience with robotic technology for thoracoscopic surgery. Eur J Cardiothorac Surg 21:864, 2002.
45. Park BJ, Flores RM, Rusch V: Robotic-assisted VATS lobectomy [abstract]. Presented at the Society of Thoracic Surgeons 40th Annual Meeting; January 26–28, 2004. San Antonio, TX, 2004:134.
46. Bodner J, Wykypiel H, Wetscher G, et al: First experiences with the da Vinci trade mark operating robot in thoracic surgery. Eur J Cardiothorac Surg 25:844, 2004.
47. Morgan JA, Ginsburg ME, Sonett JR, et al: Advanced thoracoscopic procedures are facilitated by computer-aided robotic technology. Eur J Cardiothorac Surg 23:883, 2003.
48. Ruurda JP, Hanlo PW, Hennipman A, et al: Robot-assisted thoracoscopic resection of a benign mediastinal neurogenic tumor: technical note. Neurosurgery 52:462, 2003.
49. Mohr FW, Falk V, Diegeler A, et al: Computer-enhanced coronary artery bypass surgery. J Thorac Cardiovasc Surg 117:1212, 1991.
50. Falk V, Fann JI, Grunenfelder J, et al: Endoscopic computer-enhanced beating heart coronary artery bypass grafting. Ann Thorac Surg 70:2029, 2000.
51. Loulmet D, Carpentier A, d'Attellis N, et al: Endoscopic coronary artery bypass grafting with the aid of robotic assisted instruments. J Thorac Cardiovasc Surg 118:4–10, 1999.
52. Falk V, Diegeler A, Walther T, et al: Total endoscopic coronary artery bypass grafting. Eur J Cardiothorac Surg 17:38, 2000.
53. Bucerius J, Metz S, Walther T, et al: Endoscopic internal thoracic artery dissection leads to significant reduction of pain after minimally invasive direct coronary artery bypass graft surgery. Ann Thorac Surg 73:1180–1184, 2002.
54. Bolotin G, Scott WW Jr, Austin TC, et al: Robotic skeletonizing of the internal thoracic artery: is it safe? Ann Thorac Surg 77:1262–1265, 2004.
55. Srivastava SP, Patel KN, Shantharaja R, et al: Off-pump complete revascularization through a left thoracotomy (ThoraCAB): the first 200 cases. Ann Thorac Surg 76:46–49, 2003.
56. Zimmerman-Klima PM, Philpott JM, Elbeery JR, et al: Combined minimally invasive mitral valve repair and direct coronary artery bypass: a new alternative to sternotomy. Chest 122:344–347, 2002.
57. Kappert U, Cichon R, Schneider J, et al: Closed chest bilateral mammary artery grafting in double vessel coronary artery disease. Ann Thorac Surg 70:1699–1701, 2000.
58. Aybek T, Dogan S, Andressen E, et al: Robotically enhanced totally endoscopic right internal thoracic artery bypass graft to the right coronary artery. Heart Surg Forum 3:322–324, 2000.
59. Falk V, Diegler A, Walther T, et al: Total endoscopic off-pump coronary artery bypass grafting. Heart Surg Forum 3:29–31, 2001.
60. Dogan S, Aybek T, Andreßen E, et al: Totally endoscopic coronary artery bypass grafting on cardiopulmonary bypass with robotically enhanced telemanipulation: report of forty-five cases. J Thorac Cardiovasc Surg 123:1125–1131, 2002.
61. Kappert U, Schneider J, Cichon R, et al: Development of robotic enhanced endoscopic treatment for the treatment of coronary artery disease. Circulation 104(12 suppl 1):II02–II07, 2001.
62. Carpentier A, Loulmet D, Aupecle B, et al: Computer assisted open-heart surgery. First case operated on with success. CR Acad Sci II 321:437, 1998.
63. Chitwood WR Jr., Nifong LW, Elbeery JE, et al: Robotic mitral valve repair: trapezoidal resection and prosthetic annuloplasty with the da Vinci surgical system. J Thorac Cardiovasc Surg 120:1171, 2000.
64. Chitwood WR Jr, Nifong LW: Robotic assistance in cardiac surgery. Problems Gen Surg 18:9, 2001.
65. Nifong LW, Chu VR, Bailey BM, et al: Robotic mitral valve repair: experience with the da Vinci system. Ann Thorac Surg 75:438, 2003.
66. Kypson AP, Nifong LW, Chitwood WR Jr: Robot-assisted surgery: training and re-training surgeons. Int J Med Robotic Comput Assisted Surg 1:70, 2004.
67. Nifong LW, Chitwood WR Jr, Pappas PS, et al: Robotic mitral valve surgery: a United States multi-center trial. J Thorac Cardiovasc Surg 129:1395, 2005.
68. Reade CC, Bower CE, Maziarz DM, et al: Sutureless robotic-assisted mitral valve repair: an animal model. Heart Surgery Forum 6:254–257, 2003.
69. Felger JE, Reade CC, Nifong LW, Chitwood WR Jr: Robot-assisted sutureless minimally invasive mitral valve repair. Surg Technol Int 12:185–187, 2004.
70. Greelish JP, Cohn LH, Leacche M, et al: Minimally invasive mitral valve repair suggests earlier operations for mitral valve disease. J Thorac Cardiovasc Surg 126:365–371, 2003. discussion 371–373.
71. Tatooles AJ, Pappas PS, Gordon PJ, et al: Minimally invasive mitral valve repair using the da Vinci robotic system. Ann Thorac Surg 77:1978–1982, 2004. discussion 1982–1984.
72. Felger JE, Chitwood WR Jr, Nifong LW, et al: Evolution of mitral valve surgery: toward a totally endoscopic approach. Ann Thorac Surg 72:1203–1208, 2001. discussion 1208–1209.
73. Casselman FP, Van Slycke S, Wellens F, et al: Mitral valve surgery can now routinely be performed endoscopically. Circulation 108(suppl 1):II48–54, 2003.
74. Cazeau S, Leclercq C, Lavergne T, et al: Multisite Stimulation in Cardiomyopathies (MUSTIC) Study Investigators. Effects of multisite biventricular pacing in patients with heart failure and intraventricular conduction delay. N Engl J Med 344:873–880, 2001.
75. Reuter S, Garrigue S, Bordachar P, et al: Intermediate-term results of biventricular pacing in heart failure: correlation between clinical and hemodynamic data. Pacing Clin Electrophysiol 23(11 pt 2):1713–1717, 2000.
76. Gras D, Mabo P, Tang T, et al: Multisite pacing as a supplemental treatment of congestive heart failure: preliminary results of the Medtronic Inc. InSync Study. Pacing Clin Electrophysiol 21(11 pt 2):2249–2255, 1998.
77. Abraham WT, Fisher WG, Smith AL, et al: MIRACLE Study Group. Multicenter InSync Randomized Clinical Evaluation. Cardiac resynchronization in chronic heart failure. N Engl J Med 346:1845–1853, 2002.
78. Alonso C, Leclercq C, d'Allonnes FR, et al: Six year experience of transvenous left ventricular lead implantation for permanent biventricular pacing in patients with advanced heart failure: technical aspects. Heart 86:405–410, 2001.
79. DeRose JJ, Ashton RC, Belsley S, et al: Robotically assisted left ventricular epicardial lead implantation for biventricular pacing. J Am Coll Cardiol 41:1414–1419, 2003.

80. Jansens JL, Jottrand M, Preumont N, et al: Robotic-enhanced biventricular resynchronization: an alternative to endovenous cardiac resynchronization therapy in chronic heart failure. Ann Thorac Surg 76:413–417, 2003. discussion 417.
81. Argenziano M, Oz MC, DeRose JJ, et al: Totally endoscopic atrial septal defect repair with robotic assistance. Heart Surg Forum 5:294–300, 2002.
82. Wimmer-Greinecker G, Dogan S, Aybeck T, et al: Totally endoscopic atrial septal repair in adults with computer-enhanced telemanipulation. J Thor Cardiovasc Surg 126:465–468, 2003.
83. Argenziano M, Oz MC, Kohmoto T, et al: Totally endoscopic atrial septal defect repair with robotic assistance. Circulation 108:191–194, 2003.
84. Advincula AP, Falcone T: Laparoscopic robotic gynecologic surgery. Obstet Gynecol Clin North Am 31:599–609, ix–x, 2004.
85. Diaz-Arrastia C, Jurnalov C, Gomez G, et al: Laparoscopic hysterectomy using a computer-enhanced surgical robot. Surg Endosc 16:1271–1273, 2002. Epub 2002 Jun 27.
86. Beste TM, Nelson KH, Daucher JA: Total laparoscopic hysterectomy utilizing a robotic surgical system. JSLS 9:13–15, 2005.
87. Advincula AP, Reynolds RK: The use of robot-assisted laparoscopic hysterectomy in the patient with a scarred or obliterated anterior cul-de sac. JSLS 9:287–291, 2005.
88. Melamud O, Eichel L, Turbow B, et al: Laparoscopic vesicovaginal fistula repair with robotic reconstruction. Urology 65:163–166, 2005.
89. Di Marco DS, Chow GK, Gettman MT, et al: Robotic-assisted laparoscopic sacrocolpopexy for treatment of vaginal vault prolapse. Urology 63:373–376, 2004.
90. Goldberg JM, Falcone T: Laparoscopic microsurgical tubal anastomosis with and without robotic assistance. Hum Reprod 18:145–147, 2003.
91. Webster RW, Zimmerman DI, Mohler BJ, et al: A prototype haptic suturing simulator. Stud Health Technol Inform 81:567, 2001.
92. McBeth PB, Louw DF, Rizun PR, et al: Robotics in neurosurgery. Am J Surg 188:68S, 2004.
93. Falk V, Mourgues F, Adhami L, et al: Cardio navigation: planning, simulation, and augmented reality in robotic assisted endoscopic bypass grafting. Ann Thorac Surg 79:2040, 2005.
94. Blondel C, Vaillant R, Devernay F, et al: Automatic trinocular 3d reconstruction of coronary artery centerlines from rotational x-ray angiography. In Computer Assisted Radiology and Surgery 2002 Proceedings, 2002.
95. Adhami L, Coste-Maniere E: Postioning tele-operated surgical robots for collision-free optimal operation. In Proceedings of the 2002 IEEE International Conference on Robotics and Automation, 2002.
96. Troulis MJ, Everett P, Seldin ED, et al: Development of a three-dimensional treatment planning system based on computed tomographic data. Int J Oral Maxillofac Surg 31:349, 2002.
97. Satava RM: Surgical education and surgical simulation. World J Surg 25:1484, 2001.
98. Seymour NE, Gallagher AG, Roman SA, et al: Virtual reality training improves operating room performance: results of a randomized, double-blinded study. Ann Surg 236:458, 2002.

CHAPTER 20

Melissa R. Kaufman • Lee R. Schachter • S. Duke Herrell

Financial Considerations of Robotic-Assisted Prostatectomy

INTRODUCTION

The advent of robotic surgical technology has required decades of intense innovation and the investment of hundreds of millions of dollars. Initially born from the realm of military medicine, robotic surgery has recently become a driving force in the modern management of prostate cancer.[1–3] Taking advantage of the benefits of a minimally invasive approach to radical prostatectomy, robotic-assisted laparoscopic prostatectomy (RALP) has streamlined postoperative management by decreasing length of stay (LOS) via rapid advancement of diet and minimal use of pain medication.[4,5] Thus far, the data suggest that RALP has equivalent benefit to open radical retropubic prostatectomy (RRP) in terms of cancer control, continence, and erectile function.[6,7] However, the activation energy of implementing a robotic surgery program is often viewed as prohibitive in the arenas of both time and expenditure. During the upsurge of conventional laparoscopy in the 1990s, now considered a common tool in the urologist's armamentarium, similar hurdles concerning costs of new technology had to be overcome. Indeed, in the modern era of managed care, the contemplation of costs is always a prominent factor driving treatment decisions, and robotic surgery must accommodate to this environment. However, minimally invasive surgical (MIS) options such as RALP have integrated themselves into the consumer consciousness, and patient demand for these interventions appears to have a vigorous future. Herein we review the currently available information concerning the financial aspects of robotic surgery to provide insight into the fiscal benefits, pitfalls, and outlook for this rapidly advancing technology.

COST ANALYSIS STUDIES FOR ROBOTIC PROSTATECTOMY

The primary system used for RALP is the da Vinci robotic surgical system (Intuitive Surgical, Sunnyvale, CA). This surgical robot has a master-slave manipulator arrangement using articulating robotic arms (slave) controlled by a remote console (master). Images viewed by the operating surgeon in the console are three-dimensional (3D), and instruments allow seven degrees of freedom for wrist motion to approximate the hand movements used with open surgical technique.

In addition to the surgeon, the robotic team consists of a typical operating theater circulating nurse; a first assistant at the bedside responsible for changing robotic instruments and using a working port for suctioning, irrigating, and transferring of items such as vascular clips and specimens; and a surgical scrub technician. Thus, the operating room personnel required for robotic surgery are no different than that typically used for an open procedure. However, there is a significant use of time and resources in training these personnel for facility with robotic surgery. A trained robotic team is the most important component of a successful RALP program, and one must account for the labor-intensive nature of that training process when determining initial cost structure for the robotic prostatectomy program. Because of the physical size of the robotic equipment, a larger operating theater is preferable, with all the necessary electronic apparatus stationary, although all components are mobile and can be transferred from storage with minimal difficulty.

Initial cost for the da Vinci system is \$1.2 million with an annual maintenance cost of \$100,000.[8,9] The average instrument cost is \$1400 to \$1700 per case. Because of the novelty of the robotic approach in urology, only a few robust studies are currently available to scrutinize the fiscal impact of robotics in practice. Analysis in the realm of cardiac surgery reported that although cost was significantly higher for robotic operations when accounting for the initial capital investment of the robotic system, overall hospital costs did not significantly increase.[10] Initial reports from Dasari et al.[11] comparing costs between RRP and RALP indicated that although greater operating room costs were associated with the robotic approach, overall hospital stay was 1.7 days shorter for the RALP patients, mitigating some of the operating theater expenses. This analysis reported the average cost for RRP to be $5941 and the cost of RALP to be $6191, a modest difference of $250. Updated data from the Vattikuti Institute revealed that by excluding depreciation of robot and service contract, cost for RALP was actually 2.39% lower than that for open procedures.[12]

Recent reports from Joseph et al.[13] indicate that the high fixed costs and stagnant reimbursement for robotic prostatectomy realized a net loss for the hospital for every RALP case even without accounting for the initial system and maintenance costs. Total hospital costs per prostatectomy were estimated at $9102 with $2949 and $6153 in fixed and variable costs per case with reimbursement averaging $8954. The authors conclude that without alterations in reimbursement combined with decreases in equipment costs, robotic technology can only indirectly enhance hospital profits.

A similar theme of increased cost associated for RALP in conjunction with inadequate reimbursement was presented by Bernstein et al.[14] This retrospective review of 267 consecutive patients undergoing prostatectomy compared costs and revenues for RRP, perineal prostatectomy, and RALP. A formula was devised incorporating total costs, LOS, and duration of surgery to determine the cost impact of each method of prostatectomy. The authors determined the most important determinants of revenue were direct costs and the type of insurance reimbursement. For RALP, costs averaged $7062 with revenue of $7154, realizing a profit of $92, which was substantially less than the $1060 profit seen with RRP. This analysis also did not include surgeon's fees or the initial cost of the robotic system and associated maintenance fees.

Continuing this quest for a better understanding of health care resource allocation as it relates to surgery for prostate cancer, a comprehensive computer software model was created by Lotan et al.[15] to evaluate the cost components of RRP and RALP. Hospital costs were obtained from in-house data, whereas information concerning variables such as average LOS and operative times were obtained via literature search. Using a formula integrating cost data for hospital stay, operating room expenses, intravenous fluids, blood transfusions, and maintenance fees for the robot, the authors reported a cost difference between RRP and RALP of $1155. This cost again excluded the initial purchase cost of the robot. Using a one-way sensitivity analysis the authors demonstrated that no single change in LOS or operating room time could make RALP cost equivalent to RRP. They indicate that the limiting factors in making RALP cost competitive include the initial purchase cost of the robot and the cost per case of maintenance and reusable equipment.

Common to all these studies are significant upfront outlays for the robot that mitigate profit potential during short-term application. As these primary costs are amortized over a longer time span and the use of the robotic technology expands, original expenses should be more easily integrated into a practical financial landscape.

A decision analytic model was recently described by Scales et al.[16] comparing RRP and RALP, which, unlike the previously reported studies, included the initial cost of the robot and maintenance fees. Expenditures were obtained from hospital administration and were subdivided into surgical costs (operating room, consumable equipment, perioperative anesthesia care, transfusion, and professional fees) and nonsurgical costs (e.g., room and board, pharmacy, laboratory services). The initial robot cost was amortized over a 7-year period for an average monthly rate of $20,595, which included the maintenance contract. Two base case models were constructed for RRP using the previously mentioned parameters, one in a specialist setting and one in a generalist setting. The RALP base was modeled after the Vattikuti Institute data. A series of one- and two-way sensitivity analyses were used to test the importance of individual factor deviations from the base models on cost outcomes. The data revealed that RALP is always more costly than RRP independent of the setting. In the specialist setting to attain cost equivalence, RALP operating times would need to decrease to 90 minutes. In fact, the model demonstrates that in the generalist setting, unless operative times decrease to below 165 minutes, RALP will remain more costly than RRP. To attain equivalence for LOS in a specialist setting, RALP would need to become an outpatient procedure with an LOS of 0.5 days. However, in the generalist setting, an LOS of 1 day for RALP allowed it to be cost equivalent to RRP. Also in the generalist setting, a case volume of 10 RALPs per week was needed for cost equivalency with RRP, whereas a case volume of 15 RALPs per week was required in the specialist setting. The authors conclude that the principal advantage of RALP from a cost standpoint is a decreased LOS and may be most cost competitive at high-volume specialty centers when compared with RRP in the generalist setting. At our institution, preliminary financial analysis has revealed that although some financial benefit for the institution has been achieved once expertise is established, the RALP procedure has been unable to show financial equivalency to that realized from RRP (Table 20–1).

These studies all demonstrate the intrinsic high cost of implementing robotic prostatectomy when evaluated in the current reimbursement environment. However, as discussed in the following sections, a number of factors may be applied in the future that will create a positive financial outlook for RALP.

USE OF ROBOTICS IN OTHER UROLOGIC SURGERY

As training in robotic-assisted surgery expands, so will the potential applications of this technology. The expansion of robotics into other aspects of urologic surgery, similar to the situation encountered with the rapid development of conventional laparoscopy, will theoretically drive down overall costs while improving patient outcomes. Some of the urologic

Table 20–1 Cost Comparisons

	RALP	RRP	Cost Difference
Initial da Vinci purchase	$1,285,000	N/A	N/A
Maintenance costs,	$109,000/year	N/A	N/A
disposable items	$1400–$1,700/case		
Dasari et al.	$6,191	$5,941	($250)
Joseph et al.	$9,102	N/A	N/A
Bernstein et al.	$7,062	$6,248	Cost difference ($814)
			Profit difference ($968)
Lotan et al.	$7,280*	$5,554	($1726*)
	$6,709		($1155)
Scales et al. Specialist	$8,929*	$8,146	($783*)
Community		$8,734	($195*)

*Initial robot cost included in analysis.
RALP, robotic-assisted laparoscopic prostatectomy; RRP, radical retropubic prostatectomy; ($), deficit.

applications already reported have included use of robotics for percutaneous renal access, nephrectomy, partial nephrectomy, dismembered pyeloplasty, cystectomy, adrenalectomy, sacrocolpopexy, vesicovaginal fistula repair, vasovasostomy, and a variety of pediatric urologic procedures.[9,17–19]

DISCUSSION

Available studies have indeed demonstrated that as far as direct costs and reimbursement are concerned, RALP is not currently a profitable surgical procedure when compared with RRP. However, these analyses are unable to account for many of the intangible factors that drive use of this technology. As previously mentioned, consumer demand for RALP is continually increasing, and hospitals not offering this choice are almost certainly experiencing patient migration to centers with robotic options. The aura of technology afforded by the robot may also indirectly influence demand for unrelated procedures and visits to other specialties that would be difficult to quantitate but would certainly impact overall hospital finances. It may also be feasible to imagine an augment in reimbursement by insurance carriers as patient demand for RALP increases and outcome data confirm decreased morbidity.

For the classically trained open surgeon, a significant investment of resources is required to implement and master the laparoscopic skills required for robotic surgery.[20] Although the robotic approach provides an advantage in terms of ease of use from traditional laparoscopic approaches,[21] the learning curve remains steep and with it an increased use of resources surrounding the longer operative times and potentially less optimal patient outcomes. It has been demonstrated that for high-volume surgeons, operating times progressively decline as surgeon experience with RALP increases.[22] It would be reasonable to suspect that these decreases in operating room time use will progressively drive costs down. Likewise, continual advancements in the surgical techniques used with RALP will certainly streamline the procedure and decrease operative time.

Another potentially appealing aspect of RALP is a decrease in the loss of productivity for society while these predominantly preretirement patients recover from surgery.[15] Factoring in the difference in return to work for RALP and RRP actually results in a cost advantage of $1600 in favor of RALP.

Although still in its infancy, RALP has established a firm foothold in the management of prostate cancer. In the current environment, the costs of performing RALP do not routinely result in profit for the hospital. However, as the technology expands and demand and use increase, necessary modifications to the cost and reimbursement structure must be made to ensure the longevity of this valuable system.

REFERENCES

1. Abbou CC, Hoznek A, Salomon L, et al: Laparoscopic radical prostatectomy with a remote controlled robot. J Urol 165:1964, 2001.
2. Smith JA Jr: Robotically assisted laparoscopic prostatectomy: an assessment of its contemporary role in the surgical management of localized prostate cancer. Am J Surg 188:63S, 2004.
3. Herrell SD, Smith JA Jr: Laparoscopic and robotic radical prostatectomy: what are the real advantages? BJU Int 95:3, 2005.
4. Menon M, Tewari A, Peabody JO, et al: Vattikuti Institute prostatectomy, a technique of robotic radical prostatectomy for management of localized carcinoma of the prostate: experience of over 1100 cases. Urol Clin North Am 31:701, 2004.
5. Kaufman MR, Smith JA Jr, Baumgartner RG, et al: Positive influence of robotically assisted laparoscopic prostatectomy on the collaborative-care pathway for open radical prostatectomy. BJU Int 97:473–475, 2006.
6. Menon M, Shrivastava A, Tewari A: Laparoscopic radical prostatectomy: conventional and robotic. Urology 66:101, 2005.
7. Hoznek A, Menard Y, Salomon L, et al: Update on laparoscopic and robotic radical prostatectomy. Curr Opin Urol 15:173, 2005.
8. Menon M: Robotic radical retropubic prostatectomy. BJU Int 91:175, 2003.
9. Eichel L, Ahlering TE, Clayman RV: Role of robotics in laparoscopic urologic surgery. Urol Clin North Am 31:781, 2004.
10. Morgan JA, Thornton BA, Peacock JC, et al: Does robotic technology make minimally invasive cardiac surgery too expensive? A hospital cost analysis of robotic and conventional techniques. J Card Surg 20:246, 2005.
11. Dasari R, Bhandari A, Tewari A, eta al: Comparison of costs between robot assisted laparoscopic prostatectomy (Vattikutti Institute prostatectomy) and radical retropubic prostatectomy. J Endourol 17(suppl):A120, 2003.
12. Guru KA, Bhandari A, Peabody JO, et al: Cost comparison between robotic-assisted laparoscopic prostatectomy (Vattikuti Institute prostatectomy) and radical retropubic prostatectomy. Presented at the AUA Annual Meeting, 2004.
13. Joseph JV, Rosenbaum R, Vicente I, et al: Cost-profit analysis of DaVinci robotic surgery: is it worth it? Presented at the AUA Annual Meeting, 2005.
14. Bernstein AJ, Kernen KM, Gonzalez J, et al: A cost and revenue analysis for retropubic, perineal, and robotic prostatectomy at a large community hospital. Presented at the AUA Annual Meeting, 2005.
15. Lotan Y, Cadeddu JA, Gettman MT: The new economics of radical prostatectomy: cost comparison of open, laparoscopic and robot assisted techniques. J Urol 172:1431, 2004.
16. Scales CD Jr, Jones PJ, Eisenstein EL, et al: Local cost structures and the economics of robot assisted radical prostatectomy. J Urol 174:2323, 2005.
17. Hemal AK, Menon M: Robotics in urology. Curr Opin Urol 14:89, 2004.
18. Binder J, Brautigam R, Jonas D, et al: Robotic surgery in urology: fact or fantasy? BJU Int 94:1183, 2004.
19. Hashizume M, Tsugawa K: Robotic surgery and cancer: the present state, problems and future vision. Jpn J Clin Oncol 34:227, 2004.
20. Ahlering TE, Skarecky D, Lee D, et al: Successful transfer of open surgical skills to a laparoscopic environment using a robotic interface: initial experience with laparoscopic radical prostatectomy. J Urol 170:1738, 2003.
21. Yohannes P, Rotariu P, Pinto P, et al: Comparison of robotic versus laparoscopic skills: is there a difference in the learning curve? Urology 60:39, 2002.
22. Guillonneau B, Rozet F, Cathelineau X, et al: Perioperative complications of laparoscopic radical prostatectomy: the Montsouris 3-year experience. J Urol 167:51, 2002.

INDEX

Page numbers followed by f indicate figures; t, tables.

F

G

H

I

J

K

L

M

N

O

P

R